THE URGE

THE URGE

OUR HISTORY OF ADDICTION

Carl Erik Fisher

PENGUIN PRESS
NEW YORK
2022

PENGUIN PRESS
An imprint of Penguin Random House LLC
penguinrandomhouse.com

Image credits appear on pp. 361–62.

LIBRARY OF CONGRESS CATALOGING-IN-PUBLICATION DATA
Names: Fisher, Carl Erik, author.
Title: The urge : our history of addiction / Carl Erik Fisher.
Description: New York : Penguin Press, 2022. |
Includes bibliographical references and index. |
Identifiers: LCCN 2021034504 (print) | LCCN 2021034505 (ebook) |
ISBN 9780525561446 (hardcover) | ISBN 9780525561453 (ebook)
Subjects: LCSH: Fisher, Carl Erik—Mental health. | Addicts—History. |
Psychiatrists—United States—Biography. | Alcoholics—Biography. |
Alcoholics—Rehabilitation—Biography.
Classification: LCC RC438.6.F57 A3 2022 (print) |
LCC RC438.6.F57 (ebook)
DDC 362.29092 [B]—dc23
LC record available at https://lccn.loc.gov/2021034504
LC ebook record available at https://lccn.loc.gov/2021034505

Printed in the United States of America
1st Printing

Designed by Amanda Dewey

For Cat and Gus

CONTENTS

Introduction

I'm lying in bed when I hear the commotion. I peer through the doorway of my room, and right outside, the new guy is getting in Ruiz's face. There's a phone right outside the door, one of those sturdy metal payphones—it looks like it's been carried in from the street—and Ruiz, a gentle older man with shoulders stooped by the demoralization of his nth relapse and hospitalization, is just trying to talk to his family. But the new guy has been manic and pacing since he arrived a few hours ago, and he won't take no for an answer.

I watch the new guy stalk the other way across the doorway, muttering to himself, menacing even in retreat. Then a warning shout echoes from much too far in the distance, and he appears once again—flying, near horizontal—to tackle Ruiz, dragging him off the phone.

The staff quickly take him down; thankfully, no one was seriously hurt. Shaken, I try to focus on my journal, but my mind races. My roommate—a burly middle-aged guy with a scar down the side of his head, attesting to the brain injury that's brought him back here over and over again—turns to me laconically and says, "There goes dinner."

I'm twenty-nine years old, writing in my journal in a sloppy felt-tip pen (no ballpoints are allowed), trying to understand how I went from being a newly minted physician in a psychiatry residency program at Columbia University to a psychiatric patient at Bellevue, the city's notorious public hospital. Bellevue is synonymous with the most challenging, chronic mentally ill cases, and now I'm locked on the dual diagnosis ward on the twentieth floor, near the top of the building, where they put people who have both substance use problems and other mental disorders. I've already recognized some of the faculty from when I applied here for residency, and I know from the tour I took as an applicant that the special prison ward, protected by a guardhouse with bulletproof glass and thickly barred gates, is a floor below us.

I need that phone those two men were fighting over. It's my only way to reach the outside world, that other plane of reality where I was once a psychiatry resident. I'm having trouble accepting that I belong here, not there. Day by day, it seems more likely that what the doctors have been telling me is correct—that, just like the new guy, I too have had a manic episode, in my case induced by weeks of stimulants and alcohol. But I'm still not sure what I should do.

The next day, I meet with the whole treatment team—half a dozen psychiatrists, therapists, and counselors facing me across a massive table in one of those windowless hospital conference rooms. For the first time, I truly let my guard down and recount my whole drinking history. How I grew up with two alcoholic parents and swore to myself I'd never be like them. How, even as I finished medical school at Columbia, I had the creeping sense that my drinking was out of control. How the blackouts got more and more frequent, but I didn't reach out for help, and I didn't accept the help that friends, colleagues, and supervisors had all offered, then implored me to take.

I tell them everything, even the one time that I woke up on the floor of the hallway in my building, shirtless, my skin sticking to the tacky linoleum, locked out of my own apartment. It was only by getting up to the roof and climbing down the fire escape that I made it in to work that day at all. I was late again, and so ashamed and scared by what it said about me. It was obvious that something was wrong, but I never told anyone about it, because to do so would be to acknowledge what I had long suspected.

They ask me about my family, and I tell them about my father's four rehabs and the bottles of wine my mother secreted around the house. I describe my parents as alcoholics, as I usually do, but I also finally give voice to that dangerous suspicion about myself: ". . . And I'm starting to realize that I'm an alcoholic, too," and I break down crying.

Despite all this, later that weekend, I call my friend Ravi from that payphone, looking down the disorientingly long hallway that stretches the whole length of the ward. He's helping me with all the logistics, setting up disability insurance, getting my rent paid, and generally making it possible for me to go to rehab: a place I don't quite want to go to but I'm told that I need.

We talk about how it'll be good for me, and how I've struggled for so long. His voice is strained. It's clear he's worried about me. So I hesitate for a moment—I have the clear sense of telling myself, *this is a truly ridiculous question, don't ask him this*—but then ask him anyway, even as I keep one eye down the hallway for any potential assailants: "Do you really think I can never drink again?"

I'm supposed to be headed to some specialized rehab for doctors, but I know nothing about it. I want to go, but not really. I need help, but maybe I can do it on my own, or at least find a better way. Why is this so hard?

I did go to that rehab for doctors, and in time, I returned to the residency program at Columbia. For years afterward, I was in supervised treatment. At a moment's notice, I had to be prepared to run across the medical center or across town to my "urine monitor," a woman who would watch me urinate to make sure I didn't try to pass off someone else's bodily fluids as my own. As I slogged through half a decade of this, I got more curious. I knew that the addiction treatment system was broken, having experienced it firsthand, but the *why* was mystifying: Why was there a totally separate system for addiction treatment? Why do we treat addiction differently from any other mental disorder? If everyone seems to know that the system is broken, why isn't anyone changing it?

I decided to become an addiction medicine specialist. In a surreal twist, as I studied psychotherapy and medications, I was also going to my own treatment and meetings and generally trying to work out what recovery meant to me. As I finished training and joined the psychiatry and bioethics faculty at Columbia, the worst seemed to be behind me. But as I emerged from those revitalizing yet profoundly disorienting years, the same questions lingered, insistently: How did I get here, and what exactly had gone wrong in me? Or, as patients often ask: What happened to me? Why am I like this? How do I get better?

In search of answers, I immersed myself in the field, studying the psychology and neuroscience of addiction. I wanted to find the right definition—the correct and tidy medical theory that would explain it—but I was soon overwhelmed. The field seemed to be in chaos. Scientists and other scholars seemed bitterly divided, always talking past one another. Some insisted that addiction was primarily a brain disease. Others claimed that this brain-centric view blinded us to the psychological, cultural, and social dimensions, including trauma and systems of oppression. Few other fields of medicine are so powerfully driven by cultural bias and ideology.

Everyone seemed to have their own take, as did every field of study. One summary of "theories of addiction" listed no fewer than thirty different models—from psychological concepts to neurobiological mechanisms to economic models of choice—and those are just the ones deemed respectable today. Each one of them had something useful to add, but more often than not their answers felt demoralizingly incomplete.

I began working in psychiatry, not incidentally, at a time of increasing disillusionment with the simplistic view that all of human suffering could be reduced to neurobiology. President George H. W. Bush had designated the 1990s the "Decade of the Brain," but during the 2000s and into the early 2010s, as I finished my training, there were signs that neuroscience, while useful and even revolutionary in some ways, was not sufficient to explain the complex phenomena of mental suffering. Researchers were still trying to make sense of what it meant to call something a mental disorder, and the picture was yet more complicated in the case of treatment. Antidepressants were nowhere near as useful as the first generation of heady advertisements had promised. Biotech companies were slashing funding and even shuttering their neuroscience research divisions altogether after years of failed drug discovery. There was a growing awareness that the country had been misled by pharmaceutical companies—and not just the opioid manufacturers. These developments motivated my own turn from neuroscience research to bioethics, where I hoped to incorporate a more thorough understanding of the social and political realities of mental suffering, along with the best the science had to offer.

Then, as I continued my research into addiction, I noticed something interesting. The broadest-thinking and most creative scholars kept making odd and intriguing connections to fields beyond my usual horizons. They drew on ancient philosophy to clarify the problem. They looked to sociology to show how it is impossible to separate addiction from its cultural context, now and for generations back. They even delved into theology, to trace how legacies of thinking about morality have powerfully influenced the way we think about choice and responsibility. In a short time, I became absolutely convinced that medical science alone, while important, was insufficient for understanding addiction.

Understanding addiction in the present required looking to the past. Addiction seemed to be everywhere and at every time. Starting my investigations in the midst of an opioid overdose epidemic, I learned that human society has been wracked by drug epidemics with dismaying regularity for more than half a millennium. I saw how centuries of policy, stigma, and racism are all inseparable from how we currently understand and treat, or fail to treat, addiction. We have long wielded the concept of addiction as a weapon, using it to wage war—not just "on drugs" but also on people who use drugs. I was struck by how long societies have feared the corrupting forces of technology, from opioids and smartphones and porn-on-demand to syringes and telegraphs and sugar. It was clear that addiction was not just an issue of medical science but also one of identity, power, commerce, and fear—as well as one of devotion.

I got to leave Bellevue relatively quickly. By nothing more than an accident of birth—my status as a doctor, my Ivy League education, my ability to pay, my access to a program that happened to treat addiction somewhat adequately, my whiteness, and just dumb luck—I entered recovery, returned to a good job, and eventually got to write this book. If only everyone were treated the way I was, we'd all be better off. But make no mistake. I am not an "unlikely" case. I am not fundamentally different from Ruiz, or the new guy, or anyone else on that dual diagnosis floor. The most important lesson the history taught me is how divisions between us are just a story, one that has long fed injustice, and one that comes back to harm us all. It will continue to do so, unless we start to look deeper.

This book is a history of addiction. It is the story of an ancient malady that has ruined the lives of untold millions, including not only those of its sufferers but also the lives touching theirs, and yet it is also the story of a messy, complicated, and deeply controversial idea, one that has eluded definition for hundreds of years. Addiction doesn't just cut across time and place; it cuts across fields far beyond medicine and science, to politics, spirituality, law, economics, philosophy, and sociology—not to mention all the literature and art that point toward the ineffable gaps between. Addiction is a brain disease, a spiritual malady, the romantic mark of artistic sensibility, a badge of revolution against a sick society, and all of these things at once. This book is a history of ideas: a history of addiction as an idea and a history of ideas about addiction.

What does addiction mean to you? Everyone has a preconceived notion. Do only drug and alcohol problems qualify, or can you be addicted to gambling, sex, eating, work, or even love? Is it a matter of severity, like drinking or using too much, or is it driven by how you feel, some internal sense of being out of control? Is everyone somewhere on the addiction spectrum—does not being able to put down your phone count?—or is it a clearly demarcated disease, neatly partitioned off from normal society? The point is not that these questions have easy answers, but that these are not purely scientific or medical questions; they are inextricable from our most closely held, culturally contingent, and often implicit beliefs and values. Questions about addiction are questions about what it means to be human.

As I studied the many attempted responses to the problem of addiction, I came to distinguish between four broad approaches that have recurred throughout history. A *prohibitionist* approach has sought to control addiction through punishment and other law enforcement strategies. A *therapeutic* approach has argued that addiction is best handled as a disorder to be treated by the medical field. A *reductionist* approach has sought to explain addiction in scientific terms, often seeking biology-based cures. And a *mutual-help* approach has sought community healing and grassroots fellowship—and sometimes, but not always, spiritual development—to recover from addiction. Variations on each of these themes abound, and they also overlap and blend into one another at times, but overall, they occur with surprising regularity across the centuries. What should not be surprising is that no single approach holds all the answers.

Each of these approaches has had its turn in responding to addiction—often, multiple turns. Whether a "miracle drug," a new enforcement policy, or an innovative rehabilitation program, these interventions almost always took the form of a quick fix that would ostensibly solve the problem of addiction—or sweep it under the rug, or dominate and control it. None has ever been successful for long. With the benefit of history, we can see that these attempts were doomed to fail, even when their supporters' intentions were noble.

Then what is to be done, if these cycles have repeated themselves with such crushing regularity? I've come to believe that the history, while sometimes discouraging, ultimately lights a way forward. By accepting that addiction has been and will continue to be a part of human life, we can abandon dreams of eradicating it and free ourselves to look instead at the full variety of interventions available to help. The primary goal should be not victory or cure, but alleviating harm and helping people to live with and beyond their suffering—in other words, recovery. If we want to break the cycle, we must take the best of each of these approaches—medical, social, spiritual, and so forth—and apply their lessons in a truly holistic balance, while always being sure to let the history spark humility and openness to multiple perspectives.

I don't mean to suggest that this path forward is easy. Confusion, fear, and aversion often obscure the way, complicated by the fact that forces of oppression and domination commonly co-opt the idea of addiction for their own ends. Even as addiction recovery has emerged as our era's archetypal story of self-discovery and spiritual growth, substance use problems are still portrayed as a stigmatized and "odious disease," as they were labeled when medical writers attempted to describe the phenomenon centuries ago.

What follows are two stories. The first and foremost is a story about addiction, treatment, and recovery across the ages. The second, alongside it, is the story of my own experience as a physician and person in addiction recovery. I wanted to include my own story because ideas about addiction are necessarily intertwined with personal beliefs and experiences, and I wanted to disclose my biases rather than adopt a tone of false objectivity. But I also hoped to illustrate as vividly as possible the real human implications of this history and the ways it continues to exert force on the present.

Not surprisingly, this investigation seldom yielded easy answers. Most often, it produced examples of hubris and failure, and of seemingly unending cycles of hatred and division. And yet it never stopped feeling urgent to me. It helped me understand my past and that of my family, and it helped me in my work with patients. I felt great kinship with people in years past who battled addiction, and their stories gave me hope for recovery and the possibility of change. Though the challenges ahead are daunting, I firmly believe that if we meet it with open eyes, the history will help us on our way forward.

Author's Note

The language of mental health matters. It has tremendous power to shape our policies and attitudes. Much of the old language around addiction is now considered stigmatizing by many advocates: not just "junkie" or "drunk" but also "addict" and "alcoholic," because the preferred anti-stigma approach is to use "person-first language"—for example, "person with addiction" rather than "addict." This is reasonable and humane, and there is evidence that it has a real effect on stigma.

However, the issue of language presents problems for a book that attempts to capture how people with addiction have been understood and described at various times. The language of addiction has undergone massive shifts from era to era, and those shifts were deeply meaningful to how people understood themselves and the people they cared for. Benjamin Rush studied "drunkenness" at the end of the eighteenth century, others struggled with their "intemperance" in the middle of the nineteenth, and today psychiatrists debate whether to return to the term "addiction" as opposed to the anemic and bureaucratic "substance use disorder." I do not assume that our present understanding maps neatly onto all times and cultures in the past—to the contrary, one key assertion of this book is that addiction does not exist as a permanent and unchanging fact, but rather is highly dependent on social and cultural factors. So I had to weigh the danger of perpetuating stigmatizing language against the need to clearly and accurately represent the history. Generally, my approach has been to use the historically appropriate terminology for the era under study. To the extent I use potentially stigmatizing words for people with addiction, I attempt to do so in a way that makes it clear I am representing the views of the time.

This history is necessarily selective. In particular, it is largely an American story, which partly reflects my effort to understand my own heritage and culture. However, the focus on the United States is not merely an artifact of my background. The disease idea of addiction—addiction as a chronic identity—solidified in the early United States around the time of the Revolutionary War, and it was disseminated worldwide by movements largely originating in the United States. Both Alcoholics Anonymous and the current framing of the "war on drugs" are creations of the U.S. Top doctors from countries all over the world are regularly funded to travel to the United States to learn about how we think about addiction. And so, this story is largely centered in the United States, the birthplace, in a way, of the modern notion of addiction. This is not to discount the value of cross-cultural perspectives on addiction, which I have attempted to include throughout.

My patients, simply by virtue of their humanity, have helped me immensely in this historical investigation. They run the gamut from current drug users to enthusiasts of AA and other twelve-step programs. They include people who see their behaviors around work, love, and eating as addictions, and people who hate the very idea of addiction, even as their drug and alcohol use brings them to the brink of death. They have helped me to see the problem from many viewpoints, and for that, and for the opportunity to serve, I am truly grateful. Though I have both worked in the criminal legal system and tended to the privileged, I have done so mainly in the New York City area, so they represent just one slice of life. Regarding confidentiality, I occasionally discuss my patients, but I have respected their privacy by disguising their identities, including their names (I have also changed the names of others who appear in this book out of respect for their privacy). No one in this book is a composite character.

This book is intended for the general audience. For more technical material, academic readers may wish to consult the book's endnotes, which I use to both cite supporting data and expand on certain points.

I researched and wrote this book over the course of ten years. Though I reviewed medical records, journals, and other documentary information from my life, and I spoke with many individuals about those experiences, much of my personal story was drawn from my memories and perceptions.

There is a tradition in recovery communities like AA to practice anonymity at the level of mass media. There are good reasons for this, and yet there has also been a proud tradition of self-disclosure in many addiction memoirs. Many of those personal accounts have helped me immeasurably, and I know people in recovery who credit such books with saving their lives. I've shared my own experience of recovery in this book, but it is not my intention to argue for or against any particular pathway of recovery. I speak only for my own experience, not for any recovery tradition or organization.

PART ONE

BEHAVIOR IN SEARCH OF A NAME

One

FOUNDATIONS:
BEFORE "ADDICTION"

I get an immediate sense of how Susan's doing from the moment she walks through my office door. When she's not drinking, she's meticulously groomed, hair just so, sharp business-formal blazers and crisp shirts over her tense, thin frame. But today, I can tell, she's slightly off. Over the years I've learned the tells. A little too much perfume to mask the smell of morning drinks. Hair askew. Rumpled shirt. Slightly sloppy makeup.

I've also seen her in total crisis, with dirt caked under her fingernails and alcohol fumes lingering in the room long after she leaves. But to her, just to be drinking at all feels like a crisis. She identifies as an alcoholic, she is certain that she wants to stop drinking, and yet she does not, and this is what she hates the most—the disorder, the lack of control. I can see she is struggling with this feeling now.

She tells me about the most recent relapse. Alone in her room, she felt restless, and she couldn't get the thought of drinking out of her mind. She had firmly decided that she wouldn't have wine that night. She absolutely would not go to the liquor store. Then, in a twisted compromise, she watched herself walk to the corner store and buy a few bottles of vanilla extract.

The vile liquid made her drunk, then sick to her stomach, she tells me. Eyes wide, she says, "It was ridiculous."

These days in my psychiatry practice, I mostly see people with complicated substance use problems: people who still struggle after spending thousands of dollars on rehabs and outpatient programs, people for whom the traditional treatments don't work nearly often enough. Susan has gone to those programs—both the old-school abstinence-based rehabs and the more modern and flexible treatment programs—but she's never stopped drinking. For months, she's lingered in that in-between place, still doing some minimal work in her private legal practice, making enough to get by, but well below what she could.

She is in a notable minority: the fewer than 5 percent of people in the United States with substance use problems who actually believe they have a problem and want treatment. Even so, despite the alcohol withdrawal seizure she had a few months ago, despite the blackouts, despite losing her corporate job, she has not been able to stop.

She is not in any physical danger now. She hasn't had enough to be in alcohol withdrawal. Still, she says, this is awful for her. She dwells on the last month of failed resolutions and unsuccessful attempts to cut down, and as she goes around and around, butting up against the limits of language and reason and trying to make sense of it all, a note of frustration, even desperation, enters her voice.

"I know what I need to do. I want to do it. But I don't do what I want to do. And then I'm drinking again, and I just don't know why or how."

Addiction is a terrifying breakdown of reason. People struggling with addiction say they want to stop, but, even with the obliterated nasal passages, scarred livers, overdoses, court cases, lost jobs, and lost families, they are confused, incredulous, and, above all, afraid. They are afraid because they cannot seem to change, despite the fact that they so often watch themselves, clear-eyed, do the very things they don't want to do.

For thousands of years, people have struggled with the frightening phenomenon that Susan faced. It's not always easy to find, as few ancient cultures had a term for what we would recognize as addiction. For example, the ancient Greeks had the word *philopotês*, a "lover of drinking sessions," but the word itself didn't necessarily indicate that someone had a problem.

And yet, in other times and cultures, addiction is clearly present. Teng Cen (AD 1137–1224), a Chinese poet of the Song dynasty, described how he made a pact with the gods to stop drinking, only to succumb to cravings during a banquet—he ultimately rationalized it by convincing himself that it was in his "true nature" to drink. The Chinese literature scholar Edwin Van Bibber-Orr has documented several other Song dynasty works describing *shi jiu*, a love of drinking marked by craving, desire, and thirst that bears striking similarities to what we call addiction today.

But one of the oldest examples of addiction in history concerns not substances but gambling, a behavior nearly as old as human civilization itself. In the *Rig Veda*, an ancient compilation of Vedic Sanskrit hymns from India, among the oldest surviving compositions in any language, an evocative poem known as the "Gambler's Lament" presents an unambiguous description of gambling addiction. In a text that likely dates to before 1000 BC, a fourteen-line poem captures in vivid detail the despair of a man who struggles unsuccessfully against his desire to play at dice.

At the start of the poem, we learn that the dice have already inflicted a heavy toll. The gambler has driven away his true community, his devoted wife and mother. Yet despite that wreckage, for much of the poem, he struggles to stop. He resolves not to play with his fellow gamblers—but then, at the sound of the dice's voice, he rushes to them "like a girl with her lover." His body is aflame. He feels as if the dice themselves have power over him:

> The gambler goes to the hall of play asking himself, "will I win?" puffing himself up with "I will win!"
> The dice run counter to his desire, conferring the winning throws on his opponent.
> They are just "dice"—but hooking, goading, debasing, scorching, seeking to scorch,
> giving (temporarily) like a child, then in turn slapping down the victor,
> infused with honey, with power over the gambler.

The power of the dice is mystifying. (Note: the dice acquire their own agency, going from "scorching" to "seeking to scorch.") The gambler swings between guilty excitement, anger at the dice, scorn at his weakness, and shame. The very roll of the dice evokes the gambler's own descent into the pit of addiction: "Downward they roll, and then spring quickly upward, and, handless, force the man with hands to serve them." Still, the gambler is not completely compelled, as there is a paradoxical play between the gambler's agency and helplessness; at times he is able to exert some choice; at others he is completely overpowered.

The final stanza of the poem is intriguingly ambiguous; contemporary scholars have arrived at drastically different translations. In one possibility, the man is freed from the shackles of gambling and he beseeches his friends not to resent him for it and to seek their own release. In another version, he begs the dice to have pity on him, to calm their inner fury, and to move on to another victim. In yet another interpretation, somewhat chillingly, the dice themselves speak of how it is futile to be angry at the awful, sublime, and timeless power of addiction over humanity: "Old gambling friends, be kind to us! Don't be disgusted with our power. / Calm your resentment from within, and pass us to another foe to conquer."

I've been using the word "addiction," but before going further, it's important to reemphasize that addiction is not a tumor or a bacterium but an idea—or, more correctly, a set of ideas. Addiction is not outside of the historical process, sitting there as an independent fact waiting to be discovered. The term "addiction" was not adopted until recent centuries, but the concept of addiction, loosely conceived, could include everything from the notion of addiction as a disease to sweeping philosophical formulations of will and self-control. Well before our modern notions of addiction took shape, thinkers puzzled over those concepts—in fact, they form the foundation of our ideas about addiction.

Addiction is often explained in terms of a dichotomy of free choice versus total compulsion. By claiming that addictive behaviors are simply a kind of choice, people have justified punitive measures for centuries, from putting drunkards in the stocks to imprisoning people for drug possession. If their drug use is a free choice like any other, the argument goes, people should accept responsibility for their behavior, including punishment. The opposite view, which these days is commonly presented as a compassionate counterargument by neuroscientists and advocates, is that addictive behaviors are involuntary and uncontrollable compulsions, and thus people with addiction deserve compassion and treatment, rather than punishment.

But in cases from the gambler of the *Rig Veda* to my patient Susan, this dichotomy between choice and compulsion is unsatisfying. Lived experience flies in the face of such a stark binary, and many people with addiction feel themselves occupying a confusing middle ground between free choice and total loss of control. The thing that is terrifying to Susan, and to many others like her, is that they watch themselves making a choice even while feeling there is something wrong with the choosing. It is, in other words, an issue of *disordered* choice: a problem with choice, choice gone awry.

The ancient Greeks had a word for this experience of acting against your present judgment: *akrasia,* often translated as "weakness of the will." *Akrasia* isn't just doing something that is arguably harmful, like eating too much pie or spending too much money on clothes. Everyone indulges, even though indulgence is rarely the best option according to a cold, utilitarian calculus. *Akrasia* is doing something even though you truly believe it would be better not to, of recognizing in the moment that you are acting against your better judgment.

Akrasia was a controversial concept from the start. Socrates (as depicted by Plato) developed one argument in the *Phaedrus* that dismissed *akrasia* out of hand as a simple matter of choice. There could be internal conflict—pleasure and judgment often "quarrel inside us"—but people never truly act against their better judgment. Though Socrates allowed that people could be buffeted by desires and aversions leading up to a decision, at the moment of truth, he said, people always choose what they think is best for them at the time. They might come to regret their choices later, but that doesn't mean they were suffering from a lack of self-control. As he famously declared in the *Protagoras*, "No one who either knows or believes that there is another possible course of action, better than the one he is following, will ever continue on his present course."

Aristotle, on the other hand, was deeply invested in the idea of *akrasia*. To him, it was self-evident that people sometimes acted against their better judgment. He saw more nuance in the notion of choice, and he believed there were various ways that internal conflict might interfere with that choice. Surely, he asked, emotions or misguided reason can often get in the way of one's better judgment? The contemporary philosopher Alfred Mele has described the process in terms that might sound familiar: "Fred" decides to take a month off from after-dinner snacks. Around the fifteenth, his resolve starts to waver. He sees a slice of pie in the fridge. He recognizes the temptation and says to himself, It would really be best not to eat the damn thing. Then, even as he's telling himself that it's a bad idea, Fred calmly takes it out, carries it to the table, and scarfs it down. Socrates attributed poor choices to ignorance, but in this description of *akrasia*, Fred seems to fully understand the decision he's making.

Socrates's student Plato later arrived at a different point of view. He understood the problem of self-control partly as the result of a divided and conflicted self, one he illustrated through the famous metaphor of the chariot: the intellect is the charioteer attempting to wrangle the two horses of positive moral impulses and irrational, passionate drives. The notion is also found widely in classical narrative, such as Medea's psychological struggle in Ovid's *Metamorphoses*, torn between love and duty: "But a strange power attracts me against my will—desire urges one thing, reason another."

In the study of addiction today, the divided self is a prominent explanation of how choice can be disordered. For example, behavioral economics research describes the psychological feature of "delay discounting," in which smaller but more immediate rewards are favored over larger, delayed ones—this process is universal to humankind but more pronounced in addiction. Immediate rewards are grossly overvalued, causing extreme impulsivity that feels like loss of control. This can be seen not as a "control failure" but as a breakdown in a process called "intertemporal bargaining," in which the present self negotiates with—and irrationally overwhelms—the future self.

Nudging these types of choices can be a highly effective component of addiction treatment. The most obvious example originates from the 1980s, when Stephen Higgins, a psychologist at the University of Vermont, developed a "contingency management" program to treat people with cocaine addiction. In addition to the usual counseling, Higgins added a voucher system that gave people small rewards, such as sports equipment and movie passes, for cocaine-negative urine samples, and gave them a bonus for longer stretches of abstinence. This strategy was highly successful. One of the early experiments found that 55 percent of the voucher subjects were continuously drug-free for ten weeks, compared with fewer than 15 percent of subjects receiving the usual treatment.

After decades' more research, contingency management now has strong evidence in its favor, especially for stimulant problems, for which there aren't good medication treatments. My own monitored treatment, which required regular urine screens to test for drug or alcohol use, was a form of negative contingency management. I wasn't totally committed to abstinence at first, but my license was on the line, so I chose not to drink. This powerful contingency is, in large part, why these physician health programs have extraordinary five-year success rates of 75 percent or higher, eclipsing the effectiveness of essentially all other addiction treatments.

Yet some people don't stop, no matter what the cost. There is still that nagging 25 percent of people who don't make it to the five-year mark, for example. Some of my friends and colleagues from the physician health program did relapse, and they were trying their best—none thought in the moment that it would be better to start drinking or using again. Those outcomes are a testament, I think, not to the power of a simplistic compulsion, but to the complexity of the enigmatic internal forces that lie beneath the stereotype.

During my first year out of college, as my friends were starting graduate school or their first jobs, I was in the back of a taxi weaving its way through the jumbled streets of Seoul, South Korea, any sense of direction long since lost. My new friend Ravi and I were there for a one-year fellowship, and we were supposed to have been studying Korean the whole summer, but I had mostly drunk away my stipend and enjoyed my freedom. When I left, our private Korean tutor had one last request: "If you meet anyone who knows me, please don't tell them I taught you." Now we couldn't even communicate with our driver.

It was meant to be a fun experience, and it was. The fellowship set me up in a South Korean neuroscience lab where I didn't have to work all that hard. I sang with an opera company, gladly stepping out at encores to sing songs from *The Phantom of the Opera*. I got to travel all around East Asia. Long curious about Buddhism, I connected with a Zen teacher and began exploring a spiritual practice.

But I was also struggling, and, frighteningly, I wasn't sure why. I had spent four years in the meritocracy chasing awards, but now, between college and medical school and with nothing to prove, I had no more frantic activity to medicate the internal critic who told me I wasn't enough. I tried to re-create my own meritocracy—setting ambitious study schedules, trying to teach myself cognitive neuroscience so I could get a jump on med school. Instead I picked up that great Korean pastime of StarCraft, gluing myself to my computer for hours. I deleted and reinstalled and deleted the game again. And increasingly, my nights were devolving into drinking. Most nights I was out well past midnight, or I simply picked up small emerald-green bottles of astringent soju to drink in my apartment. Most mornings I woke with crushing regret and made desperate, ambitious plans to get back on track.

The consequences began to mount. In the same week, I slept through a lab meeting where I was supposed to present a paper and, much worse, missed a commitment to help chaperone a group of orphans on a field trip to a theme park. I felt I was wasting my life, wasting an amazingly privileged opportunity. What the hell was wrong with me?

I did wonder if I was an alcoholic, like my parents, but I quickly dismissed the notion. I thought addiction meant compulsion—a total loss of control—whereas my problems weren't that bad, and my actions weren't that extreme. I decided that my problem was just discipline, or planning, or perhaps personal development. I tried to meditate, but the practice didn't take; I just wound up back at the computer, playing StarCraft, soju in hand.

It was, looking back, a crucial point in the development of my addiction: not the patterns of my behavior or the severity of the consequences, but my ideas about what addiction was, and what it wasn't. I clung to the supposed divide between my parents' issues and mine, and that kept me from responding effectively to my growing problems.

When he was seventeen years old, a gifted North African man named Augustine left his home in the Roman city of Thagaste, in what is now Algeria, to study in the bustling metropolis of Carthage (in what is now Tunisia). He was intensely moral and religious, devoted to philosophy as a way of escaping his backwater farm town and deepening his Christian faith. And yet, he soon found himself "in the midst of a hissing cauldron of lust." As he described it in his later *Confessions*, he was "tossed and spilled, floundering in the broiling sea of my fornication. . . . The frenzy gripped me and I surrendered myself entirely to lust."

Augustine of Hippo, aside from being the most important early Christian philosopher and perhaps the most important figure in the whole of Christian thought, is often cited as an early example of addiction—you could call his *Confessions* the first addiction memoir. The first twelve-step group about sex, Sex and Love Addicts Anonymous, was also known as the "Augustine Fellowship," because one member who had been reading the *Confessions* claimed, "He's obviously one of us."

Notably, however, what those Augustine Fellowship members probably missed was just how tame Augustine's "fornications" were by modern standards. For a good portion of his sexual life, he was committed and monogamous, but he felt guilty about enjoying sex. Later, he stopped having sex entirely, but he was still tortured about his lustful feelings and sexual dreams—even though he was only consenting in his sleep. In this light, it might seem odd to label his problem an addiction. "Addiction" is commonly used to imply an extreme condition distinct from the rest of human society and marked by severe consequences, but Augustine's addiction was essentially an addiction to thinking.

Augustine was working through a universal theological puzzle: God was meant to be omnipotent, yet there was still sin in the world. Today, sin is commonly associated with blame and corruption, but Augustine was struggling to understand a deeply human phenomenon: Why do people turn away from what they know to be good toward a path of suffering? In particular, Augustine was troubled by a destructive urge to sin just for the sake of sinning, what Edgar Allan Poe would later call the "irrevocable overthrow" of "the spirit of Perverseness": the "unfathomable longing of the soul to vex itself—to offer violence to its own nature—to do wrong for the wrong's sake." How could that be if God was all-powerful? Augustine's answer was that all people have a God-given will, but the will is itself burdened by the "original sin" of Adam and Eve's betrayal, saddling all humans with lustful feelings and irrational urges—in what seems like Augustine's own fantasy, he believed that before the fall, sex involved no lust, and physical arousal was under completely voluntary control. But it wasn't just lust—original sin fundamentally transformed all of human nature by weakening our will, rendering the will both free and severely limited at the same time.

Augustine did not see his "addiction" to lust as discrete from other forms of suffering—it was all of a piece with the bigger problem of that misdirected will, a central preoccupation of his life. He constantly strove to bring more discipline to his reading and studying, scribbling notes to himself: "I have no time for reading . . . I must plan my time and arrange my day for the good of my soul." As he rose through academia and his wealth and fame grew, he came to see attachment to achievement and success as a sinful misdirection of the will, one no different from what he perceived to be the lowest attachments to drunkenness.

Out walking one day in Milan, worrying about a speech he was preparing, he noticed a drunken beggar laughing in the streets, and he realized they were both suffering from the same madness. In fact, he thought, maybe the beggar had it better: they were both chasing happiness, but the beggar could sleep off his drunkenness, while Augustine was tortured by his hunger for glory day after day.

Religious thinkers have long perceived such attachments in thinking as the root of a universal suffering. The early Christian Desert Fathers removed themselves to silent retreat to quiet their thinking and render their minds "naked," trying to free themselves from "the impress of any forms." Meister Eckhart sought to practice *Gelassenheit*, a state of "letting-go-ness" and release from the external world and preconceived notions of God. Buddhist teachers, similarly, taught that the primal addiction is the mind grasping at itself, seeking certainty and relief—it was a focus of the Buddha's very first teaching, and a key component of his diagnosis of the problem of human suffering, *dukkha*. Early Buddhist sutras are replete with references to this core diagnosis in similar terms. In one, this grasping is called a "mental illness" common to all sentient beings in the world, aside from the very few who have "overcome the intoxicating inclinations" toward pleasure (or cravings for existence or nonexistence, for that matter). On this view, there's no real difference between what we call addiction and any other persistent attempt to self-soothe this inherent unsatisfactoriness and to shore up the distorted vision of the self.

A common assumption about addiction today is that it is a unique ailment neatly bounded off from the rest of the population, but in a sense Augustine and the Buddha anticipated an emerging, alternative perspective. Several contemporary psychological theories support the idea that addiction is just one manifestation of ordinary, though detrimental, psychological processes. For example, some explanations frame addiction as a manifestation of "psychological inflexibility": attempts to manipulate and avoid negative thoughts and feelings by disappearing into addictive behaviors, including not just substance use but also worry, rumination, self-stimulation, and other forms of mindlessness. Those avoidant responses are a kind of self-medication, not in the sense that addiction is the superficial expression of a "deeper" problem, but rather that substance addictions are merely one variant of a universal feature: the way our human psychology sometimes reacts ineffectively to pain.

The idea of addiction as a universal feature of psychology might seem jarring, because it is so drastically different from the usual modern idea that "addicts" and "non-addicts" are fundamentally different. That binary framing has long been a mainstay of a reductionist approach that attempts to describe addiction as a brain malfunction. But the notion that addiction is a discrete disease is complicated by a recent, larger development in psychiatric research that questions whether *any* mental disorders are discrete entities. For years, psychiatry labored under the idea that mental disorders were categorical, fixed entities—things people got—but today there is a rising recognition that all mental disorders seem to exist on a continuum. For example, substance problems are on a neatly graded spectrum, with no clear transition in the data that tells us where to draw the line between mild and severe issues. This is why the most recent version of the *DSM*, the psychiatric diagnostic manual used to classify mental disorders, has done away with the division between "substance abuse" and "substance dependence," the latter of which was a stand-in for addiction. "Spectrum" concepts have been gaining momentum, from autism to disability to many other issues, and the neurodiversity movement similarly seeks to challenge the notion that mental disorders are inherently pathological. This trend represents a major advance, not just for science but for a deeper truth: dismantling the artificially constructed barriers between "us" and "them," the simplistic dichotomy between "normal" and "abnormal" that obscures the way mental disorders are part of a complex system.

People use drugs for reasons; the banality of that statement is matched only by our constant lack of mindfulness to it. The message screams from the pages of addiction memoirs. Caroline Knapp describes how "liquor occupies the role of a lover or constant companion," creating an illusion of emotional authenticity that seemed like it granted access to more meaningful feelings. William Burroughs described how heroin "is momentary freedom from the claims of the aging, cautious, nagging, frightened flesh." Owen Flanagan, a distinguished philosopher, has written extensively about his own alcohol and benzodiazepine addiction and how it medicated "an existential anxiety involving not feeling safe in my own skin."

I think about my first drink, at a keg party at one of the cool kids' houses during my junior year of high school. I was a science-league and marching-band type of guy, so I was never welcome there, but it was a class-wide party, and everyone, even me, was invited.

It is a cliché to say one's first drink was magical, but it truly was for me. I was in a cavelike suburban New Jersey basement, drinking thin keg beer out of a red plastic cup, and it was a subtraction, not an addition, that was the trick: self-consciousness and social anxiety evaporated, and I felt free, connected, loose, joyful. I drank a beer through a funnel, and jocks who had previously shot at me with BB guns or beaten me up applauded. After walking home with my buddy from the saxophone section, I fell to the ground on my front lawn, feeling completely held by the earth. It felt so safe that I laughed, like the feeling of letting go of a deep breath.

Alcohol became my good friend and companion the rest of that year, and by the time I was applying to college, I showed up to my MIT interview hungover and late—it was my dream school, and I blew it.

Augustine's accounts in his *Confessions* resonate today because of his evocative descriptions of his internal struggle. He believed in his heart that he wanted to be chaste, but he just couldn't resist his sexual urges: "My two wills, one old, one new, one carnal, one spiritual, were in conflict and in their conflict wasted my soul." Decades ago, German physicians called *das Nichtaufhörenkönnen*, "the inability to stop," the main criterion of "true alcoholism," and today some scholars argue that *"akrasia"* is the best way to capture the mystery at the heart of addiction. Perhaps substance use disorders are on a spectrum, the argument goes, and we can't draw a clear line on the basis of problem severity, but surely we can draw a line here: the subjective experience of being out of control.

While there are several other historical figures who seem to fit a diagnosis of addiction, we don't always know if they had the same sort of inner struggle as Augustine. Their examples point toward yet another complication with the notion of addiction. Marcus Antonius (Mark Antony, Cleopatra's lover) struggled with drinking: once, while hungover and holding court as Julius Caesar's second-in-command, he was sick in public, "flooding his own lap and the whole platform with the gobbets of wine-reeking food he had vomited up." Though Antony published a book defending and celebrating his legendary drinking habits, contemporaneous commentators like Seneca the Younger call alcohol a chief factor in his downfall. Likewise, any biography of Alexander III of Macedon ("the Great") contains a litany of worsening alcohol problems: he burned the Persian city of Persepolis to the ground during a wine-saturated celebration, killed his beloved mentor, Cleitus the Black, in a drunken rage, held drinking contests that left dozens of his men dead, and, against his doctors' orders, drank heavily even while suffering from a chronically high fever, dying a month short of his thirty-third birthday.

What these examples reveal is a challenging heterogeneity to addiction. It's common today to talk about addiction as if it were one thing: not just discretely divided from "normal," but also unitary in the sense of being relatively consistent from person to person. But there is actually remarkable diversity, including at the level of one's self-concept. What about people who completely deny they have issues and perhaps even lack any sense of inner conflict, but who, to most outside observers, seem to have a serious addiction?

Present-day emergency rooms are full of such cases: people who seem gravely disabled by addiction yet deny they have a problem. One report from Bellevue Hospital described a thirty-two-year-old patient with severe alcohol addiction—who had 428 previous ER visits and nine ICU admissions—before he finally died of hypothermia. Clearly, lives are at risk, regardless of what people say about their internal conflict, or lack thereof. People like this do not fit the definition of addiction as *akrasia*, although they do fit a broader definition of addiction as "continued use despite negative consequences."

This is an extraordinarily consequential distinction. A definition of addiction "from outside," one that requires no self-report, allows others to diagnose you with it. It allows for interventions, mandated treatment, and entire systems of control for people with substance use problems. This kind of addiction definition, in various forms, has long served as a foundation for punitive approaches to addiction.

Yet the *DSM*, the psychiatric diagnostic manual, does not make this distinction. It has one umbrella diagnosis called "substance use disorder" that combines both subjective and objective criteria. You can have substance use disorder based on criteria that are essentially self-diagnosed, like whether you often use more than you intend. But a diagnosis of a substance use disorder can also be based on more objective criteria, like spending a lot of time on substance-related activities, experiencing problems at home or work, or using substances in a way that's physically hazardous.

This lumping is a deliberate trade-off on the part of the *DSM* authors, and the result is enhanced reliability for the criteria. However, this reliability comes at the expense of appreciating the heterogeneity of addiction. For example, there is a strand in addiction advocacy today that seeks to replace "person with addiction" with "person with substance use disorder," seeking a more compassionate and less stigmatized term. However, the terms are not really equivalent: "substance use disorder" includes a huge swath of people who have substance problems but do not necessarily feel like they are struggling with internal conflict or self-identify as addicted.

An alternative strategy is to draw clearer distinctions within that heterogeneity. Aristotle considered it useful to classify different kinds of *akrasia*: like the "clear-eyed" kind, as opposed to the fierier "impetuous" *akrasia* driven by passions or cravings. Likewise, in a landmark 1971 article, the philosopher Harry Frankfurt distinguished between "willing" and "unwilling" addicts—both have an immediate desire to take a drug, but the willing addict is not conflicted about it, and the unwilling addict doesn't want to have that desire. To have "unwilling" addiction is to be subjectively addicted—like Augustine, or my patient Susan, troubled by an internal sense of being out of control. Alexander, perhaps, was "willing," as are innumerable frequent ER utilizers and multiple-DUI offenders today.

Diagnosis is a subtle practice, one only made more difficult by the amount of work we ask a given diagnosis to do. Whether or not something is classified as a mental disorder is an enormously significant determination, not only for medicine but in fields like law, politics, and sociology, where insurance reimbursement might be at stake and guilt or innocence might hang in the balance, or philosophy and ethics, where a disease status implies involuntariness and absence of guilt. A disorder diagnosis means different things to different people: a scientist arguing for research funding, a doctor communicating something about risk or treatment, an advocate arguing for social change, or someone making sense of their own identity.

For the moment, it seems the only reasonable solution is to be careful and clear about using language to describe such rich and nuanced conceptual territory—which naturally prompts another question: Where did we get this complicated word, "addiction," in the first place?

In July of 1533, a young man named John Frith, only eight years out from his Cambridge graduation, was imprisoned at the Tower of London and burned alive for heresy. As a secret member of the Protestant Reformation, which was at that point less than two decades old, he had toiled underground for years to produce pamphlets and books criticizing the Catholic Church. Though he was only one of hundreds of Protestant martyrs who would die for their beliefs, as far as today's linguists have determined, he was the first to use the word "addict" in English—in a text criticizing the pope, no less.

The Latin *ad-dicere* means to "speak to" or "say to," and in classical Latin, *addicere* was a legal term meaning "given over to." One use of the word described how a debtor could be enslaved by a creditor to pay off a debt, and some modern writers eagerly cite this fact to invoke a debased sense of slavery, hijacking, and compulsion. But there is more to the word. *Addicere* also referred to augury—the divination of the will of the gods through omens and portents, like reading the flight of birds—and it referred to a strong devotion or a habitual behavior, or even more simply, a strong preference. For example, in that first text, Frith used it to say, "Judge . . . all these things with a simple eye / be not partially *addict* to the one nor to the other / But judge them by the scripture," as a way to urge the reader not to be overly attached to preconceived ideas.

For Frith and the other reformers in his circle, "addict" was a powerful word. It was a loanword from Latin, one of many at a time when English writers were eagerly vacuuming up words from other languages to expand their vocabularies and express new concepts. Many of those neologisms were short-lived, but something about "addict" stuck. "Addict" did useful conceptual work for those early Protestants; it had a depth and complexity that helped to point toward that confusing gray area between free will and compulsion.

Crucially, the word didn't refer to a condition or a status, but an action. It was not something that happened to you—addiction was not a force that overthrew the will—but something you chose. To "addict" yourself in the wrong way, like Faust, was a dire matter indeed, but to addict yourself rightly deserved to be celebrated as an almost heroic devotion and commitment.

"Addict" was powerful, but not necessarily negative. A disdainful man could be addict to pride, and an evil one could be addict to sin, but a devout one could be addict to worship. The important thing was what the word said about freedom. "Addict" pointed toward a paradoxical sense of "willed compulsion" that is simultaneously active and outside of an individual's control. It was an active process of giving over one's agency, a choice to give up choice. It was this paradox, and how it fit with a theological puzzle of the time, that made the word itself so captivating.

These early Protestant reformers, not unlike Augustine, were preoccupied with fate, freedom, and the bondage of the will. The Protestant tradition is particularly concerned with freedom, tying salvation to the idea of self-discipline. Christopher Marlowe's 1604 play *Doctor Faustus* was so fraught with competing interpretations—could Faust have done otherwise? was it a somber warning about damnation or a criticism of Calvinist determinism?—that there were legends about audience members being driven mad and actual devils appearing onstage during the "profane" play. But *Doctor Faustus* is not just a story about damnation and fate; it's about a particular type of devotion that leads to impaired freedom—notably, the *English Faust-Book* of 1592 describes Faust as "addicted."

Despite our tendency to regard the condition of "addiction" as quite narrow—a severe disorder at the furthest extremes of behavior and usually involving substances—in our everyday language we often speak of being addicted to the latest show or app, or a favorite food, or a new hobby. I know researchers and clinicians who bristle at this usage, and I used to be bothered by it, too, until I learned that this is how the word was actually meant to be used. The word beautifully captures the nuances and complexities that underlie the concept of addiction, like disordered choice and universality, while also preserving room for heterogeneity.

From the beginning, the word "addiction" was not a narrow description of a medical problem, but an immensely rich and complicated term, used to gesture toward core mysteries of the human condition. It was not just about drugs, but about willing and agency—being someone who chooses—and the related, timeless puzzle of our seeming inability to control ourselves. It is crucial to be clear in speaking about addiction, but it is also crucial to embrace the paradox around it—far better to welcome its capaciousness and flexibility than to fight against five hundred years of culture. We could look at addiction as a big mistake, a word so vague and variable that it is meaningless and misleading. Or we could look at it as a finger pointing at the moon, something gesturing toward something mysterious, confounding, but ultimately human. I prefer the latter.

Two

EPIDEMICS

By late October 1492, Christopher Columbus had grown impatient. His first expedition was going poorly: his crews were on the verge of mutiny, and the trade with the indigenous Taíno people was disappointing. Columbus was hungry for gold, or at least to make contact with China (he had convinced himself that he had arrived at the outskirts of Asia—a delusion he would carry to the end of his life). By November 1, when his crew anchored on Cuba's northeastern shore, he decided that they must have reached the mainland. He quickly dispatched a few men, including the scout Rodrigo de Jerez, to bushwhack into the lush, exotic vegetation, bearing letters of introduction to the Great Khan.

De Jerez and his companions returned five days later. They had come across a large Taíno settlement, but to Columbus's disappointment, there were no spices, no gold, no sign of the great Chinese empire. The only notable discovery was the native population's odd custom of rolling up an unfamiliar plant, setting it aflame, then inhaling the smoke—on purpose.

This practice was completely new to them—Europeans had no experience whatsoever with smoking to this point—and little did the disappointed Columbus know that he had stumbled across what would become the great American cash crop. But de Jerez took an immediate liking to tobacco, as people often do, and he brought the custom back to his hometown of Ayamonte, in southwest Spain, where his neighbors were so terrified by the sight of thick smoke billowing out of his mouth that they hauled him before the Inquisition with accusations of sorcery. De Jerez was imprisoned for seven years. By the time he was released, tobacco had transformed from a diabolical plant to a hot new trend among the elites of Europe, one that would soon spread across Eurasia and become nearly ubiquitous in modern culture.

Every human civilization on earth has developed a relationship with mind-altering substances. In cases like tobacco and Taíno society, humans and drugs coexist peacefully, because social customs and traditional wisdom keep drug use in check. At times, though, those relationships become strained, when a new drug—or a reformulation of an existing one—triggers a wave of dramatically increased use. For hundreds of years, these waves of increased use, and related problems, have been widely described and understood as "epidemics."

The way the word "epidemic" is used to describe drug crises is slippery and sometimes outright harmful. The term can variously mean increased drug availability, use, harms, or addiction, for example. The word "epidemic" also suggests a medical model, potentially obscuring the other social factors at play and suggesting that drugs are a sort of pathogen to be exterminated. These are valuable cautions, and it's important to recognize that calling a drug crisis an epidemic should not imply that the medical domain is best for addressing it, or that all drugs should be eradicated. That said, throughout this book I call these phenomena epidemics, primarily because that's how they've been understood and discussed for hundreds of years.

By looking closely at these repeated epidemics, we can better understand both the forces driving them and the ideas about addiction that have arisen in their wake. As a series of epidemics wracked the modern world with disturbing regularity, beginning with tobacco, various explanations emerged: a barbarous and dangerous drug, rapacious commercial forces, deeper societal problems. From a wider vantage point, we can see that each explanation contains some truth, as these forces often overlap and coexist, but also that epidemics often inspire panics out of proportion to their true harms.

Columbus's journey occurred at the dawn of a new age—what David Courtwright, one of today's leading historians of addiction, has called the "psychoactive revolution," marked by wave after wave of novel, powerful, and often frightening mind-altering substances. Though alcohol was common, Europe circa 1500 was completely naive to most of the other drugs that dominate society today, from cocaine and tobacco to coffee and tea. But in the years from about 1500 to 1789, the insatiable drives of transoceanic commerce and conquest yielded not just lucrative trade routes but also a host of exotic plants with powerful effects on the mind and body—and, significantly, new ideas about how to use them.

Within a few decades of their arrival in Europe, coffee, tea, and chocolate exploded as mass-produced "soft drugs," democratizing new ways of expanding consciousness and broadening the repertoire of drug use outside of socially sanctioned realms. Even sugar began as a rare medical preparation reserved for kings and aristocrats, only later becoming a bedrock staple of the modern Western diet. Likewise, premodern Europeans had tended to use opium only for medicinal purposes, but as early as the sixteenth century, an intrepid physician and botanist named Garcia da Orta sent word back from Goa that some in Indian society used opium to calm their mental troubles, too. Da Orta's report was just one of many accounts of non-medical opium use that would trickle in over the coming years, all the way up to the Orientalist explorations of the Romantics, like Samuel Taylor Coleridge, in the early nineteenth century.

As the use of a novel drug became more widespread, especially outside of socially sanctioned use, it often inspired another new feature: a drug scare. Drug scares are a form of moral panic, which are almost always stoked, if not initiated by, elite forces and often used to buttress the social order in societies undergoing rapid change. Tobacco began as a special and rare medicine, an almost supernatural panacea, promoted among the royalty by Jean Nicot, a young French diplomat. In England, Sir Walter Raleigh inspired a fashion craze for recreational smoking, initially associated with the leisure class. Dandies learned to blow elaborate smoke clouds and rings, "reeking gallants" carried boxes of gold, silver, and ivory accessories, and pipes were lit with coal passed on the point of a sword. However, as tobacco became more widely used across all social strata, it prompted intense fears and increasingly desperate attempts to control it. The Mughal emperor Jahangir forbade all smoking. Pope Urban VIII threatened snuff users with excommunication (snuff is a ground form of inhaled tobacco, and the pope was reportedly scandalized by accounts of priests having sneezing fits during Mass). Russian, Japanese, and Chinese rulers all gave out harsh penalties for tobacco use. Sultan Murad IV of the Ottoman Empire punished tobacco users in the 1620s and '30s with heavy fines and, occasionally, death—at one point executing twenty of his officers "with the severest torture." But no matter what, the drug rolled on, seemingly unstoppable. Those Ottoman soldiers whom Murad IV killed? Some smuggled pipes in their sleeves so they could sneak a few last puffs during their executions.

The anti-drug sentiments of the early modern period were closely associated with fears about foreignness, class, sin, and subversion. In England, King James I—a serious and devout man obsessed with sin and witchcraft—took aim at the new, dangerously non-medical practice, publishing *A Counterblaste to Tobacco* in 1604, castigating his subjects for imitating "the barbarous and beastly maners of the wilde, godlesse, and slavish Indians, especially in so vile and stinking a custome." Other English anti-tobacco writers followed with a panic about "a Plague intolerable." The drug scares of this time show just how little such scares have to do with actual medical harms or any fears about

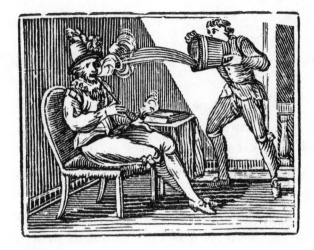

Mid-nineteenth-century woodcut of Sir Walter Raleigh smoking tobacco. According to legend, he was doused with a pitcher of water by a servant who feared he was on fire.

"addictiveness"—people did not yet perceive the health risks of smoking tobacco, and the idea of addiction as a medical problem linked to drugs hadn't even been articulated by this point in history. Though, as we know today, there were real harms, and other, more insidious forces at play.

G rowing up, I loved the Jersey Shore. I loved the expansive board-walk cluttered with carnival games. All summer, I'd play at the cacophonous Skee-Ball lanes and spinning wheels, collecting tickets to trade in for boxes of baseball cards, hoping above all to score my favorites from the Yankees' lineup. The only part I hated was the drive. From start to finish, the car was thick with cigarette smoke, both my parents chain-smoking the whole hour-long trip down.

Secondhand smoke was a well-publicized health issue in the 1980s, and even in elementary school I understood the dangers, so I didn't understand why my parents didn't. Alone in the back seat, I'd beg them to lower the window until my father, begrudgingly, would crack his an inch.

I became preoccupied with their smoking. I'd scream and rail and stomp my feet as I begged them to stop. Over time, they hid their packs, which I'd find and haughtily show them as I theatrically cut them in half.

One of the most vivid images I have from my childhood is cigarette burns in our pillowcases. Every single pillowcase was peppered with burns, like buckshot, some just a tiny hole, some long, oblong, with a stiff black fringe. I knew at the time that this wasn't normal, I suppose, but I didn't fully appreciate that each little burn came not only from cigarettes but also from alcohol. Drinking, ultimately, is how the burns happened—and why they passed out most nights in front of the TV, and why they could be so volatile and emotionally unpredictable. In a way, I knew this. I had already learned to pay exquisite attention to them: how they talked, whether their voices were slurred and how much, the quality of their attention, if they were acting goofy and whether it was simply playful or a harbinger of something more. Drinking makes a parent childlike in a way that can be deeply frightening. Smoking was safer and more tangible to my younger self.

At a pirate-themed seafood restaurant at the shore, I'd gleefully pluck their maraschino cherries from their mixed drinks and enjoy the sharp and numbing bite as I played with the flimsy plastic swords that had pierced them. Come to think of it, that was my true first drink. It was sweet, and I loved it.

Purdue Pharma, until recently a private company owned by the über-wealthy Sackler family, has emerged as the leading villain of today's opioid epidemic, and not without reason. In 1996, the company launched OxyContin with one of the largest and most sophisticated marketing campaigns in the history of the pharmaceutical industry. They engineered a surge of advertising to overcome fears about addiction, and perversely, general practice doctors were a centerpiece of that strategy. They paid thought leaders to give presentations about the purported safety of the drug and to write statements for professional medical organizations about treating chronic pain. They funded the attendance of thousands of clinicians at medical conferences, where they could absorb those carefully crafted and targeted messages. In 2001, as the country began to realize it had a proper epidemic on its hands, Purdue executives testified before Congress that their marketing was "conservative" and the problem lay in bad people abusing the medication, or perhaps in bad doctors who overprescribed OxyContin. When states started to develop laws intended to curb the epidemic, Purdue orchestrated backroom lobbying to kill the bills. At the time of this writing, the company has pleaded guilty to its role in misleading the federal government about sales of OxyContin, and it is still embroiled in bankruptcy proceedings. The Sacklers, who own the company privately, will lose it outright, and they must pay $225 million in civil penalties, but it appears that they will be able to shield much of their massive wealth, which has been estimated at more than $11 billion.

Purdue didn't create the epidemic on its own, but it did contribute significantly to it. And even though they were masters of the craft, there was nothing really new in what Purdue's leaders did—they were simply playing a role in a larger system that has existed and evolved for generations. Drug epidemics throughout history have commonly featured not just a novel drug but also a powerful industry promoting that drug.

In the words of the addiction researcher Jim Orford, companies like Purdue are participants in "addiction supply industries," selling products that by their very nature have a special hold on human desires. Psychoactive substances are consumer products with a telling feature: in economic terms, they are relatively "inelastic," meaning they are more insulated from the laws of supply and demand than ordinary products. Raise prices on soda and people buy water. Raise prices on heroin and many people just figure out how to make it work. Heavy users can have a surprisingly significant effect on the psychoactive drug market. For example, one-quarter of cannabis buyers account for nearly three-quarters of cannabis sales.*

Products with addiction potential are not ordinary commodities. They can cause far-reaching harms, but companies often don't directly bear the cost of those harms. The psychological despair of addiction, drunk driving accidents, cirrhosis, cancer, emphysema, overdoses, and so forth—these harms are, in the language of economics, "externalities": costs that aren't borne by those who create them.

It thus falls to governments and regulators to detect and protect us from these harms. Yet, from the earliest days of the addiction supply industries, this type of intervention has been undercut by financial incentives. King James I was able to issue a four *thousand* percent tax hike on tobacco back at the turn of the seventeenth century in part because the Spanish and Portuguese empires controlled all the tobacco-producing colonies, and the high cost of importing tobacco was bad for the English economy. But then, as English colonies started producing tobacco, importing the drug became a mutually reinforcing financial boon, so by 1643, Parliament had discarded prohibitionist taxes and even taken steps to encourage its trade. This helped a dangerous invader to become an accepted part of English culture, a genial pipe by the fire rather than a barbaric custom.

This pattern repeated itself over and over again for tobacco. In late-seventeenth-century Russia, when Peter the Great finally accepted that tobacco smuggling was ubiquitous, he stopped harsh penalties (which included nostril slitting and tearing off noses entirely) and instead permitted the sale and consumption of tobacco—if the government couldn't prevent it, it might as well make some money on it. From Cardinal Richelieu in France to the Italian republics and Habsburg Austria, other leaders followed suit and gave up on tobacco bans in favor of taxes,

---

* Here and throughout the book, I use the word "cannabis" instead of "marijuana," because cannabis is the scientific name of the plant and how it was described for much of history, until the word "marijuana" was deliberately used to attach negative, racist connotations to the drug.

monopolies, and other strategies to profit off the new crop. This pattern would repeat itself regularly throughout the entire history of drugs. Taxes on psychoactive drugs became the financial foundation of colonial empires: by 1885, taxes on alcohol, tobacco, and tea were close to half of the British government's gross income. Likewise, the need for tax revenue helped to defeat alcohol prohibition in both the United States (during the Great Depression) and India; in the latter case, the Indian constitution encouraged alcohol prohibition, but most of the Indian states were simply too dependent on alcohol tax revenue.

Drug revenues entice governments to overlook the other harms of these systems, including those beyond addiction. Addiction is often portrayed as a form of oppression or bondage, and it is not a coincidence that the history of addiction is linked to systems of subjugation and conquest. It was tobacco that saved the struggling Jamestown settlement in the early seventeenth century, and when the colonizers couldn't get enough indentured servants to work the fields, the first enslaved Africans were brought to Virginia to work on plantations. As the plantation system in the American colonies enabled the explosive growth of the English tobacco industry, European tobacco merchants not only promoted the tobacco trade but also prevented the colony of Virginia from levying a tax on slaves and obstructed antislavery movements at home in England. (The other important slave-farmed commodity, also considered a drug at that time, was Caribbean sugar.)

When profit is the organizing principle, addiction supply industries, of course, will do what they can to maximize sales of their products. Long before Purdue Pharma, pharmaceutical companies learned the power of promoting drugs directly to consumers and doctors: the U.S. company Parke, Davis & Co. began promoting the use of cocaine for "exhaustion" and "overwork" in the 1880s, and around the same time, the German company Merck promised that cocaine's "greatest future" was in treating morphine and alcohol problems. These methods repeatedly led to, in the phrase of one group of scholars, "industrial epidemics"—contemporary examples include alcohol, processed food, and guns—caused by the industrial promotion of harmful products and the industrial subversion of public health measures intended to limit those products' harms. This process has only intensified as corporations have become increasingly concentrated and globalized.

Tobacco is perhaps the best-known modern industrial epidemic. As the research linking smoking and cancer emerged after World War II, the tobacco industry poured millions of dollars into advertising intended to convince the public that smoking was safe. Though tobacco executives acknowledged in internal documents that nicotine was addictive as early as 1963, they vigorously fought the idea in public and in the halls of medicine. As one executive at a tobacco company described their strategy in an internal memo from 1969, "Doubt is our product since it is the best means of competing with the 'body of fact' that exists in the minds of the general public." Tobacco companies also mastered the move of putting blame back on individual consumers, capitalizing on research showing that some people could moderate or stop on their own.

These strategies—falsely advertising safety, undercutting evidence of harms, and putting blame on individuals—are not exclusive to addiction supply industries, of course, and the marketing of doubt pioneered by tobacco companies has given rise to an entire "product defense industry" aimed at subverting science to obscure the understanding of public health risks. Today, fossil fuel companies are using the same strategies to manufacture doubt about climate change, today's arch-externality, the deferred cost of centuries of economic growth fueled by coal, oil, and gas. This pattern demonstrates that what we call addiction is not simply a result of the inherent "addictiveness" of drugs or other products, but is often a feature of the system itself. It is not a matter of the occasional bad actor; addiction epidemics have been a feature of modern life for centuries. As long as industries are incentivized to sell potentially harmful products without having to bear the costs of those harms, the pattern will continue.

At the same time, societies, like individuals, often have their own reasons for using drugs.

When addiction epidemics strike, we want to know why. What is necessarily a complex web of intersecting forces is too often reduced to one simplistic story: trauma, brain disease, an evil and unstoppable drug, a bad pill-mill doctor, a hereditary taint, or a weak will or poor morals. The German brain researcher Ernst Pöppel called this impulse, jokingly, monocausotaxophilia: "the love of single causes that explain everything." People want answers, and perhaps more than that, they want villains. That role is easily satisfied by the notion of a dangerous drug, or a dangerous company pushing a drug, but sometimes the causes lie deeper, in more complex forms of social wounding.

In the 1720s, a bright young Native American boy was born into a society under siege. Samson Occom was one of only 350 remaining Mohegan people living along the thickly wooded banks of the Thames River Valley in what is now Connecticut, among the last remnants of a tribe that had once numbered in the thousands. The Mohegan people—unlucky enough to be located close to a prominent colony, just miles away from an excellent deepwater harbor that the English had christened New London—had been ravaged by years of disease, poverty, warfare, exploitation, and another of the great epidemics of early modern history, one that in this case had spread from Europe: alcohol.

Distilled spirits took a heavy toll on Native cultures. It was not just the immediate harms, like trackers freezing to death, insensible to the winter cold. Alcohol seemed to be eating away at their souls. Drunken men beat their wives. Usually solemn and respectful treaty negotiations broke down into violence. By the time of Occom's birth, Connecticut officials wondered at the power of alcohol, which seemed to be impoverishing and corrupting the morals of Mohegan culture.

Occom himself took to another significant European import:

Christianity. Occom was growing up during the First Great Awakening, a passionate, optimistic evangelical movement marked by ecstatic camp meetings all across the Northeast. Huge crowds wept and cried out as people were "born again," and Occom himself had his own profound conversion experience as a young boy. He came to believe that this new faith was the way to save his people. He convinced a local preacher, the Reverend Eleazar Wheelock, to take him on as a pupil in preparation for missionary work, and Wheelock was blown away when Occom quickly picked up English, Hebrew, Greek, and Latin.

Occom was pious, devoted, and driven. Despite suffering from chronic pain and various medical ailments, he traveled hundreds of miles to preach to other Indigenous tribes. From the Montauk people, at the eastern tip of Long Island, to the Iroquois Confederacy, in the thick forests of upstate New York, he saw alcohol problems everywhere. Soon the young man began to realize another important dimension to this foreign drug. Alcohol was a tool of exploitation—like smallpox blankets, it was not a passive invader, but a deliberate instrument of oppression. Colonists encouraged drinking among Native peoples to pacify resistance and tie them to the colonial economy. Traders promoted exorbitantly priced alcohol, then swapped whiskey for crushing debt and mortgages on Native land. Alcohol was a common adjunct to murder, as Native Americans were given free liquor, then killed while helplessly drunk.

At first, tribes attempted their own forms of prohibition. They begged authorities for restrictions on the liquor trade, as Occom himself chronicled among the Oneida of central New York, but whatever laws came were widely flouted. Tribes tried to enact their own restrictions—in one scene oddly suggestive of 1920s Prohibition photographs, the Shawnees of Pennsylvania poured forty gallons of rum into the street. Prohibition was not enough, though, to counteract the unrelenting pressures of trade and the deeper causes of cultural devastation roiling underneath. Even so, it was all portrayed as the Native peoples' fault—alcohol problems as a barbarian vice. In 1767, a desperate chief of the Tuscarora people, Aucus al Kanigut, formally petitioned the New York colonial government for "some medicine to cure us of our fondness for that destructive liquor." The British officer only replied that they ought to forsake their ways, embrace Christianity, and seek instruction in morality so they could better control their appetites.

Though he was a Christian preacher, Occom saw beyond this individualistic prescription. In September 1772, he delivered an immensely popular sermon at the execution of a Wampanoag man who, while intoxicated, had killed a white man. In colonial culture, these were considered important events for moral instruction, and Occom duly inveighed at length against the sin of drunkenness. But then he called out alcohol as an instrument of exploitation, denouncing the "devilish men [alcohol traders]" who "put their bottles to their neighbours mouth to make them drunk," and the fact that Native peoples "have been cheated over and over again." It was by far the most popular sermon of its time; the printed version rapidly went through nineteen editions, making him one of the leading authors in all of the American colonies.

By now, Occom was souring on the whole project of cultural assimilation, despite having become a proper celebrity himself. The decade prior, his teacher, Reverend Wheelock, had sent him on a tour around England, Scotland, and Ireland to fundraise for a charity school for Native boys, and on the trip Occom had won the praise of King George III and raised at least £11,000, an astronomical sum in those days (millions of pounds today). But on returning home, Occom found that Wheelock had neglected to take care of his wife as he had promised, and he had given up on teaching Occom's son—at one point, Wheelock advised him to just indenture the boy "to a good Master." Wheelock then tried to smear Occom with accusations of intemperate drinking, playing off the stereotypical image of Native Americans as dangerous, inherently out-of-control brutes. (Occom was exonerated by church authorities.)

In the end, Wheelock used the money that Occom raised to develop a school not for Native American pupils but primarily for English ones—his school grew into Dartmouth College, which graduated only nineteen Native Americans in the first two hundred years of its existence. Occom, disgusted, left to focus on the Brothertown movement, a confederacy of struggling tribes seeking to establish a new community in upstate New York as a refuge from disease and oppression. With Occom's help, they successfully founded their new home, made up of survivors from around the Northeast, though they were later pressured to move to Wisconsin, then stripped of their tribal status. They are still seeking official federal recognition today.

Occom was far ahead of his time, by centuries in fact, in calling attention to the role of alcohol in a wider project of oppression and dislocation. To this day, there are pervasive, false "firewater myths" about Native peoples' inborn vulnerability to alcohol. Such myths, dating from the earliest days of colonization, have a purpose: they disguise the use of alcohol as a weapon and provide ideological support for colonization and supremacy. For generations, similar myths about the supposedly special effect of cocaine on Black bodies have been used as ideological cover for harsh prohibitionist crackdowns.

Today those firewater myths have been roundly disproven, and Native drinking problems are far better attributed to the systemic problems that Occom identified. There is ample evidence that before European contact, many Native tribes used psychoactive drugs, including alcohol in some cases, without problems, and that even after contact they didn't develop harmful patterns of drinking until after the ravages of disease, war, poverty, and forced relocation—not to mention the industrial production and mercantile promotion of alcohol.

Epidemics are never caused solely by an inherent power of the drugs themselves, or the efforts of addiction supply industries; there is often, if not always, social wounding underneath, driving the substance use. The Opium Wars, a series of British military actions from 1839 to 1860 that forced open Chinese markets to opium, were followed by an epidemic of uncontrolled opium use in China. That epidemic was once widely interpreted as a story of a once noble society destroyed by a powerful drug, but more recent scholarship has argued that this simplistic explanation overlooks the turmoil, poverty, and widespread dislocation caused by the wars themselves, which in turn exacerbated the epidemic. Likewise, tobacco's explosive spread throughout Eurasia in the seventeenth century wasn't simply the natural consequence of a powerful substance; it was soothing humanity's suffering from an awful and seemingly unending series of plagues, revolts, and wars, what historians have called the "general crisis of the seventeenth century."

The Canadian psychologist Bruce Alexander has articulated this idea as his "dislocation theory of addiction," which asserts that the most important and fundamental cause of addiction is not the biological effect of a drug or some inborn vulnerability to addiction in individuals, but rather a society's wounds. Importantly, that pain doesn't need to be the kind of concrete loss such as the poverty and disease experienced by the Mohegan people in Occom's youth, or the physical separation of being torn from family and friends. There is also a psychological dislocation that can be just as toxic: being torn from culture and traditional spirituality, losing freedom and self-determination, and lacking opportunities for joy and self-expression. Even for those of us who are not suffering from such tangible deprivations today, we are just as vulnerable as our ancestors, if not more so, to the psychospiritual ones.

As I was researching this book, my mother, slowly wasting away from lung cancer, told me about how her own father, a Swedish immigrant, fell into a severe depression every winter. He would remember his happy childhood in Stockholm and compare it with their life in Newark: no hot water, working the night shift at a bottling plant, never seeing his wife, who worked an opposite shift on a different assembly line. Though he tried not to drink, he'd always relapse on alcohol as Christmas approached, and for months my mother, still a young girl, would be sent out into the Newark winters to trudge from bar to bar to find him so he could get a few precious hours of sleep before his next shift. From an early age, she was taught that alcohol was a way to cope with a difficult world.

I don't intend to diagnose my parents or grandparents. It is rarely useful to attempt to arrive at one major "cause" of anyone's addiction—genes, environment, trauma, the trauma of everyday life. But it has helped me immensely to see their addictions at least in part as a function of their unprocessed pain. Like everyone else, they were drinking and smoking for a reason: because those substances did something for them. Sadly, their use simultaneously helped them to cope and made their problems much worse, perpetuating a vicious spiral.

This is the core of the addiction-as-dislocation theory. Beyond soothing the concrete effects of physical dislocation, people use drugs to address an alienation from cultural supports. This kind of alienation is what Émile Durkheim, the founder of modern sociology, called *anomie*: the social condition of a breakdown of norms and values, resulting in an existential lack of connection to meaning and purpose. Both this sense of dislocation *and* the actions of addiction supply industries, some scholars argue, are the core drivers of today's opioid epidemic.

In 2014, the Princeton economists Anne Case and Angus Deaton (the latter of whom won a Nobel Memorial Prize the next year) happened upon an unexpected finding: a significant uptick in the number of suicides among middle-aged white Americans. They plugged in some other numbers to put those suicides in context, and to their surprise, they found that *all* deaths among that group were rising for the first time in decades. This was a shocking reversal of a supposedly modern trend. With the onward march of progress, death rates were supposed to be falling in countries like the United States. There was no world war, no infectious disease epidemic to explain it. As they described it, at first they thought they had hit the wrong key on their computer.

Case and Deaton soon found that death rates from three causes—suicides, drug overdoses, and alcoholic liver disease—were rising rapidly, and the increases were almost all among people without a college degree. In their subsequent analyses, Case and Deaton connected these deaths to a rot at the core of today's societal structure. True, these working-class whites were suffering some concrete losses from the globalizing economy, such as worse jobs with lower wages, but beyond that, work had become far less meaningful. People no longer had a real connection to their jobs—they were less likely to belong to a union and less likely to have any stability or structure in their work. Beyond that, there were plenty more reasons for despair. Marriage rates were declining, and religious participation was falling. More people were living alone than at any time in recorded human history. All these dislocations were fatally exacerbated by the U.S.'s stark inequality—the highest income inequality of all the G7 nations—combined with what is objectively the worst-performing healthcare system in the developed world, with its bloated costs and inefficiencies holding down wages and destroying jobs. Case and Deaton labeled these deaths from suicides, drug overdoses, and alcoholic liver disease "deaths of despair." In 2017, there were more than 150,000 deaths of despair in the United States—more than half the number of U.S. combat deaths in World War II—all in one year, and many of them among people in their twenties to forties.

It is perhaps no coincidence that addiction seems endemic among intellectuals who wrote of alienation, dislocation, and existential dread—all white people of great privilege. Dostoevsky struggled with compulsive gambling. Many disillusioned modernist writers of the early twentieth century succumbed to drugs and alcohol, such as Jack London and the "Lost Generation" writers Fitzgerald and Hemingway. In a typical day, Sartre smoked two packs of cigarettes, drank a quart of alcohol, and took two hundred milligrams of amphetamines along with several grams of barbiturates—and that's not even mentioning the coffee, rich meals, and endless parade of women he used addictively. Addiction was especially common in the Beat generation, notably with Jack Kerouac and William Burroughs, but also Herbert Huncke, who appropriated the term "Beat" to mean not "cool" in a jazzy sense but wiped out and pathetic, worn down by the conservative, conformist, materialistic postwar culture.

It's crucial to note that all these white people, me and my family included, were spared from other, more direct forces of oppression and racism that have driven deaths from addiction in Black and Brown communities for decades, even centuries. Persistent health inequities by race and social class have long dwarfed the white working-class deaths of despair identified by Case and Deaton. The "deaths of despair" narrative should not enable an exclusive focus on white problems; to do so would draw a false distinction between this epidemic, populated by images of white middle-class users who are portrayed as blameless victims, and the ongoing crisis of substance-related deaths driven by structural issues such as poverty, trauma, concentrated disadvantage, and hopelessness. In reality, these crises are deeply intertwined. The point, rather, is that the psychological dislocation driving addiction is, if not equal-opportunity, at least powerful enough to reach into all corners of human society, and it is not limited to concrete, material resources.

Alexander has argued that because the fundamental cause of addiction is social wounding, the fundamental solution must be found not in some narrow medical treatment but in community healing—and specifically, a kind of community healing that resists the dominant cultural forces causing that wounding. Strikingly, Native American communities under the onslaught of colonization and alcohol repeatedly arrived at the same conclusion. The first Native American anti-alcohol movements were not much more than the prohibitionist crackdowns Occom observed, but by the late eighteenth century, many tribes realized they needed more, and several different societies developed cultural practices that used mutual-help principles to address the problem of alcohol. Neolin, a prophet in the Lenni Lenape tribe, gained a large following in the 1760s after calling for a total break from the English and a return to traditional practices. Above all, he urged his followers to "abstain from drinking their deadly *beson* [medicine], which they have forced upon us, for the sake of increasing their gains and diminishing our numbers." After a spiritual awakening helped him to overcome chronic drunkenness, a man named Papunhank, in the Munsee tribe, started a movement emphasizing cultural traditions and abstinence from alcohol. And a Seneca man named Handsome Lake developed a new movement based on total abstinence that was strikingly similar to today's twelve-step groups: it provided a set of moral teachings centered on sobriety, called on people to meet regularly in "circles," and encouraged those struggling with alcohol to share their stories in order to enlist community support and refresh their commitment to abstinence. The "Code of Handsome Lake" spread broadly through many Native communities and helped countless people stop using alcohol; it was the first mutual-help support group explicitly focused on addiction recovery in America, predating Alcoholics Anonymous by almost 150 years and surviving to this day. What distinguishes these efforts was that they were more than mutual help for addiction only; they sought to be part of a broader project of community healing, one that has arguably been absent from much of the recovery movement and only recently reemerging as a priority in some recovery advocacy.

The social wounding theory of addiction can lead to the somewhat pessimistic notion that no approach to addiction will be sufficient and that the only true remedy is a wholesale restructuring of society. This notion is well beyond the scope of what I could possibly address in this book, but I will say that there need not be such a stark division between social change and individual recovery. Individual and local recovery can be a way to disrupt the intergenerational legacies of trauma and oppression that would otherwise reproduce oppression in future generations. This is in fact a key teaching of a major contemporary Native American recovery tradition, Wellbriety, which emphasizes healing as a way to stop the cycle of inflicting pain on others.

But back in Occom's day, European culture had no mutual-help movement for addiction, not yet. When the next epidemic struck, they would make sense of it in a different way.

On November 8, 1744, the distinguished men of the Royal Society of London convened to consider a troubling new illness circulating among the lower classes. London was by far the largest city in Europe—more than half a million people crammed on top of one another, living alongside open pits of sewage and garbage rotting in the streets—and the city was regularly rocked by outbreaks of cholera, typhus, and smallpox. This, however, was a completely new and unpredictable malady, one curiously concentrated among poor women. Sensational accounts from the popular press, and now more reputable reports, seemed to finally substantiate a still-rare but fearful new threat: spontaneous combustion.

As the solemn gathering soon heard, earlier that year, a fishmonger's daughter had awoken one morning to find her mother's charred remains, looking like a "Heap of Charcoal cover'd with white Ashes." The daughter, horrified, doused the remains with two large bowls of water, raising a thick, fetid cloud of smoke. There was no other sign of fire. She seemed to have been consumed by some inner cause. The only likely culprit seemed to be the drug that the mother had binged on the night before: gin.

From the late seventeenth to the mid-eighteenth century, several accounts of people spontaneously bursting into flame captivated the English press. The victims were mostly old, mostly poor, all women, and all thoroughly alcohol-soaked—reflecting the anxieties of a society that was simultaneously confronting a set of vexing challenges: a new urban environment, an unprecedented level of class conflict, rapidly evolving gender norms, and, most notably, a rising and seemingly unstoppable deluge of distilled spirits.

England was experiencing the "Gin Craze," the first urban drug epidemic. Newly cheap, ubiquitous, and up to twice as strong as it is today, "rotgut gin" (a distilled alcohol loaded with botanicals and other flavorings to mask its revolting taste) arose to numb the pain of the working poor and to scandalize and frighten the upper classes. Consumption doubled from 1700 to 1720, then almost doubled again by 1729, then shot to more than six times the 1700 levels by 1743. The Gin Craze brought together all the various causes and conditions that had contributed to other early drug epidemics: a novel drug, an addiction supply industry, and community wounding. It was a confusing and disorienting phenomenon to live through, and it inspired the beginnings of a new perspective on addiction.

Some called for restrictions on the newly powerful distilling industries, which had been able to make spirits on the cheap because of improved technology and a drop in grain prices. (Gin, though not completely novel, was functionally a new formulation of a drug, because of how cheap and widely available it was across the whole social spectrum.) Some railed against *"geneva"*—the Anglicized name for the Dutch liquor jenever—as a foreign invader. Overall, though, the moral panic was dominated by fears about widespread drinking among the underclass—fears that were gladly stoked by the distillers to deflect attention from their products and themselves.

The distilling industry funded pamphleteers, most notably the great Daniel Defoe, author of *Robinson Crusoe,* to defend themselves. A favored tactic was to put the onus of responsibility on the bad behavior of the poor—the problem was bad drinkers, not a bad drink. Writers blamed the "poorer Sort of People" for destroying the health and strength of society with their immoderate drinking. In reality, the Gin Craze was strongly driven by growing inequality, which in turn perpetuated the craze. England was on the forefront of a massive shift toward a mercantile, proto-industrial economy, and the reigning (and explicit) ideology sought to keep "inferiors" mired in poverty so that English goods would be competitive on the new global market. The rootless poor, in search of opportunity, flocked to London, where they crowded into slums. Separated from their normal social ties and lacking financial supports, they turned to drinking as a salve for their dislocation.

Gin was also a rare source of opportunity for the urban poor. Hawkers flooded the streets and completely overwhelmed what little police force there was in impoverished districts. Retailers were everywhere. One writer in 1736 estimated that there were 120,000 outlets selling gin in England, one for every ten households, and these were not stately bars and pubs but ramshackle stalls set up in back alleys and open-air markets, in wheelbarrows and baskets. In a twist even more shocking to refined sensibilities, gin was increasingly quaffed *and* hawked by women.

The role of poor and unattached urban women in the Gin Craze greatly exacerbated the panic, so much so that gin itself was personified as feminine and called "Madam Geneva" or "Mother Gin." Women gravitated toward selling gin for understandable reasons: it required no capital or prior qualifications, and the market was hot. Shocked observers, though, saw the unholy pairing of women and gin as a sign of the decline of society: mothers who were corrupted by this new vice would also corrupt or even destroy future generations. One sensational tale from 1734 described a woman named Judith Defour who strangled her young daughter and sold her clothes, which she had just received from the parish workhouse, for gin money. Defour was the perfect emblem for the fears of the upper classes. Not only was she a bad mother and violently degraded by gin, but she was committing the eighteenth-century version of welfare fraud to boot. The tale in part inspired William Hogarth's famous 1751 engraving *Gin Lane,* which depicts a fat, ugly, syphilitic drunkard, squatting at the center of the picture and surrounded by urban decay as her baby tumbles headfirst over a handrail.

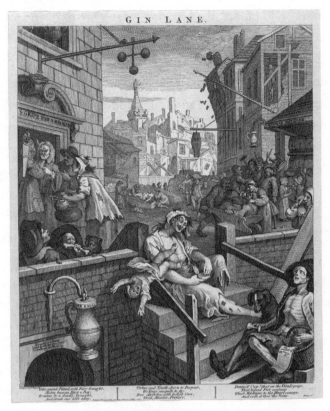

Gin Lane,
William Hogarth, 1751.

This frightful urban drug scare, fittingly, prompted a war on drugs. From the beginning, the upper class had clamored for tighter controls on the rowdy new underclass. One lord complained, "whoever shall pass among the Streets, will find Wretches stretched upon the Pavement, insensible and motionless, and only removed by the Charity of Passengers from the Danger of being crushed by Carriages or trampled by Horses." The government instituted a series of increasingly tight prohibitionist controls. Notably, the ruling class was largely composed of landowners and was hesitant to raise taxes on the commodity, so they predominantly aimed their measures at the poor, despite the fact that everyone was drinking. A 1736 act of Parliament targeted "the people of lower and inferior rank" and pushed the licensing fee to a stratospheric £50. That law also created an ill-fated policy of paying informers £5 for snitching on illegal gin shops, which backfired spectacularly, both because of people feeding junk information to the government and because of violent backlashes against informers. Drinking gin itself became an act of political protest, a symbol of opposition toward an unpopular government.

Prohibition wasn't working as planned. The question was *why?* As the panic proceeded, confused observers speculated about gin's special power over the body. Defoe—who just two years earlier had written in defense of the distillers—changed sides and railed against gin in a famous 1728 pamphlet in which he described the spirit as a contagion sweeping the city. Defoe had also written *A Journal of the Plague Year* a few years earlier, and in this light, the way he uses medical language to describe gin is striking: it "debilitates and enervates" the common people, "it curdles the blood, it stupefies the senses, it weakens the nerves," it spoils the milk of women who drink it, and it weakens the children. Amid the hopelessness and confusion, the Gin Craze began to inspire a nascent idea of addiction as a proper epidemic.

O f those doctors and scientists of the storied Royal Society, some began to describe habitual drinking as a medical problem. They called gin drinking an "infection" that "daily spreads" through the city, one unresponsive to tighter restrictions because of its physical effects. In 1734, one clergyman and scientist, Stephen Hales, published a pamphlet, *A Friendly Admonition to the Drinkers of Gin, Brandy, and Other Distilled Spirituous Liquors,* that provided a reductionist account of why the craze was out of control: spirits "extinguish the natural Warmth of the Blood," causing an insatiable thirst for more liquor. Hales argued that drunkenness became a chronic condition: "infatuated" and "inslaved" people "would go on, though they saw Hell-fire burning before them." (In a chilling foretaste of today's reports of morgues overflowing with opioid overdose bodies, Hales also described how burials were increasing "at a dreadful rate.") He worried that "the Infection is spread so far and wide" and predicted that in a few generations it would "infect the whole Kingdom with its baneful Influence."

Hales and his medical colleagues were influenced by a long line of thinkers concerned with the problem of habitual drunkenness. As early as 1576, a pamphlet titled *A Delicate Diet for Daintiemouthde Droonkardes* warned that drunkenness was a "monstrous plant, lately crepte into the pleasaunt Orchyardes of Englande." In 1606, Parliament passed an "Act for the Repressing of the Odious and Loathsom Sin of Drunkenness." Religious writers of the seventeenth century had long been describing drunkenness as a problem of "addiction": in 1609, the influential Puritan John Downame bemoaned the fates of those who "addict themselves to much drinking" and lamented how "many of our people of late, are so unmeasurably addicted to this vice." Addiction was no longer just an action one did but also a condition: people actively "addicted" themselves to something, but were also "addicted" by something else acting on them—like, of course, gin.

Medical writers during the Gin Craze drew on these developments and began using the word "addicted" to explain the impaired choice of habitual drunkenness. However, it was far from a clear formulation. The word "addicted" was usefully ambiguous and flexible. Not only was it both action and status; it also referred to both disease and sin—no one was "so far gone in the disease of drunkenness" that they could not be "cured" by "diligent and fervent prayer." Other eighteenth-century writers regularly conflated the moral and the medical, even in the same piece of writing—for example, calling habitual drinking both a form of blameless insanity and the just deserts of sinful behavior. Yet it was during the Gin Craze that the medical framing of addiction began to take shape. In short time, another thinker, working amid another epidemic, would use these ideas to portray addiction even more clearly, and enduringly, as a disease.

Three

A DISEASE IN
THE WILL

In the sweltering summer heat of 1777, with the cannon fire from the country's first Independence Day still ringing in the air, Benjamin Rush, surgeon general to the Continental Army, snuck away from Philadelphia to his wife's family farm in the country. The mood was tense throughout the young republic. More than fifteen thousand British troops were massed on ships outside New York, ready to strike at Philadelphia, at that time the nation's capital. Amid all this, Rush got to the farm just in time to see the birth of his first child, his son John.

Just a week later, the family received word that more than two hundred British ships had set sail for Philadelphia, and Rush grimly returned to his post, joining General Washington and the Continental Army. The ensuing battles were chaotic, and Rush was dismayed by the drastic shortages of medicine, food, and blankets in the hospitals. He was even more distressed by the outrageous use of alcohol, which caused his hospitals to be filled not only with the wounded and feverish but also with rowdy, drunken soldiers. Alcohol problems were rife among the fighting forces in general—on one occasion, troops drank confiscated Hessian rum and got so drunk that they fell out of their boats into the Delaware River.

Tall, attractive, ambitious, and confident, Rush had a tendency to ruffle feathers. The thirty-one-year-old physician fired off angry letters and sparred with his superiors, and he was soon made to resign because of his arrogance and combativeness. If he had proceeded more carefully, Rush might have become more of a household name, maybe even a president like his good friend John Adams. (A couple of years earlier, he had been one of the youngest to attend the Continental Congress and sign the Declaration of Independence.) Instead, he returned to Philadelphia, disgraced and dejected. The country was wracked by war, his political career was ruined, and he was unemployed, with a one-year-old son. Before long, though, Rush would create for himself a new legacy, becoming one of the most significant medical writers and teachers of the young country—and the world's first influential champion for the notion that addiction is a disease.

The first time he met Rush, John Adams reflected, "He is an elegant, ingenious Body. Sprightly, pretty fellow. . . . But Rush I think, is too much of a Talker to be a deep Thinker. Elegant not great." But Rush *was* in fact a deep thinker, schooled in the best philosophy and medicine of his day in Edinburgh, where he had met David Hume and studied with the leading figures of Enlightenment medicine. After his inauspicious dismissal in the midst of the Revolution, he won a professorship at the University of Pennsylvania's medical school and the prestigious Pennsylvania Hospital. He was also deeply optimistic and religious, which inspired him to ally with causes such as the nascent abolitionist movement, hopeful that social reform could shape the scrappy former colonies into a truly great nation. It was that reformist streak that led him to focus on what he saw as another great threat to the States: alcohol.

One day in 1784, Rush took a rare vacation through the Pennsylvania backcountry, where he was struck by the postwar poverty and social upheaval, and he worried about how it all seemed to stem from drinking: "The quantity of rye destroyed and of whisky drunk in these places is immense and its effects upon their industry, health, and morals are terrible." The country was experiencing a true alcohol epidemic. Alcohol had become a crucial commodity for the colonies, and it was rampantly produced. Cheap molasses from slave plantations in the Caribbean inundated the market, and enormously profitable distilleries were opening up and down the Eastern Seaboard to turn it into rum. Retailers competed ferociously, and the rootless American colonists, lacking one unifying culture or authority, were developing a new style of binge drinking that was creating significant disorder. The custom was so clearly harmful that the Quakers prohibited their members from selling spirits, and Benjamin Franklin compared the drunken disorder to England's Gin Craze, "for our RUM does the same Mischief in proportion, as their GENEVA."

Through his work at the Pennsylvania Hospital, Rush had come to believe that most of the mental illnesses he saw were caused by alcohol, and his backcountry trip convinced him that the problem was only getting worse. His concern with alcohol was driven in part by a simple desire to help, but also in part by a philosophical commitment connected to the very idea of Americanness itself. The Enlightenment tradition in which Rush was trained was optimistic about the force of reason and progress to tame social problems, and it put tremendous emphasis on individualism and self-control, but nowhere was that ideal of autonomy and self-determination stronger than in the young United States. This was especially so in the context of an American strain of Christianity that put special focus on willpower and demonstrating faith by works. For elite white men like Rush, who had access to that idealized freedom and autonomy, drunkenness was a threat to all they held dear in their young republic.

Upon his return, he quickly dashed off his most famous publication, *An Inquiry into the Effects of Ardent Spirits upon the Human Body and Mind*. It was an impassioned broadside against distilled alcohol and contained a new twist on anti-alcohol messaging. Not only did drunkenness cause a "temporary fit of madness," but habitual drunkenness was

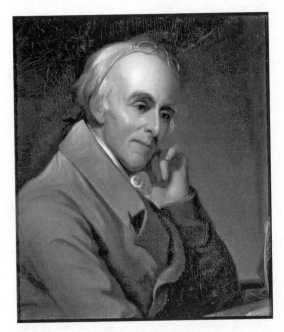

Benjamin Rush,
Charles Willson
Peale, 1818.

itself a kind of insanity. Rush described habitual drunkenness as a chronic and relapsing disease that resembled "certain hereditary, family, and contagious diseases." In other words, Rush's was the clearest statement up to that point that habitual drunkenness was a disease unto itself. As one medical historian put it, "In some ways, disease does not exist until we have agreed that it does—by perceiving, naming, and responding to it." Of Rush's many legacies—which include tireless work treating people with mental illness, a pursuit that earned him the title "Father of American Psychiatry"—his naming addiction as a disease was his most significant contribution, and one that would have an impact far beyond medicine.

What does it mean to call addiction a disease? The term is inherently slippery. By one definition, calling something a disease simply means that it is at least partially amenable to medical treatment.

This is a relatively low bar: that among all the possible approaches that might be brought to bear on the problem—legal enforcement, public health policies, mutual help—a therapeutic approach can help. But the word "disease" can also imply something much more: that a therapeutic approach is the single *best* way to address the problem, that the causes are best located in reductionist biology, or that the problem is a discrete category neatly divided from the "normal" population. None of those claims are true for addiction.

Rush, for his part, was not making any of those stronger claims. He described several medical treatments for habitual drunkenness, organized into two categories: ways to cure a fit of drunkenness (like sticking a feather down the throat to make someone vomit, or furiously whipping them, which allegedly brought blood down from the brain into the body) and ways to cure the desire for ardent spirits itself (like spiking drinks with vomit-inducing medications or "blistering the ankles," which he believed would "suspend the love of ardent spirits"). Nevertheless, he was not arguing for the sole primacy of medicine; he also contended that prayer and religion were good treatments, as was inducing guilt and shame.

Other writers were bolder about claiming medical ownership of addiction, such as the Scottish physician Thomas Trotter, who wrote a widely read essay on drunkenness in 1804. Trotter also argued that habitual drunkenness was a disease, but he explicitly asserted that doctors like him would be better suited to address drunkenness than the "priesthood" or the "moralist," who he claimed had "meant well" but missed the point when it came to the underlying problem: "The habit of drunkenness is a disease of the mind."

Trotter cheekily claimed to be the first physician to fully describe drunkenness as a disease, even though he was writing several years after Rush, and he was almost certainly aware that many other writers had preceded them both with similar arguments. Of course, it was almost a century earlier that doctors writing about the Gin Craze had begun to frame habitual drunkenness as an ongoing medical condition of impaired volition. One particularly influential English physician, George Cheyne, had also described how the habit of drinking could be progressive ("Drops beget Drams, and Drams beget more Drams . . .") and how alcohol was a "bewitching poison" that bound even the "Virtuous and the Sensible" in "Chains and Fetters." In 1724, Cheyne had published a treatise on "Nervous Diseases" that included an autobiographical section describing his own struggles with alcohol: after becoming a successful doctor, he had fallen in with "Bottle-companions" and "Free-Livers" who enticed him to "eat lustily and swallow down much Liquor." He eventually came to weigh more than four hundred pounds and suffered from a range of health problems—lethargy, fever, constipation, diarrhea, gout, shaking, vomiting, and vertigo—despite adhering to a "sober, moderate, and plain" diet (including no more than three pints of wine per day—that is, ten standard drinks). In the end, he cured himself with a diet consisting only of "milk and vegetables." Anthony Benezet, a Quaker reformer in Rush's circle, wrote an influential 1774 pamphlet, *The Mighty Destroyer Displayed*, in which he described how "unhappy dram-drinkers are so absolutely bound in slavery to these infernal spirits, that they seem to have lost the power of delivering themselves from this worst of bondage." Benezet's diagnosis was that habitual drunkenness was an enduring condition of powerlessness, and his prescription was that all people should abstain from distilled spirits entirely—a dramatic departure from the prevailing view of alcohol as healthy.

To a greater extent than ever before, though, Rush emphasized and elaborated on the disease status of drunkenness: it was an "odious disease," one that expressed itself in a "numerous train of diseases and vices of the body and mind." Rush put medicine at the center of his analysis not to claim ownership, but merely to call attention to what he saw as a long-neglected and potentially fatal malady.

One of my first patients in my internal medicine rotation during medical school was a rail-thin man with heroin addiction who had an enormous, crusted tumor sticking out more than half a foot from his jaw. He had tried to get a little nodule on his tongue checked out a few months earlier, but the clinic doctors didn't have a lot of patience for his drug use and "noncompliance," and he quickly fell out of care. By the time I met him, his tumor was the size of a small watermelon and bursting through his skin. He had no hope for recovery; his family had brought him to the hospital to die.

I was in the middle of the third year of medical school—the dreaded "clinical year," when students rotate through different specialties in the medical center as part of the teams directly caring for patients—and it was wearing on me. That man seemed to embody everything wrong with modern medicine: not our inability to cure the cancer, but how easily patients could be left by the wayside. The churn of the system was demoralizing. We'd patch up acute conditions and dump people back into nursing homes or even onto the streets, with little opportunity for working with the human problems so often at the root of unhealthy behavior. As the winter rolled on, I got tired of waking up at 4 a.m. just to tackle checklists of tasks that didn't seem to be helping anyone.

I started drinking more—much more. I started crying unexpectedly. After taking an online quiz that said I was severely depressed, I met with a bushy-bearded psychoanalyst in a cramped cinder-block office at the medical center, though at first I hid the extent of my distress behind safe, professional language, claiming I was there because I wanted to develop as a future psychiatrist and learn about myself. He was gentle and kind, and eventually I opened up about the drinking and my general sense of malaise. We spun theories about the root of my suffering: My drives were in conflict. After growing up with alcoholic parents, I was struggling to parent myself. The drinking was an attempt to manage existential fears, trying to annihilate time so I wouldn't have to die. (In the words attributed to psychoanalyst Otto Rank, which I copied into my journal: "Refusing the loan of life in order to avoid the debt of death.")

After limping through the year of clinical rotations, I spent an extra year completing a research fellowship in brain stimulation. Having done research in genetics as an undergrad, I hungered for the flexibility and anarchic hustle of laboratory work after the hierarchical, buttoned-up year of clinical practice. I was also genuinely fascinated by the prospect of using new technologies in powerful magnetic stimulation and brain surgery to directly alter people's thoughts and feelings. I loved the lab itself: the antique dentist's chair someone had seemingly pulled out of a dump for our transcranial magnetic stimulation "rig," getting to try it myself, the huge figure-eight electrical wire pressed against the side of my skull, the tingling shock as it stimulated my motor cortex to make my finger jump. It all represented tremendous possibility: the chance to precisely target an aberrant brain circuit and tone down someone's OCD or severe depression, a tangible and specific intervention seemingly light-years beyond the blunt instrument of psychiatric medications, with all their side effects.

It takes a special kind of desperation, or perhaps faith, to volunteer for these types of futuristic experiments. For a trial of deep brain stimulation (DBS) surgery for depression—one that implants a sort of pacemaker in the chest, runs a wire under the skin up to the skull, and drills a thin electrode down into the center of the brain—some people were calling and asking to get the surgery for relatively mild depressions. They didn't qualify for the trial, of course—the inclusion criteria required very severe, intractable depression and multiple unsuccessful attempts at other treatments—but their interest stood out to me, and I was amazed at how much blind trust some people put in the promise of reducing psychiatry to neurobiology alone.

Even during the comparatively relaxed research year, my drinking got progressively worse. I set countless limits for myself, then immediately violated them. After telling myself I wouldn't drink at a scientific conference in Miami, I passed out against a palm tree, then puked in a cab. I wondered if I was an alcoholic, but I quickly dismissed the possibility.

I had gone to an AA meeting as a med student—we were all required to go as an educational exercise—and it seemed clear that I wasn't like those people, or my parents. My problem, I thought, was more sophisticated, something more complex and existential than a "disease" like alcoholism or a psychiatric disorder like suicidal depression or debilitating OCD. Patients facing those conditions were the ones really suffering; they were the ones who needed treatment. I just needed to grow up.

And yet, as the consequences mounted, I started to believe that I might have a problem. My psychiatrist fired me as a patient because of all the sessions I missed, and I poured a full bottle of gin down the sink and swore to myself that I'd really cut down this time. I didn't realize then, but I do now, that I was doing the same thing I had tried with my parents once I got old enough to recognize just how bad their drinking was: searching the house for cached bottles and demonstratively pouring them out in front of them. It worked just as well.

In July 1793, a flood of European settlers from the Caribbean arrived in Philadelphia, fleeing slave revolts and epidemic disease. By the end of the month, the first cases of a severe strain of yellow fever had spread, and fear shot through the nation's capital. The people who could leave did so, and the surrounding communities barricaded bridges and roads to divert refugees. In the end, an estimated 9 percent of the population died, and as much as half the total population fled. Rush stayed.

By this point, Rush was a leading figure in the Philadelphia medical community, and he turned his home into a makeshift clinic staffed by five of his students (three of whom died in the epidemic). He personally saw as many as a hundred patients in a day, giving them enormous doses of laxatives and subjecting them to copious bloodletting. He called it "depletion therapy"—also known as "heroic medicine"—and it was a popular approach of the time, intended to calm the excited blood vessels and relieve the fevers and headache that marked yellow fever. Rush thought that as much as 80 percent of a person's blood could be removed; in time, so much blood was spilled on his front lawn that it stank and perpetually buzzed with flies.

Rush was, and continues to be, rightly criticized for this "heroic" treatment. His efforts during the yellow fever epidemic undoubtedly killed hundreds of Pennsylvanians, and, even worse, another kind of overconfidence in racist science doomed hundreds of Black people to death. Rush claimed that Black people were immune to yellow fever and encouraged Black workers to care for the sick, so, during a massive shortage of healthcare workers, Black nurses worked around the clock caring for delirious patients vomiting blood; scores of those nurses died as a result. (For that matter, Rush believed that the dark pigmentation of Black skin was itself a disease—the effect of leprosy—and though he was an abolitionist, he owned a slave.)

Rush had been led astray by reductionism, a theme I identify throughout this book, though not always to criticize it. A reductionist approach is not necessarily problematic, as many scientific challenges need to be unpacked by examining lower levels of organization— studying viral genetics to develop vaccines, for example. But frequently throughout the history of medicine, and especially the history of addiction, overly simplistic attempts to reduce complex phenomena have often misled more than they have helped.

Rush was not all that reductionist in his thinking about addiction, as he took a relatively balanced and humble perspective on the role of medicine to explain it. Future thinkers, however, used his disease idea to promote a myriad of useless and often harmful "cures." The more complicated and difficult the malady, the more fertile the ground for grandiose and outsize claims, and the addiction treatment field is no exception, where unending processions of would-be heroes have proposed endless, bizarre treatments founded on overconfident, reductionist theories.

Though it's a crowded field, Leslie Keeley, a late-nineteenth-century addiction entrepreneur, probably takes first prize. He was certainly first among the "cure doctors," the nontraditional practitioners of his day who promised a kaleidoscopic range of nostrums, powders, and bottled cures for just about anything under the sun—such as the White Star Secret Liquor Cure (ninety-four cents for a box of thirty cocaine capsules) and the Hay-Litchfield Antidote, which promised to eliminate the appetite for drink with a noxious brew of ingredients including beef gall, eel skin, codfish, milk, cow's urine, and alcohol. After the Civil War, Keeley announced that he had discovered a "bi-chloride of gold" cure for addiction, but he refused to reveal the composition of his medicine. He opened a massively successful series of treatment institutes, where his solution was injected (through a red, white, and blue syringe!). He crowed that his proprietary technology not only detoxified people from their addictions but also "liberate[d] the will" and served "to give the opium user will power." His company made millions of dollars, more than 500,000 people with addiction took his cure between 1880 and 1920, and his name became known to all, with massive billboards and wall-size signs in every modern city.

A key component of Keeley's marketing genius was his use of the notion of disease to sell his product. He declared, simply, "Drunkenness is a disease and I can cure it." The corollary seems simple; obvious, even. This pattern of using an exclusively scientific explanation to sell treatment has repeated itself incessantly. Until recently, one of the fanciest rehabs on the "Rehab Riviera," in Malibu, California, notoriously promised an "Alcoholism and Addiction Cure," advertising cure rates as high as 60 percent after its thirty-day program, available for $112,000.

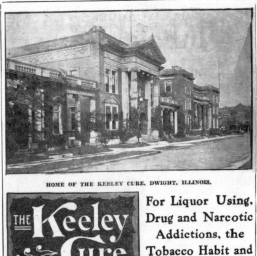

HOME OF THE KEELEY CURE, DWIGHT, ILLINOIS.

THE Keeley Cure

For Liquor Using, Drug and Narcotic Addictions, the Tobacco Habit and Neurasthenia

successfully and continuously administered for more than thirty years.

All correspondence confidential. Printed matter sent on request in plain, sealed envelopes. Address

THE KEELEY INSTITUTE, DWIGHT, ILL.

Advertisement for "The Keeley Cure," a popular late-nineteenth-century "miracle cure."

Though he clearly looks like a quack today, much of Keeley's language about disease sounds surprisingly modern: "The physiological action of opium is to diminish the natural forces of the nervous system." If the drug use is continued for long, it changes the "structure of the nerve and its action" to cause the disease of "morphinism," or morphine addiction. This, too, is a theme that has recurred over a striking length of time: in framing the problem as one originating in the nervous system, Keeley sounded like he was describing a brain disease.

Addiction Is a Brain Disease, and It Matters." Published in 1997 by Alan Leshner, director of the National Institute on Drug Abuse, the provocative and influential editorial was neuroscience's rallying cry to the problem of addiction. Leshner argued that two decades of studies, from meticulous molecular characterizations of neurotransmitters and receptors to the relatively new science of brain imaging, had established that the brains of addicted people were different from those of others. A single common neurobiological pathway was disordered in all cases of drug addiction. Not only that, but chronic use changed the brain itself. (Leshner assiduously avoided the term "brain damage," opting instead for the less charged "long-lasting brain changes.") The science was settled, he maintained, but policymakers and the public hadn't yet grasped that fact, and researchers needed to spread the word—not just to muster more funding but also to combat stigma. The brain disease model of addiction, he predicted, would present a new, compassionate alternative to the reigning models of addiction: calling people either victims of their environments or weak and immoral.

Leshner's editorial was a resounding success. It has been cited by other researchers more than two thousand times, a staggering number by any criterion. The brain disease idea helped to get congressional funding for addiction research. Today, the idea of addiction as a brain disease is taught everywhere, from treatment settings to professional schools. I heard lectures on the model both at medical school as a student and in rehab as a patient.

Yet almost from the beginning, the brain disease idea has also been the subject of intense debate. Its detractors worry that it prioritizes the brain over all the psychological, social, and political issues that matter so much to addiction. In 2014, ninety-four scholars from diverse fields wrote a blistering critique published in the journal *Nature*; signatories included not just social scientists but also major biomedical researchers, including Carl Hart and Jerome Jaffe, Richard Nixon's first drug czar. The letter called it "myopic" to present addiction as a brain malfunction and warned that such a framework trivializes the broader human context.

The "brain disease model of addiction" can mean different things. The most modest claims are reasonable, bordering on uninteresting: neuroscience can help us to understand addiction, including ways of helping with medical treatments, but it is not necessarily the only way to understand the problem. Leshner offered the caveat that "addiction is not just a brain disease," and said it is also necessary to investigate the social components of addiction. But ultimately, he made a stronger claim and put the brain first: in his conception, addiction is "fundamentally" a brain disease, it "results" from the effects of drugs on the brain, and "the brain is the core of the problem." The concept was taken up in the American Society of Addiction Medicine's own definition of "addiction," as "a *primary*, chronic disease of brain reward, motivation, memory and related circuitry."

Scholars in Benjamin Rush's day were occupied with similar debates about the physical causation of mental illness. Rush had trained at the University of Edinburgh, at the time both the leading medical school in the world and the epicenter of a particular take on the mind-body problem. Following the philosopher John Locke, most scholars there believed that the human mind was a tabula rasa, a blank slate, and that therefore everything that a person was—his character, knowledge, morality, and very sense of self—relied on sensory stimuli from the outside world. Medical thinkers in the Edinburgh school therefore prioritized mind over body: as Locke wrote, "Madness seems to be nothing but a disorder in the imagination." Similarly, Thomas Trotter insisted that because drunkenness was a disease of the mind, the proper treatment was not physical cures but rather mental treatments that sound almost like today's psychotherapy: gaining patients' confidence and helping them to unlearn their habits. Philippe Pinel, a contemporaneous pioneer in promoting more humane treatment for mental illness, also stressed mental treatments—such as kindness and meaningful recreation—over physical ones, like medications and the often brutal physical manipulations used in those days, such as sensory deprivation and physical restraints.

Over Rush's lifetime, though, medical thinking increasingly turned toward a more physically oriented view. The medical world's center of gravity was shifting from Edinburgh to Paris, where the French Revolution moved the control of the hospitals from the church to physicians.

New techniques of bedside examination and autopsy opened a new world of physical evidence, visualizing in stunning detail exactly how the body worked. This next generation of clinical scientists, themselves infused with revolutionary spirit and skeptical of authority, put "bodies before books" and demanded physical correlates to all diseases, including mental ones.

Biologically inspired scholars of the time argued that because mental problems were ultimately rooted in physical causes, they should be understood and treated at the physical level. For example, in 1819, a German physician living in Moscow, Carl von Brühl-Cramer, proposed the disease of *"Trunksucht"* ("drink obsession" or "drink thirst," but often translated into English as "dipsomania"). Brühl-Cramer saw how Napoleon's 1812 invasion of Russia had left deep scars on the Muscovite psyche and seemingly caused a spike in alcohol problems. (Alcohol, incidentally, had been used as a weapon: as the French advanced, the Moscow governor withdrew the fire pumps and used the city's copious vodka supplies like firebombs, setting storehouses and boats loaded with alcohol aflame and burning three-quarters of the city to the ground.) Yet while Brühl-Cramer noted that drinking problems were associated with social stresses like Napoleon's invasion, he insisted that dipsomania was fundamentally a biological problem and therefore should be treated physically—for example, with bitter herbs, iron, and diluted acids. Following the quantifiable and precise ideals of biological medicine, Brühl-Cramer painstakingly described a variety of different subtypes of dipsomania and claimed to have uncovered their underlying medical laws.

The error in this reasoning is that the nature of causes should not necessarily dictate the nature of remedies. Writers of the time recognized this; the French physician Jean-Étienne-Dominique Esquirol, one of Pinel's pupils, argued that even if all psychiatric disorders could be traced to biological causes, physicians could still help the most by focusing on social triggers and psychological treatments. Rush himself was an enthusiast for extreme physical treatments like cold-water plunges and his particular favorite, copious bloodletting, but he used mental treatments too, because, after all, mental treatments indirectly healed the body through their effects on the mind. Today's critics of the brain disease model would take that argument a step further and say that the mind-body dualism underlying these debates is untenable. If you accept that the mind is what the brain does, the division is meaningless, and it is misleading to try to reduce a complex phenomenon such as mental distress to a single "fundamental" cause. To say that a brain region or activity "underlies" a mental experience, for example, only substitutes one level of explanation for another, rather than explaining how one gives rise to the other.

Reductionism can be helpful. I have a good friend who is an art conservator. She works with lasers and chemicals to restore old tapestries and sculptures, so she needs to think about art as molecules. Still, no one would claim that this is the best level for people to understand art. Likewise, reductionist neuroscience has its uses for understanding addiction. Neuroscience can help to clarify important questions: What are the different factors that push someone toward addiction? Are there different kinds of addiction? How and why do some get better but not others? Research can help to develop new medications or determine where to put surgical electrodes. But calling addiction *primarily* a brain disease goes too far. It is a setup for that old, recurrent problem: an attachment to a single scientific explanatory model that cannot possibly explain the essence of a complex system. Neuroscience is not the only way to describe addiction, and it is hardly ever the best way. I suspect that even the most dyed-in-the-wool scientists don't actually mean to argue that it is, but the implication is there, and it does have consequences.

While classifying addiction as a brain disease has helped to get research funded, some scholars have documented a long and worrying drift of U.S. federal research on alcohol and drugs toward reductionist biological research and away from social, epidemiological, clinical, and policy investigations. What's more, a reductionist framing may not actually reduce the stigma attached to addiction. Some studies have found that biological explanations for mental disorders reduce self-stigma and blame, but others have found that biological framings promote the belief that psychotherapies are ineffective. Overall, the largest and most rigorous studies of this kind show that biological explanations increase aversion and pessimism toward people with psychological problems, and that they feed into the stereotype that people with mental disorders are especially dangerous.

By this point, the term "brain disease" is so overused and ideologically freighted that it has become misleading, if not entirely meaningless. Perhaps its greatest harm is that it reinforces the false dichotomy between choice and compulsion. For example, Leshner claimed that a "switch is thrown" as a result of prolonged drug use, making addiction involuntary and compulsive. His successor at the National Institute on Drug Abuse, Nora Volkow, has put it in stronger language, saying that the "brain [of an addicted person] is no longer able to produce something needed for our functioning and that healthy people take for granted, *free will*." All the vagaries of human action and volition cannot be simplified to such a binary—perhaps this is why the stigma research suggests that the brain disease narrative erodes hope. Even the reductionist Brühl-Cramer stopped short of saying that dipsomania obliterated people's power for voluntary action—as opposed to struggling with a difficult impulse. Likewise, Rush refused to say that mental illness completely eradicated free will. "How far the persons whose diseases have been mentioned, should be considered as responsible to human or divine laws for their actions, and where the line should be drawn that divides free agency from necessity, and vice from disease, I am unable to determine."

By 1809, Rush's prodigious energy was flagging, and his family life dealt him a serious blow. Several years after his good friend John

Adams lost his son, who had struggled for years with habitual drunkenness, Rush received word that his own eldest son, John, was starting to lose his grip on reality.

John had always been different: brilliant but impulsive, given to fits of anger and recklessness. He worried his parents enough that when he went off to Princeton, his protective father didn't allow him to live in the dorms. Unlike his brothers, who seemed cast from the mold of their serious father, John had flitted between different professions, eventually landing in the Navy. No one would have called him mentally ill in those days, but Rush and his wife urged him to stay sober and be careful about his difficulties with self-control.

Now John was stationed on the other side of the country in New Orleans, where, in the context of heavy drinking, he had been derelict in his duties: the son of an abolitionist, he had commanded a boat that fired muskets on slaves along the riverbank. He became manic and attempted to take his own life with a gruesome razor slash to the neck. He would have been called dual diagnosis today—the term for people with addiction plus another mental disorder, which is a population that still suffers from a relatively poorer prognosis. In those days, the treatment options were profoundly limited. The Navy doctors thought they had no choice but to send him back to his father, the eminent Dr. Rush of the University of Pennsylvania's medical school. As they wrote to him, "Your acquaintance with the 'anatomy of the human mind' will enable you to do more for him than any man on earth could."

When John finally walked through the threshold of their Philadelphia home, Rush was horrified at his son's long, matted hair and clawlike nails. Hoping that he could coax him back into some semblance of sanity, he kept John at home for three days, trying desperately to connect with him, but John wouldn't even let them clean him up. Rush, defeated, admitted his son to his own mental hospital. He wrote ruefully to Adams, "It is possible he may recover, but it is too probable he will end his days in his present situation." To Thomas Jefferson, he was blunter: "He is now in a cell in the Pennsylvania Hospital . . . where there is too much reason to believe he will end his days."

This gloomy outlook reflected Rush's world-weary cynicism about treating mental disorders in general. After decades of working at the University of Pennsylvania in a specialized wing for insanity that he himself had helped to build, he was no longer as confident as he was in his younger days. In particular, he was far less hopeful about the prospects for a therapeutic approach to habitual drunkenness. In 1812, he assembled his psychiatric magnum opus, *Medical Inquiries and Observations, Upon the Diseases of the Mind*, in which he noted how habitual drunkards, suffering from a "disease in the will," often become "irreclaimable," even when they seemed to have it all: neither family, friendships, reputation, work, nor "religion and the love of life" could protect them. He described the case of one habitual drunkard who, when urged to quit, said, "Were a keg of rum in one corner of a room, and were a cannon constantly discharging balls between me and it, I could not refrain from passing before that cannon, in order to get at the rum."

Other medical thinkers were increasingly skeptical of Rush's notion that habitual drunkenness was a disease at all. They were interested in phenomena like delirium tremens—the condition of severe alcohol withdrawal marked by seizures, hallucinations, paranoia, and death—but less so in the psychological features of habitual drunkenness, and many doctors doubted whether habitual drunkenness belonged in the medical field in the first place. Just a few decades later, a successful Swedish physician named Magnus Huss wrote the first treatise on a disease he termed *Alcoholismus Chronicus*, giving birth to the word "alcoholism," but only in the sense of a physical and mechanistic description. Huss saw chronic alcoholism as nothing more than the tangible consequences of habitual drinking (such as organ failure), and the idea of habitual drunkenness as a disease of the mind fell completely out of favor in the medical world.

Rush, toward the end of his life, had also become pessimistic about the potential for social reform to overcome the country's alcohol epidemic. He yearned for prohibition but suspected it would fail. In a letter to Adams, he wrote of an elaborate dream in which he was president and banned all liquor, but the people rose up in protest and he was booted from office, back to his "professor's chair." In the dream, one of his councilors explained that men everywhere would reject the "empire of Reason" and instead "yield a willing, and in some instances involuntary, submission" to the "empire of Habit."

Rush had devoted his life to treating mental illness and, along with others like Trotter and Hales, had made a valiant effort to force the medical field to take addiction seriously. As he weakened toward the end of his life, exhausted from years of a taxing schedule and what was likely chronic tuberculosis, he thought he had failed. His son was confined in Pennsylvania Hospital's locked wing for the insane, and after Benjamin Rush died in 1813, John spent most of his remaining twenty-four years pacing back and forth, muttering to himself, wearing a deep gutter into the floors that came to be called "Rush's walk." And yet, as the elder Rush lay dying, a movement was already afoot that would adopt his ideas and change the world.

PART TWO

THE AGE OF INTEMPERANCE

Four

POSSESSION

A medical student and I were crammed into a closet-size, curtained-off square of the emergency room, talking with our new admission, a fifty-five-year-old construction worker who was still a little loopy on sedatives. Jackson had been remodeling his apartment with his teenage son when he fell to the floor in a full-body, two-minute-long seizure. In monosyllables, he told us that he had been drinking at least two six-packs a day, but though he was fully alert, we couldn't seem to get any further than that. We had already gleaned from his medical record that this was just the latest in a long history of alcohol problems. For five years, Jackson had been swinging between the poles of constant intoxication and the total bodily revolt of alcohol withdrawal.

After taking a brief history, I showed the medical student how to measure the size of the liver by tapping on Jackson's right abdomen, our fingertips easily sounding the borders of the swollen organ: his liver was double the normal size, and his blood, as the labs soon showed, was flooded with abnormally elevated enzymes leaking from his damaged liver cells.

We stepped outside the exam area to meet with his son, who, stoic and prematurely jaded, filled us in on the rest of the history. The last time his father was admitted to the hospital, he had started drinking again as soon as he was discharged. Their family didn't know what to do. His father was a calm, kind, good man. That morning, they had joked as they passed tools to each other, working steadily side by side. But other times it seemed as though someone else took over. Most nights he was angry and unpredictable, when he wasn't completely unconscious. If he didn't agree to go to rehab, they weren't sure they could take him back. They simply didn't know who would be coming home to them.

It was a Saturday evening in October, and I was a resident physician— it was well into my intern year, the grueling first year of hospital-based training after medical school. I was on a q3 rotation, meaning every third night I took a twenty-four-hour shift, covered the other interns' patients, and admitted new people to the hospital. The pace and routine were crushing. The pockets of my long white coat were stuffed with little reference books, a few medical tools, and, most importantly, the sign-out lists, scribbled with marginalia and on-the-fly notes about the forty human lives for which I was responsible. We were on the infectious disease service, which, aside from a few serious flu and tuberculosis cases, was largely the de facto medical home for patients with more complicated social problems. The vast majority of our cases—on this service and on all internal medicine services, really—seemed to be plagued with substance problems, alcohol chief among them.

There were people projectile vomiting bright red blood from violent esophageal tears. Others were shaking and delirious with unstable alcohol withdrawal. In one gruesome case, a huge alcohol binge had dealt the patient's pancreas such a powerful blow that his digestive enzymes spilled out into the abdominal cavity, literally eating through his internal organs and turning the fat around his intestines into soap. And though I wasn't talking with anyone about it, every time I cared for one of those folks, I felt a twinge in my gut—more precisely, under my lower right ribs, where my own liver was.

I knew my own alcohol intake had shot way into the unhealthy range. Some mornings, I imagined that I could feel my own swollen and aching liver. One slow afternoon while on call, I asked my supervising resident to draw my blood for liver function tests. I could tell she thought it was odd, and I tried to play it off as a joke, but I secretly wondered if I was doing real harm. When the labs came back showing only some minor, transient liver damage, I was relieved, but also a little disappointed, because I knew it wasn't enough to make me change. I wondered what would be enough.

I no longer considered getting real help from a therapist or anyone else. Instead, I got Adderall. I found a primary care doctor and told him that I needed more energy to write; he shrugged and wrote me a prescription, cautioning me that it was an off-label use. I also started smoking weed more regularly. I didn't use either drug very often, but when I did, I used them primarily to counteract the negative effects of drinking, the habit that was actually worrying me.

My eye twitched if I went too long between drinks. Even on nights I didn't want to drink, I joylessly downed a few shots of whiskey to put my body to sleep. More and more often, I was waking up late, panicked and hungover on the couch, not remembering how I got there. Huge swaths of time were disappearing: one moment I'd be drinking at the bar or at home, and the next it was half a day later.

The fear, shame, and strategizing were exhausting. I had to devote a huge portion of my brain to keeping track of the various consequences and complications of my addiction—not just my excuses for the missed shifts and sick days, when I slept through my alarm and pager, but managing my body's increasing need for ethanol, too.

One night, at a panel discussion hosted by one of my faculty advisers at a gorgeous apartment overlooking Central Park, I felt my heart start to pound. I was light-headed and sweaty. I glanced at my hands and saw a subtle tremor. I imagined having a seizure, there, in front of all my colleagues, being taken to the ER, the attending physician ordering a urine toxicology screen and finding the amphetamines and weed in my system. I'd be put on probation or, worse, forced to stop using. I was terrified, trapped. In the middle of the talk, I awkwardly stood up and shuffled over to the bar to refill my laughably small plastic cup of wine. I filled and refilled it for the rest of the night, trying to pace myself, fearfully studying the others' faces to see if they noticed.

In the weeks after that scare, I tracked my own drinking to try to regain control. I set moderation goals for myself, then blew right through them. The next morning, I'd look back amazed, wondering at how it had happened yet again. I told a friend from medical school that I had a "burgeoning addiction," and she responded compassionately but also admitted that she herself felt stranded in intern year, hating it all and thinking of leaving medicine entirely. We commiserated for a while, and I felt heard and understood, but also like there was no escape for any of us. It was as though we were two shipwreck survivors on separate life rafts, drifting together but not yet in sight of shore, nothing to offer each other. I told her that I would make a real try at cutting down this time. Later that night, I fixed myself a huge manhattan, and because I made it with top-shelf rye and vermouth, and because it was delicious, and because I told myself I needed it to get to sleep, I decided that it was okay.

Within days, I went out drinking, and I blacked out again. I felt stuck, trapped, possessed. There was plenty of fear, but there was also a blithe indifference, as though I were looking out through glass on the accumulating wreckage of someone else's life. It was like I was becoming a different person.

In the twelfth century, during the Song dynasty, a scholar named Zhang Bin felt that his drinking was getting out of hand. Every night, he stashed several liters of liquor beside his bed to stave off withdrawal. One night, after blacking out, he forgot where he put his drinks, and he woke up, tremulous and panicked, before vomiting up a little piece of meat. It was yellow and smooth, almost like a piece of liver, but it was quivering oddly on the floor—as he described it, like a "bee's nest." He tried soaking the meat-thing in alcohol, and it made a satisfied little sound. Disgusted, he threw it in the flame, where it sputtered and burned away. He never drank again.

Is addiction part of me, or is it something apart from the self? Addiction is often personified as an opponent: inside the body yet still apart from someone's "true nature," like an alien spirit or demon. In rehab, I was taught that my disease was a malevolent force doing push-ups in the basement of my mind, that it was a sleeping tiger I had to be careful not to wake by dabbling with any mind-altering substance. Mexican American heroin users in Southern California speak of the *tecato gusano*," an indestructible junkie worm living in their guts and forever threatening a relapse. Many brain researchers locate the "other" elsewhere: a "midbrain mutiny" where the warped and unnaturally powerful brain circuits of addiction rise up to overcome rational efforts at cognitive control.

This language has less to do with medicine than with mythology: internal conflict between the true self and a corrupt invader, a fight over good and evil, addiction as possession. These possession stories render both drugs and addiction the enemy; they often rely on the idea that drugs have an inherent power to cause progressive and inescapable ruin. It is a powerful image of addiction present across cultures and times. One particularly influential form emerged out of the impassioned religious tradition of the young United States, during the earliest days of the nineteenth-century temperance movement, its champion an influential preacher named Lyman Beecher.

Stern and serious, Beecher was a zealous believer even for an era of zealous belief. The descendant of a long line of blacksmiths, Beecher studied divinity at Yale at the close of the eighteenth century, during the early years of the Second Great Awakening, a massive wave of religious activity sweeping the country. The Second Great Awakening was a fervent rebellion against religious formalism characterized by a simpler, more democratic folk religion. It was a populist, grassroots movement that promised not only to save individual souls but also to reform society. In 1798, after graduating from Yale, Beecher took his first assignment as a preacher at the Presbyterian Church of East Hampton, at the eastern end of Long Island, where he cultivated his own reformist inclinations.

At that time, East Hampton was little more than a small collection of farming villages, with the main road no more than two ruts through green turf. Once a week, the local townspeople would come by wagon to church, and once a week a small schooner ran to New York to buy provisions (there was not a single store in town). It was a simple, agrarian existence, the kind idealized by many in those early days of the young nation. But Beecher, who had read English anti-vice tracts, imagined something darker: a community beset by skepticism and sin, with him doing battle for their souls. Significantly, he read Benjamin Rush's *Inquiry*, which catalyzed his most significant inspiration.

That part of Long Island was also home to the Montauk people, and Beecher was alarmed by how one local settler used liquor to entice them into dependence. The town "grog-seller," himself a notorious drinker, would get the Montauks drunk on whiskey and rum, then buy up all their corn. One bitter winter, as icy winds blasted their seaside community, Beecher watched as the Montauks trekked twenty miles just to buy back their own crops, going deeply into debt to avoid starvation. The moment stuck in Beecher's mind for the rest of his life. As he recounted much later to his daughter Harriet Beecher Stowe (author of *Uncle Tom's Cabin*), "it was horrible—horrible! It burned and burned in my mind, and I swore a deep oath to God that it shouldn't be so." That night, he went home and drafted a sermon against alcohol, one that he would write and rewrite over the coming decades.

Beecher was horrified at how alcohol was used as a weapon against Native Americans, but he also saw in their example the extent to which all of society was afflicted by alcohol. The epidemic first noted by Occom, Rush, and Benezet was in full swing. Americans drank morning, noon, and night, on stagecoaches and steamboats, from farms to manors to factories. They drank alcohol, not coffee, to wake up before work—then for the "elevens" (at 11:00 a.m.), then again in mid-afternoon, before dinner, and so forth—not to mention at meals themselves, as water was thought to be unhealthy. By the 1820s, drinking had reached its all-time high: the average American drank around seven gallons of *pure* alcohol a year, well more than five standard drinks daily for everyone aged fifteen or older—almost three times the average today.* And it wasn't just the overall volumes but also the patterns of drinking that were out of control. Group and solo binges increased in the decades after independence, leading to widespread alarm about public disorder. John Adams worried that Americans exceeded all other nations in "this degrading, beastly vice of intemperance." Foreign visitors agreed, from English reformers deploring the extent of intemperance to a Swedish visitor who reported a "general addiction to hard drinking."

Beecher returned home to Connecticut in 1810 with the conviction that something had to be done. He joined a church committee and urged his brethren to get involved in the burgeoning anti-alcohol movement, increasingly known as a movement for temperance.

The word "temperance" has an odd history. That American crusaders took the word and shaped it into a militant, almost fanatical movement for total abstinence—one so powerful that it spread outward to captivate huge swaths of the globe—is one of the great linguistic ironies of our time. Aristotle and Plato defined temperance as moderation, equilibrium, or harmony. Christian thinkers like Augustine and

---

* Women and enslaved Americans drank far less than average, so the actual numbers for regular drinkers were almost certainly much higher.

Aquinas listed it as one of the four cardinal virtues. The Jews and the early Christians mostly had no problem with alcohol. Like the Stoics, Saint Paul condemned drunkenness, but wine, as a creation of God, was inherently good and perfectly appropriate for moderate—or temperate— drinking. As factions jockeyed for power in the early days of the Christian church, some small sects called for abstinence, but the mainstream church responded by insisting that not only was drinking acceptable, but it was heresy to despise alcohol. Only excessive use was a sin.

Likewise, the Puritans of the American colonial period, such as Increase Mather, had preached against drunkenness as a sin, but generally they had hailed alcohol as the "good creature of God"—in any talk of sin, the focus was on the person and their behavior. The next generation of religious thinkers, such as the preacher and theologian Jonathan Edwards, rejected the idea that alcohol was some sort of irresistible force. In his work *The Freedom of the Will*, Edwards instead attributed excessive drinking to a "Moral Inability" in the will.

Like these predecessors, Beecher and other early leaders of the temperance movement in the 1810s were only arguing for moderation, not yet total abstinence. Even with that modest goal, Beecher had to work mightily to convince the other leaders in his own church, the Connecticut Congregationalists, who had formed a committee to investigate whether to join the temperance cause. The committee initially decided that the cause was hopeless and declined to get involved, but Beecher, incensed, gave impassioned speeches about the church's duty to reform drunkards, working all night by candlelight to compose his arguments.

While Beecher was haranguing his congregation, a broader movement was afoot. Shortly before he died, in 1813, Benjamin Rush gave an address on temperance to an important meeting of church leaders in Philadelphia, and it was almost as if the doctor was passing the torch from medicine to religion, just as a religious revival was gathering in strength and influence. The Second Great Awakening was dawning— between 1776 and 1845, the estimated number of preachers per person in the country tripled. Aided by that energy, small temperance societies were springing up around the Northeast, eagerly quoting Rush on the dangers of spirits to warn against the disease of drunkenness.

By the 1820s, Beecher had become massively influential as one of the foremost preachers of the day, drawing huge crowds at revivals across the region. He sensed that the nation was finally ready for his message, and he pulled out that lecture he had written in East Hampton all those years ago, a lecture that he had been polishing for decades.

Around 1826, Beecher delivered *Six Sermons on the Nature, Occasions, Signs, Evils, and Remedy of Intemperance,* which, upon their publication, became an instant hit and a major milestone in the temperance movement. While at one time he had advocated for moderation, now his simple and radical prescription was complete and total abstinence from liquor. (Of note, distilled spirits were thought to be uniquely dangerous, unlike beer, wine, or cider, a division that collapsed later during the temperance movement.)

To Beecher, alcohol was simply too dangerous to use in any quantity; it had to be exorcised entirely from the social body. In his sermons, he described how alcohol eroded your very ability to perceive the danger until it was too late. Intemperance began with "smiling deceptions" but ended with an irresistible "serpent-bite." Alcohol was unsafe in any quantity; people might speak about the prudent or moderate use of spirits, but Beecher said we might as well speak of "vipers and serpents introduced prudently into our dwellings, to glide about as a matter of courtesy to visitors, and of amusement to our children." Alcohol was the vicious enemy strangling the country and cutting down entire branches of family trees. Imagine, Beecher said, if a snake were to coil around your child, "wreath about his body his cold, elastic folds—tightening with every yielding breath his deadly gripe, how would his cries pierce your soul—and his strained eye-balls, and convulsive agonies, and imploring hands, add wings to your feet, and supernatural strength to your arms!" Yet, "You can only look on while bone after bone of your child is

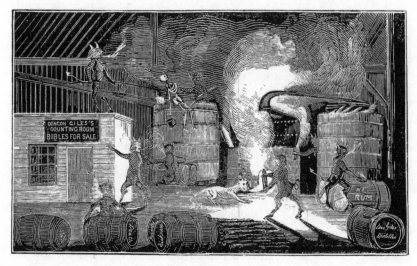

Deacon Giles' Distillery, illustration by George Barrell Cheever from a
temperance pamphlet of demons manufacturing casks labeled
with "poverty," "sickness," and "death," 1835.

crushed, till his agonies are over, and his cries are hushed in death." If
the drug was so demonic, the only answer was total abstinence.

Other temperance reformers quickly picked up on this language, referring to alcohol as a corrupting, seducing, boiling, poisoning, diseasing, or invading entity. These possession stories, relying as they did
on the notion that alcohol had an inherent and irresistible power unto
itself, made both alcohol and intemperance into devils. It was not just
the substance, but the condition it produced. They were one and the
same: the spirit was taken into the body and became the "giant-
wickedness" of intemperance, an "insatiable desire," a "moral ruin" in
the soul.

Beecher's movement for temperance constituted a remarkable shift
for the United States. In the space of just a few decades, the "good creature of God" had become, in the words of a popular reverend preaching
soon after Beecher, "a poisonous foe." Alcohol was personified as Satan,
its footsteps "marked with blood," threatening the precious new country
and its hard-won freedom. Sociologists would later call this "demon

drug" concept "pharmacological determinism"—the idea that a specific drug is endowed with uniquely addictive or "enslaving" powers strong enough to determine human behavior, with all the power residing in the substance. An 1835 illustrated pamphlet, *Deacon Giles' Distillery,* captures it perfectly: demons manufacturing casks labeled with "poverty," "sickness," and "death." Before long, the core belief of the temperance movement was perfectly encapsulated in its new label for alcohol: "Demon Rum."

Benjamin Rush's fantasy of an alcohol-free nation was starting to look like a reality, and the "empire of habit" was crumbling. Beecher's sermons marked the start of an organized, popular temperance movement against alcohol, and specifically a crucial transition in American thinking about alcohol use from an ideal of moderation to one of abstinence.

Beecher had called for vigorous local action: educational campaigns and the establishment of local temperance societies to persuade people to stop drinking and to advocate for broader change. He was not disappointed. By 1833, there were more than five thousand local temperance societies, with an estimated 1.25 million members (almost a full 10 percent of the nation's population). By 1835, more than two million people had renounced distilled liquor. In part because of advances in beverage chemistry, and in part because of the lived experience of reformers who saw how weaker drinks like beer and wine still led reformed drunkards to relapse, the distinction between distilled spirits and fermented drinks began collapsing, and the "teetotal" movement urged abstinence from all forms of alcohol. Eventually, the movement would rock the country in successive cycles, sparking prohibitionist policies toward alcohol and other drugs, inspiring similar international movements, and resulting, much later, in the total prohibition of alcohol for more than a decade. But despite all those enormous changes to come, American drinking habits have never changed more than they did in the years after Beecher's sermon.

In the ten years from 1830 to 1840, the amount that Americans drank dropped by almost half, the biggest decrease in the nation's history—more even than the decline caused by Prohibition in the 1920s. In fact, though the early temperance movement could be called "prohibitionist" in the loose sense that it was an anti-drug movement seeking to forbid alcohol, no legal prohibition was required; reformers simply changed hearts and minds about the nature of drinking. Organizations like Beecher's American Temperance Society papered the country with tracts, pamphlets, and printed sermons full of cautionary tales. Popular writers picked up on the idea, and soon the country was awash with temperance stories: poems, how-to books, novels, plays, songs, paintings, and drawings—all of which contributed to a significant transformation in how people understood alcohol problems. Out of these efforts, a new and important character soon rose to the forefront of the national consciousness: a consistent and abiding story about the "drunkard" and the nature of intemperance.

In 1843, Edgar Allan Poe published "The Black Cat," the tale of a kind and gentle man who is slowly, insidiously warped by drinking. His beloved cat Pluto watches sadly as the man becomes moody and irritable, then violent. Possessed by "the Fiend Intemperance," he beats his dog, his rabbits, his monkey, and his wife. ("My disease grew upon me—for what disease is like Alcohol!") He viciously cuts out Pluto's eye, then drowns his guilt in wine. Overthrown by the "spirit of perverseness," he hangs the poor creature from the limb of a nearby tree. Soon a demonic, doppelgänger Pluto appears and goads the man into burying an ax in his wife's head. With shades of Poe's better-known "The Cask of Amontillado" and "The Tell-Tale Heart," the story culminates with him bricking up her body in the wall of his basement.

Poe, sadly, was drawing on a deep well of personal experience to craft this allegorical tale. His older brother had died after years of alcohol problems, and he himself struggled with addictive behaviors for much of his life. He gambled his way out of the University of Virginia, lost editing jobs because of his drinking, and repeatedly estranged his colleagues with his uncontrolled binges—he was even satirized as a drunken literary man in the 1843 temperance novel *Walter Woolfe, or, The Doom of the Drinker.* Some six years later, he was found delirious in the streets of Baltimore. He died four days after that.

Though "The Black Cat" is Poe's most obvious treatment of addiction, much of his work is shot through with related themes: the divided self, a descent into insanity, a supernatural struggle against a seductive, shadowy, and irresistible evil. Just five months after his brother died, he published one of his earliest stories, "Metzengerstein," about a debauched nobleman whose "perverse attachment" to a "demon-like" horse drives him to insanity and death.

Poe had ample reason to be preoccupied with alcohol, but his stories were just one drop in a flood of writing about the drunkard, a new character in American writing. Around this time, a remarkably consistent story about intemperance came to prominence, portraying the drunkard as overcome by the irresistible desire for drink and experiencing a total loss of control. According to this "drunkard narrative," if the person is redeemed, it is only because salvation has come from a powerful external influence. Crucial to the drunkard narrative is a predictable, inevitable downward arc, one graphically displayed in a famous 1846 lithograph, "The Drunkards Progress," which shows a man descending into desperation, crime, and death by suicide, framed by the sad tableau of his wife and child huddled in front of their burning house. It was a parable of downfall in which alcohol is the fatal flaw, and it proved to be remarkably popular.

In 1842, temperance advocates commissioned Walt Whitman to write *Franklin Evans*—his first novel and his bestselling work during

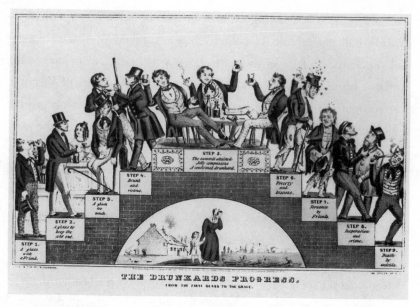

The Drunkards Progress: From the First Glass to the Grave, Nathaniel Currier, 1846.

his lifetime—describing an innocent young boy who is ensnared by intemperance. (Whitman later denounced the book, claiming he wrote it in three days *while drunk* and calling it "damned rot—rot of the worst sort.") Herman Melville won praise from a temperance journal for his 1850 novel *White-Jacket,* in which he insists that sailors are predestined to be "driven back to the spirit-tub and gun-deck by his old hereditary foe, the ever-devilish god of grog." Timothy Shay Arthur's *Ten Nights in a Bar-Room and What I Saw There*, a graphic tale of the horrible consequences of intemperance, was the second-most-popular book of the era, after *Uncle Tom's Cabin*. Many of the most popular stage plays in all of nineteenth-century American theater were based on stories like this, culminating in long scenes graphically illustrating the horrors of delirium tremens.

The country, so saturated by alcohol itself, was now saturated with stories about drunkards. One researcher has estimated that during the 1830s, 12 percent of American novels had temperance themes. A critic writing in 1837 was already bemoaning the "hackneyed" stories and "literary or clerical mediocres" clogging up the temperance genre, without "a single original idea" between them.

These pervasive stories were extraordinarily effective, spreading far and wide the notion that to be possessed by "the Fiend Intemperance" was to be destroyed by a progressive and inexorable loss of control. There is no drunkard narrative without the pharmacological determinism of Beecher's demon rum: the idea that the power resides in the substance itself. Once a hard-drinking nation, a vast portion of the country soon agreed that alcohol was inherently and irresistibly dangerous. Pharmacological determinism presents an intensively powerful image that can be invoked for all sorts of social and political purposes, and it has had remarkable endurance, so much so that, 150 years later, almost the exact same story about the possessive power of a drug was being told about crack cocaine.

Bill Moyers—the venerable journalist, one of the most trusted newscasters of his generation, and onetime press secretary to President Lyndon B. Johnson—was sitting in a van with an "intervention team," including armed off-duty policemen, driving through steady rain to collect his son, William Cope Moyers, from an Atlanta crack house. It was October 1994, and his son was thirty-five years old and going through the most recent in a string of relapses. Moyers wondered: Why would this time be different? Why should he have faith? With every possible advantage and privilege, why did this keep happening to his son?

The group successfully got the younger Moyers out of the crack house and into treatment, and something stuck: he never used again. But Bill Moyers retained an interest in exploring the why, and in 1998 he aired a five-part documentary, *Moyers on Addiction: Close to Home*, in which he presented his answer. After a full year of production and intensive interviews with the leading scientists and policymakers of the 1990s, Moyers had learned that his son's brain had been "hijacked."

In the opening scene of the documentary, after Moyers briefly reveals to the audience that his son had been swept up into addiction, he promises that "scientists will show us how drugs hijack the brain." The camera then cuts to a brain scanner as we hear the Harvard researcher Steven Hyman explain, "Literally, what this allows us to do is get an image of desire in the brain." The entire second episode in the series was titled with this new, gripping metaphor: in "The Hijacked Brain," researchers outlined how drugs "fool the brain" and "usurp" the "pleasure circuit" to cause addiction.

This idea of "hijacking," which got its first wide public airing with the Moyers documentary, was a key component of the idea of addiction as a brain disease. It was the *how* to the *what* of disease: a detailed description of what actually happened to those warped brain circuits. To this day, it remains the leading popular metaphor for addiction, partly because it reinforces the older stories of pharmacological determinism, but also because it draws upon legitimate advances in brain science dating back decades.

In 1954, a researcher named James Olds discovered that an electrode planted deep inside a rat's brain could activate a circuit seemingly so enjoyable that the animals would stimulate themselves instead of eating or sleeping, which in at least one case led to death from exhaustion. Olds took to calling this brain area the "pleasure center." This finding was bolstered by the work of the now largely forgotten neuroscientist Robert Heath, the founder of Tulane's Department of Psychiatry and Neurology, who experimented widely with deep brain stimulation surgery in the 1940s and '50s. Heath, in a series of studies, few of which would meet today's ethical standards, implanted electrical stimulators in the brains of patients with schizophrenia, violent behavior, and, in one especially reprehensible case, homosexuality to attempt a brain-based "conversion therapy." In the process, he found that one of his patients would press a button up to 1,500 times in a three-hour period to stimulate a particular brain center. Yet this discovery wasn't well recognized in addiction science at first. What was missing was a link between the purported pleasure circuit and drugs, a development that didn't materialize until years later.

In 1975, the researcher Roy Wise and his colleague Robert Yokel reported in the prestigious journal *Science* that they had discovered such a link: an obscure molecule named dopamine. Dopamine didn't have the celebrity status it has now. People knew that it was associated with Parkinson's disease, especially after Oliver Sacks's 1973 book *Awakenings*, but researchers doubted whether it was even a neurotransmitter (a type of molecule that transmits information between nerve cells) in its own right. Wise and Yokel, however, used dopamine-blocking chemicals, or "antagonists," to show that dopamine was responsible for the rewarding effects of amphetamines. In a subsequent series of papers, Wise put forth a provocative hypothesis that brain dopamine systems were responsible for the good feelings produced by food, sex, and drugs, because of dopamine's role governing the "pleasure center in the brain." The research community took some notice, though it had little effect among the lay public. Ten years later, though, the crack cocaine epidemic hit.

In the 1980s, crack cocaine sparked an extraordinary drug scare in America. Seemingly overnight, the media exploded with pieces about an unimaginably powerful new drug that was ubiquitous in the poor, Black, urban neighborhoods labeled "inner cities." The visibility of crack among the urban poor, along with the visuals on television, combined to paint a menacing picture. Across the nation, but especially in the urban Northeast, the evening news was saturated with ominous footage of Black and Brown men being arrested for crack-related crimes. In 1986, drug use was the "issue of the year," according to *Time* magazine. Rudy Giuliani, the U.S. attorney for the Southern District of New York, purchased crack on camera to show the brazenness of street corner sales. Later that year, CBS aired *48 Hours on Crack Street*, promoted by Dan Rather as a look inside "the war zone, for an unusual two hours of hands-on horror."

Make no mistake: crack caused true devastation. People went on crack binges for days, not stopping until their money ran out or they simply collapsed. Dealers viciously exploited and degraded women with addiction, whom the media labeled "crack whores." Because crack was so easily made and distributed, and therefore cheap, there was violent competition for market share in cities across the nation. But the popular images didn't fit the reality, as most crack users were white, and the racially charged panic left the public with a twisted portrayal.

Newspapers, magazines, and television networks used coded racist language to sound the alarm about dangerous Black and Brown users infecting white America. *Newsweek* warned that crack "has transformed the ghetto" and "is rapidly spreading into the suburbs." In a series of high-profile articles, *The New York Times* warned that crack was infecting "the wealthiest suburbs of Westchester County," culminating in a fearful declaration on the front page of June 8, 1986: CRACK ADDICTION SPREADS AMONG THE MIDDLE CLASS.

Wise's dopamine hypothesis, now a decade old, was suddenly thrust into the center of the national conversation about the nature of addiction. Physicians and researchers described crack as a sort of superdrug, "the most addictive drug known to man," one that would cause "almost instantaneous addiction." Dopamine was the reason why: one psychiatrist described how crack "appears to stimulate the brain's most primitive neural reward circuits" to "create an intense and unrelenting drug hunger," making him fear that "crack caused compulsive use in everyone." In a 1988 *New York Times* front-page story about "The Crack Plague," researchers described how they were struggling to understand the "nearly unbreakable habit" of crack addiction, and experts called it "the most troubling drug we have studied," one that was "nearly impossible" to stop using because of its dopamine-related neurochemistry. Roy

Wise himself declared that "if I knew that my daughter was going to try either heroin or crack, I'd prefer that she try heroin."

Through the 1990s, dopamine only grew as a source of fascination in the medical field and the media. New microdialysis experiments that sampled the concentrations of dopamine in rat brains seemed to show that a wider range of drugs, including opiates, alcohol, nicotine, and cocaine, increased dopamine release. This finding prompted a theory of addiction that said that addictive drugs release dopamine but non-addictive drugs don't. Stronger neuroimaging technology only made the idea of a pleasure center more compelling. A *Time* cover story from 1997 described how dopamine was the "master molecule of addiction" and painted a vivid picture of dopamine neurons radiating out from a brain area called the nucleus accumbens to influence widespread neurological activity. Featuring the work of a rising star in the neuroimaging research world, Nora Volkow (the current head of the National Institute on Drug Abuse), who had recently published a noteworthy study on dopamine in the journal *Nature*, the article explained that drugs work through dopamine, "hijacking a natural reward system that dates back millions of years."

The story of those "hijacked" brain circuits has proven to be enormously influential—the reason that dopamine is a near-household word today. The "hijacking" metaphor is omnipresent, in everything from YouTube explainers about how addiction takes over the brain to communiqués from leading institutions in neuroscience and addiction, including the National Institutes of Health and Harvard Medical School. After more than two decades of media coverage, dopamine is synonymous with pleasure—the "dopamine hits" in your brain are supposed to be the reason that alcohol, other drugs, social media notifications, and that jolting sip of morning coffee all feel good. Silicon Valley biohackers even go on "dopamine fasts," abstaining from any activity with the slightest hint of pleasure, including eye contact, in order to "reboot the brain."

However, this narrative is an oversimplification. Dopamine is an enormously important molecule in addiction, central to the experience of learning and reward prediction, but its functioning is far more complicated than it is commonly portrayed. In a way, the popular stories about dopamine still rely on a circa-1980s level of understanding, overlooking the tremendous strides that have been made in research since then. For one thing, dopamine is not a "pleasure" molecule: it has more to do with the feelings of desire and "wanting," not enjoyment and "liking." After a series of experiments in the mid-nineties bore this out, even Roy Wise retracted his hypothesis that dopamine was at the root of pleasure. Furthermore, not all drugs "bombard" the brain with dopamine by tapping directly into that circuitry: Wise worked largely on stimulants, which do powerfully and directly release dopamine, but cannabis and opioids do not. To the extent that those other drugs affect dopamine, they do so indirectly, by acting on upstream circuits, not by directly influencing the dopamine circuit.

Dopamine functions in the hijacking story just like demon rum: it is supposed to explain why drugs have such a special power, like agents with their own malevolent volition, and why they cause addiction. But this is not how drugs work; addiction does not proceed inevitably from use. Most people who use drugs—including crack, methamphetamine, and heroin—do not develop significant problems. In studies spanning decades, no more than 10 to 30 percent of people who use drugs develop significant substance use disorders. Drugs are not "addictive" in themselves; they don't cause addictions in isolation.

Science can be a powerful tool in social movements, and scientific stories about substances are easily twisted to fit the dominant prejudices of the time. From the very beginning of the temperance movement, in his *Six Sermons*, Beecher spun medical stories about how the stomach was the source of "pleasurable and painful vibrations to the nerves" and "vigor to the mind," and how it was warped by the repeated stimulation of alcohol, resulting in a vacuum "which nothing can fill" and thus a deadly habit. The temperance movement, driven predominantly by religious leaders, subsequently rallied physicians to their cause to speak against alcohol. Later in the nineteenth century, the movement established a Department of Scientific Temperance Instruction that screened textbooks for schools and colleges, insisting, for example, that books stress the points that alcohol creates an uncontrollable craving and that alcohol is a poison and toxin in any amount. The actual science didn't really matter; it was all retrofitted onto the existing story of possession. Science was just being used to bolster claims that seemed self-evident.

In the 1990s, the "hijacking" story followed a similar pattern of reflecting the predominant social concerns. The very word suggests violence and force. (Not incidentally, the late 1990s were a time of escalating fears about both carjacking and terrorism; in 1997, Osama bin Laden gave his first television interview, and Louisiana passed "Kill the Carjacker" legislation that allowed motorists to kill anyone they believed to be carjacking them.) In putting all the power in the drug itself, such demon drug narratives provide good cover for law-and-order crackdowns; the anti-drug frenzy was used to justify increasingly punitive policies in the war on drugs. Just like the "firewater myth" that said Native Americans have a special vulnerability to alcohol, this story simultaneously obscured the true causes of the problem and the violence of the oppression.

The crack epidemic is better seen as the result of powerful, intersecting causes, not the least of which is systemic oppression. Black and Brown neighborhoods were impoverished from decades of redlining, discrimination, and other ways of systematically excluding people from prosperity. Then, as deaths-of-despair researchers Case and Deaton have described, free-market globalization and job loss hit urban Black people particularly hard in the 1970s and '80s—they were the canaries in the coal mine of a changing national and global economy. It was a preview of the same forces that would hit working-class whites in the

2000s, a common social factor underlying both the crack and opioid epidemics: a growth in inequality that was increasingly leaving less-skilled workers behind.

The idea of hijacking easily slips into dehumanization. Yes, in some circumstances the "hijacking" idea does allow for more compassion. It helped Bill Moyers make sense of his son's problems, explaining how he wound up repeatedly relapsing on crack, and similarly, in her book *Dopesick*, the journalist Beth Macy described how in recent years, community activists have helped to muster compassion for people with addiction by talking about how "free will becomes hijacked." But this particular portrayal comes at a cost. In the *Time* issue from 1997 that contained the early use of the word "hijacking," the front cover portrayed addiction as a gruesome caricature of a primordial fish-human mindlessly chomping at an empty hook. Perhaps this is how biological explanations of mental disorder lead to pessimism and hopelessness: by portraying people as passive subjects, totally taken over by the drugs, even devolving into a lower life form.

Pessimism was also the result of the nineteenth-century drunkard narrative. Almost all of the focus was on keeping people from becoming drunkards in the first place, rather than saving people with drinking problems. There were some attempts at helping people to swear off alcohol, but if they lapsed, they were largely written off as hopeless cases. One co-founder of Lyman Beecher's American Temperance Society put it starkly: "All who are intemperate will soon be dead, the earth will be eased of an amazing evil."

Six craftsmen—a tailor, a carpenter, two blacksmiths, a carriage builder, and a silversmith—were gathered in a spare, depressing tavern in Baltimore, doing what they did nearly every night: drinking heavily. It was 1840, and the nation was in the middle of a massive depression, one that would last for years. As banks collapsed and thousands of workers lost their jobs, the newly emergent middle class of craftsmen was hit particularly hard.

They had all heard that a famous preacher was coming to town that evening to give a much-anticipated temperance lecture, but these men were skeptical about the elitist tone of the temperance movement and bored by the hours-long lectures about sinfulness. Just for kicks, but maybe with a little hopeful curiosity too, four of them decided to attend. As anticipated, they didn't like the lecture, and they mocked the uppity preacher—the temperance leaders were "all a parcel of hypocrites"—but to their surprise, they were inspired about the possibility of changing their relationship to alcohol. They hated the medium but were intrigued by the message.

They came up with their own club. It met each week and prioritized a more egalitarian spirit. To keep things interesting, the men took turns standing and describing their own problems with alcohol plainly (not unlike the structure of modern-day Alcoholics Anonymous meetings), concluding each meeting with a shared abstinence pledge and a resolution that each of them would bring a new man to the next meeting. In a nod to their battles against "King Alcohol," they named themselves the Washington Temperance Society. The Washingtonians were born.

It was a movement by and for drunkards, but all were welcome, and non-drinking supporters also flocked to the meetings as they grew exponentially. The Washingtonians' egalitarian leanings helped: unlike nearly all other temperance organizations, they accepted Irish and German immigrants, Catholics, Black Americans, and women. "Martha Washingtonian" meetings were the first place in the New York temperance movement that women actively began to speak in public settings, and such meetings provided a refuge not only for female drunkards but also for women suffering from the ravages of male drinking, thus forming an important preview of the essential role of women in the temperance movement to come. All told, more than a tenth of Baltimore's population and greater than 7 percent of New York City's were members of the Washingtonians. By the end of 1841, nearly 200,000 people had signed their pledge, and by 1843 they reported millions.

The Washingtonians represented an important departure from the rest of the temperance movement. They still demonized alcohol, but they had much more hope for redemption; crucially, they did not see drunkards as doomed in the way that the predominant stereotype did. Instead, their language was shot through with references to effort and agency. With the right community support, people had the power to choose, to exercise their will to save themselves. As one speaker declared, "This is a new era, my friend, a new power is at work; and what was once considered hopeless is an every day occurrence." A young Abraham Lincoln, early in his political career, congratulated their "powerful moral effort" in an 1842 celebration of the movement. One famous Washingtonian speaker explained his transformation by saying, "I had exerted a moral power, which had long remained lying by, perfectly useless." Another would turn to the audience at the climax of his routine and exclaim, "Poor drunkard! there is hope for you. You cannot be worse off than I was, nor more degraded, or more of a slave to appetite. You can return if you will. *Try it—Try it.*"

There were still cautions about the demonic, enslaving force of the "enemy" lurking in the cupboard—but now they could beat it. As Lincoln noted, the temperance movement was "suddenly transformed from a cold abstract theory, to a living, breathing, active, and powerful chieftain. . . . Drunken devils are cast out by ones, by sevens, and by legions; and their unfortunate victims, like the poor possessed, who was redeemed from his long and lonely wanderings in the tombs, are publishing to the ends of the earth, how great things have been done for them."

It was a bottom-up, populist mutual-help movement, a novel approach for temperance. Drunkards themselves could identify with one another's struggles, bear witness, confess and resolve their shame, find support in the group, and make restitution for their long and often catastrophic drinking careers through concrete, useful outreach work.

Unlike much of the temperance movement, the Washingtonians were tolerant of relapses and patiently worked with people to support their sobriety. Not only could drunkards be saved, but they could turn the battle against demon rum into a heroic story, one over which they had ownership. This was a major strength at both a rhetorical and an organizational level.

The Washingtonians' rigorous focus on drunkenness was a significant factor in their success. They banned prayers, hymns, and drawn-out sermons, instead speaking directly from their own experiences. In a way, they were translating the religious revival movement of the Second Great Awakening into secular terms, keeping the personal testimony and the standard fall and rise of the drunkard narrative but discarding all the religious baggage. Instead, they held sober concerts, balls, picnics, fairs, and parades. During a massive celebration in New York City, Walt Whitman, a huge fan of the movement, reveled in the pageantry and wrote enthusiastically about the "grand blow out at night to cap the whole." Above all, at a time of awful dislocation and national stress, it was a movement founded on sincerity and hope.

The accounts of the most famous Washingtonians, such as John Bartholomew Gough, a trained actor who became rich from paid speaking gigs, survive to this day, and there's something beautiful about their detailed personal narratives. Their stories linger on the irrational and befuddling conflict at the heart of addiction, not mindlessly taken over by a demon but wrestling with effort and cravings. Gough wrote at length of how his denial had grown in him. Sometimes it was an active process of convincing himself that he wasn't really a drunkard, as he would "plead my own cause before myself" and, as his own "judge and jury," win a "willing acquittal." Sometimes he'd resolve to take the pledge but put it off to a "more convenient season." And sometimes, he'd simply seem to forget, even though later he recognized it was more a result of the "master passion" of drink crowding out any opposing feeling. This is what made the Washingtonians so compelling—not explicitly religious or medical stories, but simple, personal, and deeply identifiable ones. And yet, seemingly just as quickly as they appeared, the Washingtonians were gone.

The Washingtonians were good at drumming up enthusiasm and getting people to sign the abstinence pledge, but they didn't offer much beyond the initial quasi conversion experience, and they struggled to keep up their momentum—in the words of one AA cliché, there's a world of difference between getting sober and staying sober. Critics soon complained that the format was stale. People were getting sick of the endless recitations of drunken stories: the "narration of horrible 'experiences'" by "the scurrilous army of ditch-delivered reformed drunkards." Backsliding was a big problem, including among the most famous. John Gough had multiple relapses, culminating in a weeklong binge in New York City in September 1845 that ended with his being found at a brothel. (He later claimed the enemies of temperance had drugged him.)

What's more, the Washingtonians made enemies. Their anti-religious stances had attracted the ire of the church, and, more significantly, at a moment when reform sentiment was boiling over into acrimonious disputes, they had strayed far into politics. Around that time, competing reform movements were jockeying for position. (In counterpoint to the burgeoning abolitionist movement, some temperance advocates even claimed that drinking was worse than human slavery, because it "fetters the immortal mind as well as the body.") The temperance movement itself was splitting into warring camps, primarily divided along the question of whether there should be legal prohibitions on alcohol. Although the Washingtonians had initially pledged to stay out of that debate, Gough and other prominent members of the group eventually came out in favor of alcohol prohibition, subjecting them to attacks from other temperance advocates.

The Washingtonians collapsed in a matter of years—by 1847, almost none of the societies were active—but at a time when nothing seemed to be able to help, they raised important and provocative questions that rehumanized people with addiction: What could we expect of its sufferers? How much control did they have? In the coming years, other mutual-help organizations inspired by the Washingtonian model kept the tradition alive: Sons of Temperance, the Temple of Honor, the Good Samaritans, and many more.

In the meantime, the temperance movement continued to fragment. Law-and-order enthusiasts demanded prohibition, and they won laws entirely outlawing drinking in some states. Religious leaders developed their own variants on mutual-help groups. And at this fractious time, as the country itself was headed toward civil war and fracturing along deep divisions—free soil versus slave states, immediate versus gradual abolition, and North versus South—the medical profession started to grow in power and influence, armed with powerful crystals that had recently been extracted from the tarry, opioid-laden juice of the poppy: a little-used but soon-to-be-blockbuster drug, morphine.

Five

THE FIRST AMERICAN
OPIOID EPIDEMIC

O ne dreary, dull Sunday in London in 1804, a young aspiring writer named Thomas De Quincey woke up, yet again, to piercing pains in his teeth and face. He was prone to such attacks—searing, lancing, and all-encompassing—but this one ranked among his worst, and it had already been going on for almost three weeks. In a vain attempt to distract himself, he went out for a walk. He ran into a friend who suggested, fatefully: *Why not try opium?*

In De Quincey's day, opium was a commonplace, even banal drug, stocked not only by pharmacists but also by bakers, tailors, and other basic retailers. The simplest storefronts kept a large block of raw opium on the counter, a sticky brown mass made of the juice of the poppy, shaving off penny portions and folding them up into little paper packets for all comers, no prescription needed. That day, though, De Quincey found his way to a druggist who gave him another popular form of the drug: laudanum, a ruby-red tincture of opium dissolved in alcohol, often seasoned with spices. He returned to his lodgings and took the draught.

De Quincey's pain evaporated, but more importantly, the opium sent him on a flight of artistic inspiration, giving him amazing visions and heightening his powers of perception. The physical was totally overshadowed by the psychic: "that my pains had vanished was now a trifle in my eyes."

De Quincey was just shy of twenty years old, enrolled at Oxford and dreaming of becoming a writer like his heroes William Wordsworth and Samuel Taylor Coleridge. Their poetry was the only thing that had assuaged his troubled mind to that point—when he first read Wordsworth, it gave rise to a mystical experience in him, granting him "an absolute revelation of untrodden worlds, teeming with power and beauty, as yet unsuspected amongst men." Now, opium opened that door even wider. In the coming years, he took laudanum in increasing doses, stepping fully into a new imaginative consciousness. In a drug-fueled reverie, he wandered London's streets, reveling in his transformation. Sitting in the cheap seats at the opera, he could see the intricate harmonies unfurl in front of his eyes like a tapestry.

In time, he did in fact work his way into the circle of Wordsworth and Coleridge. Yet as his opium use progressed, he had trouble translating his imaginative experiences into art. By his own account (which, it bears noting, is often unreliable and contradictory), he was well and truly addicted to opium by 1813: "From this date the reader is to consider me as a regular and confirmed opium-eater, of whom to ask whether on any particular day he had or had not taken opium, would be to ask whether his lungs had performed respiration, or the heart fulfilled its functions." His dose soon reached astronomical levels: around 1817, as high as 320 "grains" daily, which would equal more than 20,000 milligrams of morphine a day. (By comparison, a starting dose for severe pain is around 15 to 30 milligrams of morphine every four hours, or 180 milligrams of morphine a day.) He aspired to be a great writer, but his productivity had stalled, and as he himself acknowledged to his editor, the supposed miracle drug might itself be the problem: "Opium has reduced me for the last six years to one general discourtesy of silence."

In the closing years of the 1810s, De Quincey decided that he would write his way out by focusing on opium itself as his subject, composing a grand work with the drug as the main character. The result, published in 1821, was his *Confessions of an English Opium-Eater,* a fragmentary, passionate, bizarre work, by his own admission lacking "any regular and connected shape," bounding between dreams, philosophy, memory, social commentary, and (anti-)medical speculation. Yet it was a massive sensation, met with near-universal praise and rapidly going through multiple printings. Today, his *Confessions* still stands as a true landmark in the literature of addiction: the first literary text devoted to drug use and the first drug addiction memoir.

De Quincey gestured toward the dangers of habitual use—a section titled "The Pains of Opium" described his powerlessness to stop and his feeling of being trapped in a "gloom and cloudy melancholy." Nevertheless, he declared later in the book that he had quit the habit relatively easily, and as such *Confessions* is ultimately a celebration of opium: a love letter, a polemic, even a religious text. He was there, he wrote, to preach the "doctrine of the true church on the subject of opium," and the drug was no workaday tool but a gateway to the transcendent. For the opium eater, "the diviner part of his nature is paramount; that is, the moral affections are in a state of cloudless serenity, and over all is the great light of the majestic intellect."

De Quincey's work championed a particular kind of drug use: recreational use, or, as it was called in those days, "luxurious" use. In today's dry clinical language, we would say "non-medical," and De Quincey would have supported this distinction from medical use. The notion that opium was a simple clinical tool was anathema to De Quincey—according to him, medical writers offered only "Lies! Lies! Lies!"—they were the "greatest enemies" to the divine truths the drug revealed.

Recreational, luxurious, non-medical, abusive—the history of addiction is littered with labels and euphemisms for drug use outside of medically sanctioned contexts. The distinction between "medical" and "non-medical" is an artificial one, because the instrumental use of intoxication long predates modern medicine. From the hallucinogenic drugs in Mayan and Aztec ceremonies to the mysterious drink soma that appears in the ancient Indian *Rig Veda*, various cultures have used intoxicants to communicate with the spiritual world—are these uses "therapeutic," in terms of spiritual healing, or recreational? The ancient Greeks understood alcohol intoxication as a beneficent form of possession, not a physical process: they thought that drinking changed thoughts and feelings because the drinker literally became one with the god Dionysus, taking the "god within": *entheos*. That supposed medical/recreational divide also demands close scrutiny because it is commonly used to excuse some types of drug use while vilifying others, and since the time of De Quincey, drug problems among the privileged have evoked humane and sympathetic reactions. The ultimate effect is often to obscure the true extent of drug harms on both sides of the divide.

In the end, the transcendence that De Quincey sought was not so much spiritual as aesthetic, so perhaps the best word for his opium use is the same one used for Coleridge and Wordsworth's art, the movement he believed had saved his life and breathed inspiration into him in the first place: "Romantic."

D e Quincey was the prototypical addiction-tortured genius, presenting himself as a sort of Orpheus figure who charted a course into his own psychic hell and back, coming out with special insights into an otherworldly realm. It was a message tailor-made for the Romantic tradition—a loose term referring to European authors from the late eighteenth to the mid-nineteenth century who revolted against the science, philosophy, and generally stiff rationalism of the Enlightenment to instead celebrate imagination, subjectivity, and feeling. Romanticism implies spontaneity, individuality, and intense emotions, and it puts a priority on subjective, interior experience, which opium only heightened, or so De Quincey claimed. Opium, largely produced half a world away in British-ruled India, was also the perfect embodiment of the

Romantics' Orientalist preoccupation with the nebulous "East" as a mysterious, supernatural, and often subtly dangerous source of new experiences. The Romantics were interested in escaping the discipline of the Enlightenment, especially through sublime aesthetic experiences, and De Quincey fashioned drug use into exactly that: an aesthetic experience. He portrayed opium use as a way to shake off the limitations of worldly rationality and to directly and powerfully explore inner space.

There's a long list of British Romantic figures who developed significant opium habits: Elizabeth Barrett Browning, Sir Walter Scott, Lord Byron, John Keats, Percy Bysshe Shelley, Branwell Brontë, and many more. They were not blind to the dangers of opium: in the 1868 novel *The Moonstone,* a habitual opium user declares, "The progress of the disease has gradually forced me from the use of opium to the abuse of it." (The author, Wilkie Collins, was himself a habitual user who carried his supply of laudanum in a silver flask wherever he went.) The only one who could match De Quincey in opium use, though, was Coleridge, whose own Orientalist poem *Kubla Khan* was inspired by an opium dream after he had read about Xanadu, the summer palace of the Mongol emperor. Coleridge's poem captured the dual nature of this romantic drug, depicting pleasure and pain as intertwined—for example, in the metaphor of a river flowing down into a "sunless sea." De Quincey, too, portrayed the ambivalent nature of opium's pleasures and pains in his *Confessions*, presenting opium as both the holder of the "keys of Paradise" and a "dread agent" from the East, even personifying the drug as a ferocious, turbaned "Malay."

This personification of opium points to De Quincey's genius. Opium, back then, was a simple commodity; after all, you could just stroll into a store and buy it. To render it dangerous and exotic, he first had to create a taboo to break. By playing up the sensual pleasures of opium and anthropomorphizing the drug into this Asian "other," he invented a luxurious, romantic, indulgent form of non-medical use. As the cultural historian Mike Jay puts it, it was a "double game: baiting the moralists and middlebrow public opinion while delighting the elite with the invention of a new vice." In the process, romantic use became not just a tool for insight but a mark of the counterculture.

D e Quincey inspired many imitators in his time, and though he defended himself by claiming that "no man is likely to adopt opium . . . in consequence of anything he may read in a book," in fact many young literary men followed his example, and there was at least one report of a fatal overdose. (In the 1842 essay "An Opium-Eater in America," one writer glumly recounted that he had taken up the drug because of De Quincy's book, but "the latter part, the 'miseries of opium,' I had most unaccountably always neglected to read.") Substance use often serves as a mark of manly or sophisticated achievement: Jack London learned early in life that "drink was the badge of manhood," and Charles Jackson's alcoholic protagonist in *The Lost Weekend* idolized "Poe and Keats, Byron, Dowson, Chatterton, all the gifted miserable and reckless men who had burned themselves out in tragic brilliance early and with finality."

But De Quincey inspired more than individual experimentation. In the exuberantly artistic Paris of the 1840s, some of the leading creators of the day, including Honoré de Balzac, Victor Hugo, and Alexandre Dumas, began gathering in a hotel for an unusual salon. They met not to share new art or hear music, but to sample an exotic new drug from the Orient, hashish. France had received an early introduction to cannabis when Napoleon's army returned from Egypt earlier in the 1800s, and like opium, the drug was first used for relatively bland medical purposes. These psychonauts, however, were interested in exploring their own consciousness. They named themselves the Club des Hashischins (from a legend about a renegade Middle Eastern warlord who supposedly used hashish to shape young men into assassins), and many went on to write about their drug use, including Charles Baudelaire, who was particularly influenced by De Quincey. Though Baudelaire used both hashish and opium, in his 1860 book *Les paradis artificiels* (*Artificial Paradises*), he wrote only about his own experiences with hashish, and he simply retranslated sections of De Quincey's *Confessions* for the opium section of the book, claiming that De Quincey had already said all that needed to be said about the drug.

If De Quincey embodied the prototype of the addicted, tortured genius, the Club des Hashischins represented a new, bohemian counterculture, one that has itself influenced the experience of taking drugs for decades since by promoting a connection between drug use and art. Later in the nineteenth century, a clique of proto-punk writers called the Decadents took Baudelaire to an extreme, openly romanticizing and embracing morphine use. The legacy of the *club* also includes the early-twentieth-century Parisian salons where Salvador Dalí, Jean Cocteau, and Pablo Picasso smoked opium, the Harlem "tea pads" where people gathered to smoke cannabis in the 1920s, the mid-twentieth-century jazz communities awash in heroin, and many other artistic groups incorporating drug use.

Some of the most celebrated and successful art in the world seems born out of addiction. Cocteau's films, innumerable jazz masterpieces, the Sex Pistols, Nirvana, the paintings of Jackson Pollock and Jean-Michel Basquiat, the comedy of Richard Pryor. Why should there be such a connection between art and addiction? The first and most straightforward explanation is that intoxication does serve a purpose: creatives seek to quiet the discursive mind and access a deeper inspiration. But drug use, and even addiction, can serve a social purpose, too. As the philosopher Owen Flanagan has said, addiction is "not just an odd dosing regimen with respect to some substance," but also it often becomes an identity and a lifestyle, a "deep self" identification woven into the fabric of one's life. Red Rodney later said of heroin's popularity among jazz musicians that it "was our badge. It was the thing that made us different than the rest of the world." Drug use, by virtue of its transgressiveness, signifies membership.

It's important not to confuse drug use with drug addiction, and it's seductive to believe that our artistic heroes have received more than has been taken away from them—that their addictions gave them access to some sort of special insight. Drug use might give insight; addiction rarely does. Even William Burroughs warned against the notion that addiction spurred creativity and inspiration—he specifically called out De Quincey as wrong in this regard. It's a warning borne out not just by Burroughs's own life but by De Quincey's too.

Despite his section on the "pains of opium," De Quincey ended the *Confessions* on a triumphant note, declaring that he had simply reduced his dose on his own, then quit for good. In reality, he never stopped using, and for the rest of his chaotic life, he teetered on the edge of ruin. One of his biographers puts it plainly: "In the last decades of his life he was spending £150 a year on the drug (from an income of £250), permanently in debt and pursued by creditors, continually adopting false names and shifting lodgings (he would simply abandon his rooms when they overflowed with his books and papers), often dressed in castoffs and writing barefoot (a friend observed 'an army coat four times too large for him and with nothing on beneath'), and largely unable to support an ever-growing family of eight children and a suicidal wife."

He always planned to write a third part of the *Confessions* to elaborate on his problems—but he never quite got around to it. The result was a legacy of a new kind of addiction story. His was not the clear-cut temperance narrative with a predictable fall and rise, or even the type of lurid, sensationalistic, dark temperance narrative from the likes of Whitman and Poe, but the elite, romanticized drug history—the complicated, introverted, literary, scholarly, aesthetic figure, a highbrow fable that masked a devastating reality.

Toward the end of medical school, my drinking was starting to have serious consequences. I was living with my first serious girlfriend, and every time I drank, I picked bitter, vicious screaming fights with her. She threatened to break up with me if I didn't tone it down, and she told me that I clearly had a problem, but I dismissed it out of hand, chalking it up to my immaturity or the stress I was facing.

One drunken night I watched myself cross a series of lines, from argument to mistreatment, from mistreatment to outright verbal abuse. I can't remember the details—frankly, they were always hazy, and I often woke up the next morning not remembering why we fought in the first place. That night, though, when I started bellowing and calling her a bitch, I knew it was over.

The next morning, I left for a rotation at a hospital in Paris. I was hurt about the breakup, as well as insecure; my now ex-girlfriend was a cultured graduate student who called me "raised by wolves," because I knew so little beyond medicine or science. In Paris, I compensated by rushing headlong into my own romantic fantasy of drugs, alcohol, and culture. When our group of four medical students met our sponsoring doctor, he was smoking a cigarette right outside the main entrance of the hospital, a jolly, mustachioed Frenchman wearing a black turtleneck under a white coat. He told us not to worry about working too hard and gave us some restaurant recommendations. Perfect.

I spent my days strolling around the city, visiting every museum and gallery and opera I could. I also began drinking every day, earlier and earlier in the afternoon, sipping liqueurs through the evening and then going out to dinners where apéritifs, wine, and digestifs were the real main courses for me. A few times, I made myself throw up afterward so I could go back out to the bars, trying to clear the ethanol out of my system so I could drink more. By the end of the trip, I was thrilled to make a connection for cocaine, even though I had hardly ever used the drug before—not even all that thrilled to use it, but thrilled to have it, to be the kind of person who could get it.

My drinking and drug use at this time were not just about stress reduction or being taken over by the substance. Part of me was greedily grasping after a new identity for myself. I seized on the surface-level signifiers, hoping that drugs and alcohol could serve as a shortcut to becoming cultured. But there was also a harsh internal dialogue dogging me with every step I took in the city. I had ruined a two-year relationship despite trying harder than I ever had in my life, and I knew my relationship to alcohol was a big part of it. I was weak; I had no follow-through. I was stupid, plastering over my lack of culture or serious intellectual development with frantic activity, trophy collection, and, now, vapid partying. Most of the time these thoughts hovered vaguely on the edge of my consciousness, lingering more as stinging, acrid feelings than as clear ideas, but they never left me. I was restless; I couldn't sit still with myself, and soon I was drinking a bottle of cheap wine each night, alone in my hotel room.

I fell for one of the other med students there. When it was working, it was magical, romantic, the moonlight glinting off the Seine as we had our first kiss. When it wasn't working, it was painful in every way; one night when we were out together, I fell down the Métro escalator the wrong way, all six feet three inches and 190 pounds of me crushing her under me for several interminable revolutions of the stairs, flopping around slowly and stupidly like a damp stuffed animal in a dryer. I tried to laugh it off, but we were also covered in bruises and scrapes, and underneath I was terrified.

I knew by this point that my drinking was a real issue, but writing about it in my journal, I tried to justify the constant nausea and stomach upset as too much rich food, and I came up with elaborate euphemisms for the other consequences I noticed, like the made-up phrase "counter-sedative effects of alcohol rebound" instead of simply calling it what it was, the tremors of early-stage alcohol withdrawal. Back in New York,

I connected with a cocaine dealer, and right before intern year started, I placed a huge delivery order for high-end cocktail ingredients, telling myself that even if I wasn't in Paris, at least I could continue my cultural education by studying mixology. Hard drinking and drugs were a viable shortcut to some kind of counterfeit sophistication. It wasn't just an excuse for drinking more; it was a sad and painful process of trying to become someone I wasn't.

In the early 1850s at Princeton, a young man studying medicine decided that if he really wanted to deepen his education, he should start sampling some of the drugs he was studying. Fitz Hugh Ludlow was a brilliant but odd boy, fitted from a young age with enormous spectacles and inclined to describe his favorite pastimes as "books, ill health, and musing." At college, he was drawn to the local apothecary's shop and its little library tucked away behind red curtains, its air pungent with the smells of the medications stacked on the oaken shelves, and he set out to try "every strange drug and chemical which the laboratory could produce."

In 1856, at the age of twenty, Ludlow published a confessional magazine article about the new drug he had discovered, one that had brought on "a sublime rapture" and "voluptuous delirium which suffused the body with a blush of exquisite languor." The drug was cannabis, in the form of hashish, and he quickly followed with a book-length treatment called *The Hasheesh Eater*, describing his self-experimentation in turgid prose. (To be an "eater" of opium or another substance meant to take the drug orally, but it also carried the connotation of an unbreakable habit.) Ludlow, often described as a "minor De Quincey," was a total convert to the romantic aesthetic of drug use, promising that cannabis "unlocked the secret" to the "storm-wrapped peaks of sublimity which hover over the path of the Oriental story."

This writing bought Ludlow entrée into New York City artistic culture, and he became a frequent contributor to all the literary touch-stones of his day: *Harper's* magazine, the *Evening Post*, and the *Atlantic Monthly*—eventually, he became one of the first editors of *Vanity Fair.* But within a decade of his debut, his drug problems were becoming apparent.

At the end of *The Hasheesh Eater*, Ludlow claimed to have stopped using all intoxicants, but as in De Quincey's tale, that was a lie. Before long, he was spooning the new opioid medication, morphine, into his whiskey every day.* Unlike De Quincey, though, Ludlow wrote about the ongoing horrors of opioid addiction, which he described in an 1867 article as a "horrible mental bondage" and a "spiritual thralldom," rue-fully predicting that "the man who voluntarily addicts himself to it would commit in cutting his throat a suicide only swifter and less igno-ble." He traveled far and wide searching for a cure, and in 1870 he pub-lished a celebratory letter from Europe in *Harper's*, claiming that he had found a way to cure opioid addiction just like "any other chronic dis-ease." But that was wishful thinking. He died that same year, 1870, at the age of thirty-four, likely from the combined weight of chronic tuber-culosis and his many lifelong addictions.

Ludlow's rapid shift from pharmacological enthusiasm to alarmism was ahead of its time, but not by much: his experience anticipated the first American opioid epidemic, a massive and fearful surge of drug problems that had been building for decades.

Americans were arrogant about opioids at the start. One early Amer-ican reviewer of De Quincey's *Confessions*, writing in the midst of tem-perance activism in 1824, claimed somewhat confidently that good, practical Americans were unlikely to indulge in De Quincey's kind of disreputable drug use: "We believe that very few persons, if any, in this

---

* "Opioid" versus "opiate" can sometimes be confusing. While the terms are often used interchangeably, "opiate" tends to imply naturally occurring compounds, such as morphine, while "opioid" includes all synthetic chemicals, like oxycodone. To avoid switching back and forth in the manuscript, I generally refer just to "opioids."

country, abandon themselves to the use of opium as a luxury, nor does there appear to be any great danger of the introduction of this species of intemperance."

In the coming years, however, the United States did become entranced by drugs. The science of chemistry isolated wave after wave of new "specifics": purified, standardized drug extracts that were easily measured and dosed. Chloroform and ether revolutionized dentistry and surgery. Cannabis, too, enjoyed a brief period of therapeutic enthusiasm. But by far the most significant was morphine. This was decades before aspirin or any other decent pain relief was available, so a reliable, dependable, and powerful therapy for pain was a meaningful boon for the medical profession.

In the competitive and entrepreneurial culture of mid-nineteenth-century America, mainstream, professional physicians were at war with competitors from countermovements like folk medicine and homeopathy. One way the mainstream doctors distinguished themselves was by championing modern scientific medicine, especially new drugs. The field of medicine was shifting from a holistic, humoral idea of *dis-ease* to a categorization of specific diseases with biological causes, and targeted drug treatments were advertised as "more scientific."

A succession of devastating epidemics of cholera and dysentery in the 1830s through the 1850s only increased the enthusiasm for opioids, which calmed gastrointestinal symptoms. Also powerfully catalyzing the opioid epidemic was another technological advance: the hypodermic syringe. Developed in Britain in the 1840s and first brought to the United States in 1853, the hypodermic syringe was a dream for scientifically minded physicians. Here was a device that could deliver precise doses of medication directly into the body for near-instantaneous and predictable results, a perfect embodiment of the promised new precision. The hypodermic needle was professional and respectable, an ideal counterpoint to the tools of quacks and herbalists. A syringe is not itself a drug, of course, but the new delivery system essentially transmuted morphine into a new, more potent, and faster-acting form, one that was further popularized by the scientific story attached to it.

A change in the potency or dosage of drugs, or a new method of drug ingestion, can often be a significant factor in sparking an epidemic of harmful use—take the broader availability of more potent spirits that catalyzed the English Gin Craze or the development of the machine-rolled cigarette in the late nineteenth century. In 1996, Purdue Pharma's patent on MS Contin (extended-release morphine) had run out, and the company introduced OxyContin: a sustained-release formulation of the inexpensive and already widely available generic oxycodone. The largest dosages were massive—as high as 80 milligrams and 160 milligrams, far above any of its competitors, like Percodan and Percocet. It wasn't just the aggressive marketing campaigns that sparked today's opioid overdose epidemic.

The hypodermic turned the slow burn of morphine problems into a raging fire. In Parisian hospitals, where some of the better records were kept, morphine prescriptions increased by more than thirty-six-fold from 1855 to 1875, from 272 to well over 10,000 grams yearly. In the United States, according to one historian's estimate, the number of people with opioid addiction increased sixfold from 1842 to the 1890s.

The Civil War itself compounded the problem. As a percentage of the total population, more than three times as many Americans were killed in the Civil War as in World War II, and more than thirteen times as many as in World War I. Morphine made this unthinkable devastation tolerable—not just for soldiers, but for others affected by the conflict. As one book of the time described it: "Maimed and shattered survivors from a hundred battle-fields, diseased and disabled soldiers released from hostile prisons, anguished and hopeless wives and mothers, made so by the slaughter of those who were dearest to them, have found, many of them, temporary relief from their sufferings in opium."

So it should be no surprise that for years, historians have explained the first American opioid epidemic as a consequence of the Civil War, both from that national trauma and from army doctors liberally giving out prescriptions of opium and morphine to traumatized war veterans. This explanation was so popular and widely accepted that opioid addiction was called "the army disease" or "the soldier's disease." But while the war was certainly a factor, there's evidence that even before the first shots were fired, the epidemic was already developing, and it was inspiring a nascent idea of habitual opium use as a kind of intemperance.

For one thing, there are Ludlow's own words in *The Hasheesh Eater* in 1857, where he had warned that "opium-eating in all countries is an immense and growing evil." The *New York Daily Times* and *Scientific American* also warned about the explosion in morphine use as early as the 1850s, and in May 1860 the former dean of Harvard Medical School, Oliver Wendell Holmes Sr., relayed a troubling observation to the Massachusetts Medical Society. A doctor practicing out west had written to Holmes about a disturbing new trend: some doctors were prescribing so many opioids that there was an outbreak of intemperance; you could see how bad the "frightful endemic demoralization" was by all the "opium-drunkards" shuffling through the town's streets.

Calls for caution intensified in the coming years. Ludlow's essay about opioids was published in an 1868 book, *The Opium Habit*, which anthologized several firsthand accounts of people "enthralled" with the "pernicious habit" and was one of the first books to call serious attention to opioid addiction. But doctors themselves, seized by technological optimism, were slow to catch on. Even after broader public recognition of the problem took hold, many physicians still believed (or at least advertised) that injected morphine was entirely safe and that only oral morphine was habit-forming.

These events follow a classic pattern of drug epidemics: a honeymoon period of uncritical use, only later followed by a backlash, much like the example of OxyContin in the 1990s and 2000s. In the mid-nineteenth century, the same sequences played out in the case of cocaine, after it was isolated in a more easily used alkaloid form. Cocaine was soon widely sold in casual, popularly available formulations—such as the French Vin Mariani, a "tonic beverage" that combined Bordeaux wine with the drug—and, especially in the deregulated medical marketplace of the United States, cocaine was an enormously popular addition to invigorating "tonics," decongestant snuffs, and other common products. Though no prescriptions were necessary, it was widely used as a medicine, too, recommended by doctors and druggists alike. Drug manufacturers promoted cocaine directly to physicians, and it was enthusiastically accepted as a treatment for everything from hay fever to the "morphia habit"—the honeymoon was over for opioids, and by the 1880s there was a large and desperate market for opioid addiction treatment. One doctor in Kentucky wrote proudly about how he had prescribed twenty-five pounds of coca extract in the span of two years to treat morphine and alcohol problems, and he included an account from a woman who said she had no more desire for morphine, but could she please get two more pounds? (He seems to have considered this a good thing.) Other physicians, though, were inclined to look more closely at the problem of addiction.

There were almshouses, workhouses, churches, lunatic asylums, and jails, but that was about it: treatment options for people with drug or alcohol problems were limited in the mid-nineteenth century, and there certainly wasn't anything like today's rehabs or other specialized treatment centers for addiction. At its conclusion, though, the book *The Opium Habit* called for a new therapeutic approach to addiction, including the establishment of a medical institution to treat "the opium disease," and it wouldn't be long before physicians answered the call. Temperance had failed to reform the intemperate drunkard, the Washingtonians had dissolved, and state laws prohibiting alcohol hadn't curbed drinking. The church, the law, and early mutual-help movements had all had their chance. It was medicine's turn, and as the medical profession gained in power and influence, it began turning its gaze toward the problem that was increasingly being called "inebriety."

In 1870, fourteen doctors met at the New York City YMCA to establish a new group, the American Association for the Cure of Inebriates (AACI), the first medical society devoted to the idea that drug and alcohol problems deserved to be treated like any other disease. The temperance movement had given society a *concept* of addiction—the drunkard narrative, the widely understood story of irresistible loss of control caused by drink and redeemable only through external forces—and now medicine was ready to step in to further disseminate that concept and offer itself up as a redeeming force. In the coming years, a broad-based "inebriety movement" spread, for the first time, the notion that addiction was a medical disease. Benjamin Rush, Thomas Trotter, and others had laid the intellectual groundwork, but there had never been a true mobilization of the medical profession like this one. It was an optimistic and even passionate movement. The dream was evident in the AACI's name: "Cure."

From that small beginning in 1870, papers and treatises issued forth against "drugs that enslave," reflecting and steadily spreading the recognition of inebriety as a medical problem. Bartholow's *Manual of Hypodermic Medication,* the key reference text of its time, devoted fewer than two pages to the "morphia habit" in its first two editions, in 1869 and 1873, but the same entry expanded to its own eighteen-page chapter in the 1879 edition, echoing Ludlow's 1857 warning in almost his exact words: "this abuse is becoming a gigantic evil." In 1877, Edward Levinstein, a German physician, wrote an influential paper on habitual morphine use as a disease, the first detailed medical treatise of its kind, prompting greater awareness of what was variously being called "morphinismus," "morphia-delirium," or "morphia evil."

Treatment options multiplied. In the 1860s, an energetic but arrogant physician named J. Edward Turner had opened the New York State Inebriate Asylum—a sumptuous neo-Gothic facility in Binghamton, equipped with bowling alleys, a 100,000-plant conservatory, "all the

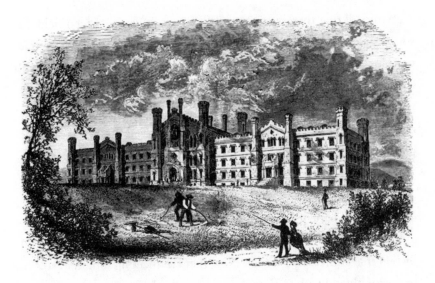

New York State Inebriate Asylum, 1882.

appliances of the Russian bath," and many more luxurious amenities. It catered predominantly to the rich and required advance payment for at least three months of treatment. It was the first of its kind in the world, a purpose-built medical facility solely for people with drug and alcohol problems, and other therapeutic institutions followed quickly behind. Six more "inebriate asylums" were built in the next decade, and by 1878 there were thirty-two in operation or planned. There were also "Washingtonian Homes" (inspired by the movement), which bear stronger resemblance to today's rehabs—they emphasized non-medical means of rehabilitation through structured daily life, discipline, moral and religious education, and mutual help. Also gaining traction was a religiously rooted "Gospel Temperance" movement—a grassroots evangelical Christian approach to reforming the drunkard, which developed both residential programs and mutual-help communities of "ribbon clubs." There was considerable overlap between these efforts. Though many nonprofessionals worked in the "homes" movement, experienced lay counselors from homes sometimes migrated to work in asylums, while asylums offered programming in moral and religious education.

Amid all that therapeutic activity, though, it was a divided field. Institutions jockeyed to position their treatment as the best and gain traction for their addiction theories. For an individual suffering with inebriety, it was hard to know how to make sense of the competing explanations. It wasn't clear how to think of the problem, where to get help, or even what counted as a legitimate medical problem—a battleground on which we still fight today.

My new patient Chris is guarded, even cagey. Over the phone, he was only willing to say that he was looking for help with an addiction that wasn't about drugs. Now that I'm meeting him in my office, he seems thoughtful, but barely contained: a lanky young man struggling to get each and every word right, fighting an urge to hide so that he can get the help he needs.

The story trickles out: porn. Newly engaged, he's worried about his sex life with his fiancée, but no matter what, almost every day he looks up porn on the internet. It's a delicate topic for anyone, let alone two guys in their early thirties in a small office in downtown Brooklyn, so I proceed slowly. Sometimes taking an addiction history is more like receiving a confession than gleaning mere information, and I try to communicate that I don't judge, knowing that this can serve as therapeutic in itself.

There's more. Chris has trouble limiting himself to his own porn collection, or to the mainstream sites. He feels driven toward novelty, and though he tries to resist this impulse, too, he often finds himself crossing a line and scrolling sketchy, unregulated online forums, looking for amateur porn that feels new and authentic to him. The search itself is intoxicating, sometimes taking up hours each day. This is dangerous, because even though he's not looking for revenge porn or anything with a hint of illegality, he has seen a lot of "horrible shit" by accident. Gore, bestiality, child porn. He says it's not at all what he's looking for, and I believe him. He clearly hates the cycle of searching that inevitably exposes him to those awful images. It feels like an addiction within an addiction: a time-obliterating fixation on porn coupled with a lottery-like drive for *more*.

He's tried blocking software, locking away his personal electronics in a kitchen safe with a timer, and other countermeasures to prevent his future self from crossing the line. But he can't seem to stop. One day, he orders a cheap laptop with same-day delivery, uses it for a search session, then destroys it and throws it in the trash.

He doesn't know what to do, what's wrong with him, or even whether to think of his struggle as an addiction at all.

In a medical context today, "addiction" implies substances, and it is only relatively recently that the field has been willing to consider whether behavioral addictions—sex, food, exercise, video games, or just the internet in general—qualify as "true" addictions. Only in 2013 did the editors of the *DSM*, the psychiatric diagnostic manual, reclassify "pathological gambling" as a "gambling disorder" and place it alongside substance addictions. Critics worry that we are over-pathologizing everyday life; a former editor of the *DSM* has said that behavioral addictions should not be labeled mental disorders "merely because we like doing them a lot and miss them when we stop."

What's missed in those debates is that these are not new addictions, but rather a reemergence of an older way of looking at addiction, dating from the inebriety movement of the late nineteenth century. The movement cast a wide net, and a variety of behavioral problems were understood as inebriety, including habitual problems with many substances: not just opioids, cocaine, alcohol, tea, coffee, hemp, and tobacco, but also things we'd consider food today, like chicory and lettuce (which was supposed to have mildly soothing properties). Writers frequently made reference to the addicting properties of other foods, and *The Journal of*

Inebriety, the flagship publication of the AACI, used the word "addiction" for the first time in reference to chocolate.

Medical thinkers were far more willing to reclassify behavioral problems as diseases as they became more interested in the old idea of "partial insanity"—a phenomenon of interest to Benjamin Rush, who had described in his later works how compulsive lying, stealing, and alcohol use could be classified as a "disease in the will." There was a rush of works about gambling as a medical problem, which was mirrored by increasing popular acceptance of what we consider gambling addiction today in works like Dostoevsky's *The Gambler* (1866) and Tchaikovsky's *Queen of Spades* (1890, itself based on an 1834 Pushkin story about a man obsessed with the game of faro). Sexual behaviors, too, were increasingly pathologized, culminating in the 1886 work of the Austro-German psychiatrist Richard von Krafft-Ebing, *Psychopathia Sexualis*.

Amid all that theorizing, though, the inebriety movement was marred by acrimonious infighting over treatment philosophies and methods. There was no coherent theory and no clear explanation—and more profiteering and individualism than organized advocacy or attempts to set up a true treatment response. It was not long overlooked that the epidemic of morphine and cocaine problems was caused by medical "progress" in the first place.

In a footnote to his *Confessions*, De Quincey bragged that only one man had exceeded him in opium use: likely a reference to his hero, Samuel Taylor Coleridge. Indeed, Coleridge did have a considerable opium problem—at one point, in an arrangement remarkably similar to today's sober companions, he paid a man to follow him around and block the doors of druggists. Unlike De Quincey, though, Coleridge saw his habit both as a problem for the medical profession to treat and specifically as the result of medical overprescribing; he lamented that he had been "seduced into the ACCURSED Habit ignorantly." The term

we use today for this type of explanation is "iatrogenic addiction"—
"iatrogenic" meaning a problem caused by medical treatment itself.
There are true victims of iatrogenic addiction, such as the people on the
receiving end of too-liberal prescriptions during our current opioid overdose epidemic, but the idea of iatrogenic addiction is also a convenient
and powerful narrative often deployed to make sense of the drug use of
privileged people.

During the late nineteenth century's opioid epidemic, medical and
popular writers alike raised the alarm about iatrogenic addiction. One
of the most popular accounts of opioid addiction was William Rosser
Cobbe's 1895 memoir *Doctor Judas*, in which he described how "medical
carelessness" with the loose use of opium, from "opium cordials" used to
quiet him as a baby to adult prescriptions for morphine, had trapped
him in "a nine years' slavery to opium." As cocaine became more widely
used, critics again blamed inattentive medical providers for spreading a
drug even worse than morphine. A key theme of these accounts was the
notion that middle- and upper-class drug users were the morally blameless victims of these new drugs and, perhaps more than that, victims of
the massive societal change underway.

Industrialization was rocketing forward at breakneck speed: U.S.
steel production shot past that of Great Britain and Germany combined,
railroad track increased from 35,000 to nearly 200,000 miles, and the
telegraph and telephone—not to mention widespread electrification—
were not far behind. Cities doubled in size or more, and a newly emergent middle class rushed to office and factory jobs. According to some
inebriety doctors, all that supposed progress was contributing to the
problem of inebriety.

Observing these emerging trends, George Miller Beard—a founding
member of the AACI and one of the country's most famous neurologists—
developed a theory of the "American disease" of "neurasthenia," a
disorder caused by the increasing complexity of modernity and one predominantly afflicting the middle and upper classes. According to Beard,

the profusion of information, the "flurry of in-door life," the fast-paced and competitive work, and the constant pressure of progress were over-loading the American brain, and this was the root cause of inebriety. He also speculated that women's brains were particularly weak and vulnera-ble, which was his explanation for why so many morphine "eaters" were women—fully 80 percent of the inebriate population in some towns. (These are the women of Eugene O'Neill's *Long Day's Journey into Night*—based on the morphine addiction of O'Neill's mother, which began around 1888 after she was indiscriminately prescribed morphine after a difficult childbirth.) Of course, the simpler explanation for this phenomenon is that doctors saw more female than male patients, and they treated women's symptoms aggressively with palliatives like opium, but the notion of supposed female infirmity was a better fit with social anxieties about progress.

Further evidence of the price of progress was the fact that doctors themselves were widely succumbing to the "great evil" of inebriety, an epidemic within the profession. (Though it was not widely known at the time, this was when the renowned surgeon William Halsted became addicted to cocaine, and later morphine, resulting from his own self-experimentation with the drugs.) In 1883, the noted American physician J. B. Mattison announced that the majority of people with habitual morphine problems were doctors, and another observer even claimed that doctors made up 90 percent of such "habitués." Spectacular stories proliferated of professionals' seduction and fall, such as one doctor who had taken the Keeley "Gold Cure" treatment ten times for alcoholism and four times for morphinism, only to relapse on fistfuls of cocaine, cannabis, and other drugs within easy reach. The clear subtext was that the drugs themselves *were* dangerous industrial products, the dark side of this era's Faustian bargain.

There cannot be a drug scare unless the stories being told about the drugs challenge something we value. American elites had long put great focus on self-determination and self-control, which is why drunkenness was so ominous to Americans like Benjamin Rush. Now it was even more ominous to see entirely new drugs sweeping the country and undermining those values, at the same time that modernity was causing such profound changes in daily life. The new industrialized economy demanded new heights of self-control and self-discipline, to the point that those attributes were enshrined as the height of middle-class virtue. Middle-class Americans thought drugs like morphine and cocaine would help them to cope with the emergent industrial order, but the drugs were actually undercutting those values.

For upper- and middle-class Americans, the reductionist narrative of neurasthenia helped to explain inebriety as the blameless result of societal and technological changes. Nevertheless, the therapeutic approach to addiction quickly lost steam. The inebriety movement, burdened by a profusion of theories and explanations for addiction, as well as the back-biting and competition, began a remarkably rapid decline in the closing years of the century. In 1893, one influential member of the AACI noted that of the first fifty institutions, only thirty were left standing, and most were not doing a good job of it. Some inebriate asylums had been chartered but never opened, and others were converted to general insane asylums before a single patient walked in the doors.

Another force was on the rise: anti-vice activism, a broad-based campaign against what reformers saw as a huge range of social misbehaviors, including prostitution, sexually transmitted infections, obscenity, pornography, crime, gambling, corruption, and, of course, the non-medical use of alcohol and drugs. Their solution to this crisis of modernity was not treatment, but restraint and punishment. Moral reformers were bold about their perspective on the new disease of inebriety, as seen in the straightforward title of the 1882 book *Drunkenness a Vice, Not a Disease.* The therapeutic approach was all well and good when inebriety was an upper-class concern, but increasingly, the problem seemed to implicate the wrong kinds of users, and with them in mind, prohibition was on the march.

Six

JUNKIES

In 1839, a few workers in Guangzhou, China, were given an odd assignment: to haul opium to the middle of town so it could be destroyed. Guangzhou was a crucial port city near the head of the Pearl River Delta, more than ninety miles inland from the South China Sea, and it was the epicenter of a tense trade standoff. The British wanted to force Chinese markets open to opium imports, which the Chinese government had sought to ban. As tensions escalated, the Chinese government maneuvered to seize all of the unwanted foreign drug in the region, which they now planned to eradicate. The laborers carried baskets full of opium to a set of massive trenches, protected by a wall of bamboo stakes and crisscrossed by planks on top. Day after day, they carefully walked out onto the planks, where they stamped the opium balls into pieces and kicked them into the water below. Workers dumped salt and limestone on top, and others down below mixed it together with seawater in a briny mess, which was then flushed out into the river. The whole process took weeks, and in the end they destroyed millions of pounds of confiscated opium.

Later that year, two enormous British warships opened fire on several Chinese war junks, sinking three, blowing two more entirely to smithereens, and showing that the British were prepared to use their superior firepower to get their way. In the ensuing Opium Wars, indiscriminate bombing killed thousands of Chinese soldiers and civilians. China capitulated and was forced to pay a huge indemnity to the British. This left the country impoverished and politically destabilized, on the brink of total ruin. There were no jobs. There wasn't even food. People were starving by the millions.

In the nineteenth century, the destruction wrought by the Opium Wars was one of several interrelated and powerful forces fueling Chinese immigration to the United States, along with a peasant revolt, rampant inflation, and Western pressure on the Chinese government to relax its emigration policies. Chinese laborers traveled abroad in search of economic opportunity, especially to the American West, to participate in the Gold Rush, and though many of those pioneers were free, a significant number came to the United States with onerous debt contracts, which forced them into a system of virtual slavery. Responding to the hunger for workers, Chinese immigrants died by the thousands on the difficult passage to the United States. Once there, from backwoods mining towns to urban metropolises, Chinese people collected in "Chinatowns," sometimes the only places where they were allowed to live.

Chinese workers were often lonely and bored young men in a foreign land, forced into mind-numbing, low-paid, and dangerous work: digging mines, completely remodeling the land for agriculture, and building the first great transcontinental railroads in the United States and Canada. In Chinatowns, opium smoking became a popular form of recreation for these dislocated and stressed men. Smoking opium helped laborers to get by (while also serving the labor system well by keeping a laborer pacified, eating up his wages, and impairing his ability to pay off his debts). Not all suffered from what we would call addiction. But as anti-immigrant sentiment grew, especially after a sharp economic depression in the 1870s, Chinatowns, and opium dens in particular, became the focus of concerns about labor competition and dangerous drug use. Perversely, Chinese immigrants, so many of whom were driven to

America by the Opium Wars, themselves became the focus of a drug scare about opium.

In the late nineteenth century, inebriety didn't remain an upper-class malady for long. A frightening and ultimately much more powerful story was emerging about how dangerous drug users—the wrong *kinds* of drug users—were driving epidemics and ruining society. As the modernizing world brought people and cultures together, racism and nationalism inspired intense fears—fears that in turn became enmeshed with ideas about addiction.

Stigma is often cited as the biggest obstacle we face to a compassionate response to addiction—the reason we still have a segregated and grossly insufficient addiction treatment system and why we have yet to respond adequately to the decades-old opioid epidemic. That stigma has often been more about the people using the drugs than about the drugs themselves, especially during the moral panics of the late nineteenth century, from which many of those negative attitudes and beliefs originated. Stereotypes about vicious and morally culpable users formed the prototype for stigmatized portrayals of drug users and addiction: dangerous, indolent, contagious, irredeemable, and addicted by choice.

There is considerable overlap between the intellectual history of addiction and the broader cultural history of drug policy, and the governing image of addiction is often revealed in policy responses to drugs. Especially since this era, these threads have been closely intertwined, if not inextricable. The drug scares beginning in the late nineteenth century culminated in national systems of prohibition and created a divide between good and bad drugs that has remained with us ever since.

In Chinese immigrant communities, what was called an opium "den" was usually more akin to a Chinese social club, where people enjoyed opium smoking and other activities such as gambling. However, there were also low-end dens catering to working-class people with meager

resources, and these were the ones that formed the early American stereotype of opium smoking and became a target of anti-Chinese sentiment. Reporters ventured into opium dens and returned with stories of
Chinese people laid out on filthy beds or in dirty rooms, seemingly ruined by the drug or turned into a fiend by it, or perhaps both—regardless,
opium was increasingly portrayed as the root of all the vice allegedly
located in Chinatowns. These menacing portrayals were entangled
with the growing anti-Chinese attitudes in the United States. In journalism and politics, the Chinese were described as an invading presence
taking jobs and ruining cities amid a rapidly changing economy and
cityscape. The stereotypical opium den, and the opium inside, perfectly
encapsulated that fear of contagion: a frighteningly exotic place full of
unsavory, dangerous characters, all using a drug that threatened to infect the rest of society. Riots broke out all across the West, and mobs
burned Chinatowns to the ground and committed outright murder.
Chinese people, often operating out of opium dens, soon became the
favored stock villain for pulp novels and penny magazines. (In the novels, they seemed to have a particular penchant for seducing and kidnap-
ping white women.)

English society experienced a similar panic in the last decades of the
century. Dickens's unfinished 1870 novel *The Mystery of Edwin Drood*
marks the beginning of this melodramatic representation of opium as
invading, seducing, and ruining white society. The choirmaster John
Jasper is turned into a despicable, lustful, and possibly murderous
habitué by the corrupting force of Chinese opium. (The very first scene
of the book has him stumbling out of an opium den.) The message was
clear: even upstanding middle-class stock could be corrupted.

Nowhere was this opium drug scare stronger than in the United
States, though, where the latter years of the nineteenth century marked
the advent of the Progressive Era. Increasingly fervent reformers set
about suppressing vices like gambling, prostitution, sexually transmitted
infections, crime, and of course alcohol and drug use. These moral

crusaders were responding to real problems caused by industrialization and urbanization. In particular, many women were taking a central role in the movement for alcohol temperance—now a movement for full-on alcohol prohibition—because of their experience of the trauma, abuse, and abandonment caused by alcohol (sometimes combined with populist anticapitalism directed against liquor companies). However, the arc of many reformers' activism, especially activism relating to alcohol and other drugs, increasingly bent toward repressive prohibition.

Reformers often drew rhetorical fodder from medicine to support their prohibitionist leanings. Around this time, the new science of microbiology was enrapturing the medical field, revealing a hidden world underlying formerly mysterious diseases. In 1882, the German microbiologist Robert Koch reported that tuberculosis was caused by a bacterium, not inherited, as was previously believed, and two decades later other researchers identified the bacterium *Treponema pallidum* as the true cause of syphilis—an infection once called "the great imitator" for its ability to cause far-flung symptoms in different bodily systems. Yet the public health efforts related to these discoveries were infused with moral judgments. Because of its associations with sex and the lower classes, syphilis in particular captivated the imaginations of anti-vice reformers, who made binary distinctions between guilty and innocent sufferers: sex workers, the deplorable sources of the disease's spread, were punished and quarantined, but wives with syphilis were labeled blameless and given treatment. (Presumably, no one asked where the husbands had picked it up.) Progressive Era reformers similarly divided the poor into the "worthy" and "unworthy": widows and orphans were given charity, but the supposedly unworthy were blamed for their own bad decisions. Soon, certain drug users were consigned to that latter category, and their association with Chinese immigrants only added to the moral condemnation.

There was a widening gap between the right and wrong kinds of users: namely, medical versus "recreational" use. At the same time that

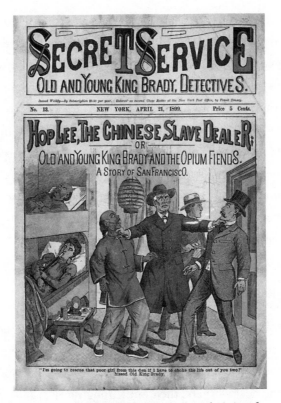

"Hop Lee, The Chinese Slave Dealer," one depiction of
Chinese villainy from an 1899 pulp fiction magazine.

opioid use in the white population was being classified as a medical
problem—as "accidental" drug users who had been led into iatrogenic
opioid addiction by unscrupulous or incompetent physicians—a different set of negative accounts depicted Chinese opium use as non-medical
and more fit for social control. These depictions ushered in the American prototype for non-medical drug use as a degraded, dangerous, and
contagious form of substance use. Journalists denounced opium smoking and its association with Chinese immigrants, calling the practice an
"Asiatic vice," one "rooted and grounded in the Chinese character."
Opium smoking was condemned as self-indulgent, unlike morphine,
with its purportedly medical uses, even though they were merely

different ways of using the same drug. (Also consider that medical indications for morphine at that time included insomnia, anxiety, overwork, masturbation, and "female complaints.") Moral associations also drove responses to addiction treatment: people having problems with morphine injections or opium preparations were largely diagnosed with the disease of inebriety and given compassionate care, while physicians and other commentators denounced opium smoking as a purposeless vice entered into voluntarily and therefore the fault of the user. Cities passed a spate of prohibitionist laws, not against opium but against opium *dens*. The importation of opium for smoking was banned outright in 1909, the first federal "exclusion act" aimed at a substance.

The same story repeated itself over and over again. In the American South, in the busy ports of the Gulf Coast, newly emancipated Black Americans working hard at menial labor were among the first to encounter the invigorating properties of cocaine. Cocaine spread among New Orleans dockworkers, then out through a distribution system of railway personnel, shoeshine boys, porters, bellhops, and other service workers. In time, the myth of the "Negro cocaine fiend" followed.

Though most people at the time considered cocaine a relatively benign drug, no worse than tea or coffee, the story changed when the users were Black Americans. One pharmacist testified before the House of Representatives that cocaine made Black people physically strong, morally weak, temporarily insane, grandiose, confident, and prone to commit rape. It is a classic racist trope that some bodies receive drugs differently—recall the "firewater myths" about Native Americans and alcohol—and in this case, the supposed special effects of cocaine on Black bodies invoked all of the greatest fears of white America. A media frenzy about "cocainized" Blacks painted lurid and frightening scenes about murder and sex. One official reportedly said, "The cocaine [n——] is sure hard to kill." In response to a myth that cocaine made

Black people invulnerable to .32 caliber bullets, many police departments switched to the .38 Special, the standard cartridge of most police departments for decades to come.

The cocaine story is particularly striking because, unlike opium smoking, cocaine was widely used by huge swaths of the population. Everywhere you looked, people were taking cocaine to dull the pain of crushing labor—not just stevedores in the South but also miners in the West and textile mill workers in the Northeast. Cocaine was on the rise in general, in fact, because it was being widely manufactured and promoted by early pharmaceutical companies as a topical anesthetic and general cure-all. But in the Jim Crow era, stories about deviant drug users played to the racist stereotypes of violent and sexually aggressive Blacks as well as the racist notion that Black Americans were especially vulnerable to the drug.

In the late-nineteenth-century South, the move to regulate drugs was completely intertwined with efforts to control Black people. Cities passed ordinances restricting the sale of cocaine. Police cracked down on Black users, at a time when police forces, prisons, and the general criminalization of Blackness were expanding rapidly. From 1880 to 1910, the southern convict population grew ten times faster than the rate of overall population growth, largely from mass Black incarceration. The dangers posed by Black men became a key justification for regulating cocaine: the chief of detectives for the Memphis police force claimed that cocaine's effects were "much more violent than that of whiskey" and described how cocaine threw its users into a "wild frenzy." The narrative was remarkably effective at stigmatizing the drug: in 1910, President William H. Taft told Congress that cocaine was the most serious drug problem the nation had ever faced.

Similar "drug fiend" associations drove negative stereotypes of heroin users. Heroin was first widely produced on a commercial scale in 1898, by the Bayer company, and initially praised as a safe, modern alternative to morphine. As this claim was swiftly disproven and non-medical use in cities grew, and especially as local restrictions made other drugs like cocaine harder to obtain, physicians and reformers began to describe a new kind of heroin user. The stereotypical portrait of heroin addiction of the time became a poor teenager, often of immigrant parents, unintelligent, greedy, and rude, and increasingly joining forces with others like him in the new urban phenomenon of menacing "gangs."

Racist and classist stereotypes widened the gap between the right and wrong kinds of use: namely, medical versus non-medical. In a self-fulfilling prophecy, unequally applied prohibitionist restrictions intensified the division. In reaction to these drug scares, medical providers controlled access much more tightly, which pushed people with fewer resources toward smaller, informal markets in vice districts—poorer, racially mixed urban neighborhoods where authorities segregated gambling, prostitution, saloons, and other disapproved trades. Substances of all sorts were always more available to the "doctor-visiting class" with more resources, but poor urban drug users had to go through non-medical channels like street peddlers.

It's notable that this was the era in which the word "addiction" was first widely used, because it was also the era when so much racist stigma was attached to the condition. To this day, white people are called "unlikely addicts," the victims of bad drugs that have spread to white suburban or rural communities, and human-interest stories profile football captains and cheerleaders, asking, as if in a horror movie, "Why is this happening?"

Likewise, during the drug scares of the late nineteenth century, a series of popular addiction memoirs, case histories, and journalistic accounts told sensationalistic stories of middle-class users turned into dangerous lower life forms by drugs. One opium user told a physician in 1881, "Truly, the name 'fiend' is aptly used. It will make a villain of the best of men." This vision of addiction was a dire threat to what it meant

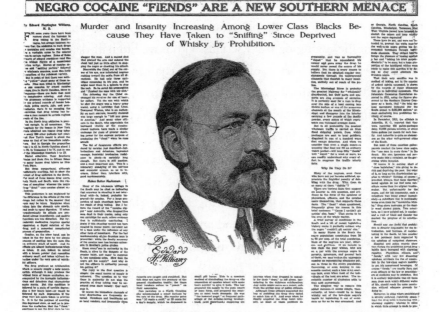

Fearful press coverage of Black cocaine users, *The New York Times*, 1914.

to be a respectable American. Increasingly, it seemed, the only answer was outright prohibition.

During my intern year, one of the New York tabloids published a vicious article about one of our regular patients. Francisco was a grizzled, homeless Dominican man who swept the sidewalk in front of a bodega for a little extra cash, then spent the rest of the day drinking cheap liquor on the corner. More nights than not—sometimes five or six times a week—he'd call 911 and report chest pains, and an ambulance would take him to the hospital, where he'd sleep it off. The article called him a "bum" who was "mooching off Medicaid," and estimated his annual cost to the system at hundreds of thousands of dollars.

We forwarded the article around and talked about how it was sad to see him painted as some sort of devious cheat who was gaming the system. He was obviously deeply troubled. No one would consciously choose that life, swinging from serious withdrawal to half-dead intoxication, sleeping on the street or upright in a chair in the brightly lit and chaotic ER. Outwardly, I said all these things to my co-residents, about how villainizing him wouldn't help. On the inside, though, there was a part of me that just didn't care anymore.

When I started intern year, I saw the experience as a tremendous privilege. Every day on the long train ride uptown, I pored over medical journals and clinical guidelines, trying to do right by my patients. I thought of myself as one of the good ones, someone more awake to and tolerant of the structural problems in medicine. In medical school, I had helped to start a free clinic for homeless people and taught a seminar about the social determinants of homelessness. And yet, in the constant grind of intern year, with my drinking getting worse and in the face of a seemingly endless parade of intractable problems, I started to lose hope. Gangrenous feet from diabetes. Occluded cardiac arteries from unhealthy diets. Torn esophagi, battered pancreases, and life-threatening withdrawal from alcohol. People just kept going out and eating harmful foods and relapsing. The problems seemed impossible, and I didn't seem to be helping anyone. I just wanted it all to end. I stopped reading. I stopped caring. Then I even stopped getting in on time.

Some portion of this feeling was burnout: the existential dread and moral injury of participating in a broken medical system, plus the simple exhaustion of months of crushing call schedules and frantic twenty-four-hour shifts. But a good portion of it was my drinking, and I was getting scared.

I was increasingly showing up late to work. Midday, hungover, I'd wake up to concerned calls telling me that I was supposed to be in the ER for a shift. I'd rush downstairs and catch a cab, chewing gum and chugging water on the ride uptown, hoping they couldn't smell last night's whiskey on me.

I struggled through to the second year: the beginning of the psychiatric residency proper. Now that I was done with general medicine and training for what I actually wanted to do, I told myself, my problems would get better. I was really, truly looking forward to it. Then, on the first day, I slept straight through the orientation session, waking up with a throbbing headache, sunlight slanting ominously through the window. I bolted from my bed to see tons of missed calls on my phone, my pager sadly chirping away next to it with worried messages asking where I was.

A few days later, the chief resident pulled me aside in the hallway to give me a warning. Everyone had noticed all the chronic lateness and unexplained absences. He told me to be careful and to pull it together. If I kept being so unreliable, I'd fall under greater "scrutiny." I tried to laugh it off as the fault of an unreliable subway system—maybe I shouldn't have moved ten miles downtown, ha ha. He looked back, stone-faced, and suggested that I was a doctor now, and I could come in a little earlier and get a jump on my work for the day. As he walked away, I resolved to try harder, but I also worried that it might be impossible, that I might be a hopeless case.

In July 1989, a Florida woman named Jennifer Johnson made legal history by becoming the first woman convicted for "delivering" drugs to her own infants. For the first few moments after the births of her son and daughter, the argument went, she had transferred cocaine to them through the umbilical cord. Johnson, who had no prior convictions and had sought treatment for crack addiction earlier in her pregnancies, was sentenced to one year of house arrest and fourteen years of probation.

The country was in an uproar about "crack babies": infants who, according to provocative research reports, were born with severe emotional, mental, and physical disabilities after being exposed to cocaine in the womb. During the crack scare, more than two hundred women nationwide—most of whom were Black—were charged with various crimes for using drugs while pregnant. Later research showed that the simplistic label "crack babies" obscured the stronger contributions of poverty: homelessness, lack of medical care, poor nutrition, abuse, and trauma accounted for most of the observed disabilities. But the story of crack babies played perfectly to the crack scare, and even more, it tapped into older fears about the power of drug use to corrupt heredity itself; to create, in the words of one columnist, a "bio-underclass, a generation of physically damaged cocaine babies whose biological inferiority is stamped at birth."

These fears had been at their apex a hundred years earlier, when the science of addiction was dominated by the idea of "degeneration," the late-nineteenth-century idea that vices like heavy drinking could cause madness in future generations. Reformers worried that inebriate women were bringing droves of "mentally useless children" into the world, who would in time become "the future criminal, drunken, and lunatic army." Francis Galton himself, who had coined the term "eugenics," warned that "the fluids in an habitual drunkard's body, and all the secretions, are tainted with alcohol; consequently the unborn child of such a woman must be an habitual drunkard." This idea was scientifically outdated by the time of the Progressive Era, but a reductionist narrative was easily co-opted to fit the prejudices of the time. As society struggled, and failed, to meet the challenge of addiction, reformers and physicians alike decided that the problem was hopeless.

Degeneration theory painted a dire picture of the biological roots of vice. It asserted that a host of vices could imprint themselves on biology and transmit negative characteristics to future generations, in a sinister process of de-evolution. It was a massively influential idea in its time. Émile Zola wrote a twenty-novel cycle, *Les Rougon-Macquart*, to trace how one family's appetites and vices led to sexual depravity, incest, murder, and insanity down the generations, and there are echoes of the same themes in Thomas Hardy's *Tess of the d'Urbervilles* and Henrik Ibsen's *Ghosts*. Bram Stoker's 1897 *Dracula* draws heavily on degeneration and name-checks the trendiest eugenic science of the day, such as the criminologist Cesare Lombroso, to explain how Dracula lacks a full "man-brain" and is biologically predestined to his criminal behavior. The theme of degeneration was also a way to express nationalist and racist concerns about threats to civilization; notably, Dracula is also a blood-sucking immigrant from Transylvania who parasitizes English society while he spreads the undead curse. (Likewise, at several points in Robert Louis Stevenson's *Strange Case of Dr. Jekyll and Mr. Hyde,* Hyde is described as "ape-like.") Anti-vice reformers described a frightening cycle that would cause nothing less than the collapse of civilization: vices caused degeneration, and the resulting degenerates would engage in even worse vices, including criminality, insanity, homosexuality, and of course alcohol and opioid problems.

The result of this ominous portrayal, combined with the outright failure of medicine to help those with addiction, was a creeping sense of pessimism about the problem. By the closing years of the nineteenth century, for all the efforts of the American Association for the Cure of Inebriates, medical science had failed to accomplish much at all, and instead the marketplace was crowded with shoddy "miracle cures." People made fortunes, but the therapeutic approach appeared to have done nothing for vice. The optimism of the inebriety movement died out— the association even struck "Cure" from its name—and many inebriety doctors abandoned therapeutic responses for prohibition. One of the group's members, concerned about the apparently unremitting flow of opium, asked if it was time to "throw up some wall . . . around our beleaguered city, that shall more effectually shield us against those noxious invaders that are, year by year, floated to our shores from the lands of the prolific Orient?"

Inebriate asylums became places for quarantining hopeless cases rather than reformation. Some doctors pushed for "inebriate colonies" where people could be incarcerated indefinitely, perhaps for the rest of their lives, so as not to corrupt future generations. Eugenics demanded they go a step further: alongside tens of thousands of people with intellectual disabilities and other mental illnesses, many people with addiction were sterilized. In the absence of a satisfying medical explanation or viable therapy, the only possible response seemed to be prohibition.

I n August 1902, Bishop Charles Henry Brent, later called "one of the most intrepid and gallant ambassadors of Christ the world has known," arrived in Manila as the first Episcopal missionary bishop to the Philippines. He was appalled to find the islands flush with opium. For more than fifty years, Spain had kept opium use under relative control with a regulated monopoly on sales, but in the process of taking control of the islands during the Spanish-American War, the United States had unleashed years of guerrilla warfare. Amid the chaos, opium imports flooded the territory. The resulting widespread drug use, Brent thought, was a dire threat to the souls of his new charges.

The new governor general of the Philippines (and future president) William Howard Taft wanted to reinstate a monopoly of opium sales to provide a regular, regulated supply, but Brent and other religious leaders were aghast. Brent had traveled across the Pacific to spread Western values and fight vice, not to enable the sale of an enslaving toxin—and of all the vices, Brent considered opium "the greatest evil in Filipino society." Brent and other reformers protested Taft's proposal. The government caved and banned opium outright. It was the birth of the international movement for modern drug prohibition.

Brent threw himself into work against the "drug problem," soon becoming the president of a 1909 opium meeting in Shanghai—the first international conference on drug control. A physician named Hamilton Wright was there with him, and before audiences first in Shanghai and then in The Hague, Brent and Wright inveighed at length about the anti-vice perspective on addiction: drugs were powerful, automatically addicting, and evil, so the only sensible policy measure was a total ban.

(An observer described the Americans as "direct, idealistic, uncompromising, and unpopular.") Other countries weren't ready to adopt the American perspective, but fatefully, Wright went home to the States to lobby for domestic anti-drug laws.

Wright was a forceful, ideologically driven man unencumbered by any felt need to stick to the facts. He readily resorted to racial scare tactics to win over lawmakers—for example, emphasizing the dangers of Black cocaine users to white women. He played fast and loose with statistics to inflate the risks of lower-class and criminal use, claiming a whopping 25 percent rate of addiction among the Chinese American population, followed closely by a rate of 22 percent among "unfortunate women and their hangers-on." In a favorable 1911 profile in *The New York Times* (Wright was described as "earnest, energetic, nervous and magnetic"), he reported that, "of all the nations of the world, the United States consumes most habit-forming drugs per capita," especially opium, "the most pernicious drug known to humanity." The headline screamed, UNCLE SAM IS THE WORST DRUG FIEND IN THE WORLD.

Wright's bogus statistics were contradicted by those from careful researchers, but from a political standpoint his approach was highly effective, and Wright set the tone and the strategy for generations of anti-drug prohibitionists. Despite concerted opposition from pharmaceutical companies, which were benefiting greatly from the deregulated market, Wright slowly built a consensus for drug prohibition. There was also hesitation to allow federal law to extend so far into the regulation of medical practice, a matter that was traditionally left to the states, but stories about Black and poor drug users helped alleviate worries about the constitutionality of a federal drug ban. After years of Wright's tireless campaigning, Congress passed an anti-drug law: the 1914 Harrison Narcotics Tax Act.

The Harrison Act, though, was a complex beast. It was a roundabout form of prohibition: it didn't ban drugs outright but rather regulated the production, importation, and sale of opioids and cocaine (now labeled with the term "narcotics"). People who sold those drugs had to register and pay a tax, so possession without registration—or, for the general public, without a prescription—made people presumptively guilty. Even so, it was a questionable move, legally speaking, to use the power of the Treasury as a backdoor move to criminalize drug possession. Even more confusing—and more dubious—was the question of what it meant for medical practice.

J in Fuey Moy was not a sympathetic character, especially considering the racial attitudes of the time. One of the first Chinese Americans to graduate from medical school, he had been arrested multiple times—first for eloping with an underage white woman, then for smuggling Chinese laborers into the United States. More recently, Moy had been writing morphine prescriptions to addicted people, and his practice was shady, to say the least. After a superficial examination, or no examination at all, he would prescribe huge quantities of morphine (up to sixteen drams at a time, which is a bit more than twenty-eight grams, the usual starting dose being around fifteen *milli*grams), and he charged patients not by the visit but by the quantity of drug.

Yet, though this practice certainly seems questionable, it wasn't quite clear what the Harrison Act allowed in terms of prescribing opioids. Technically, the law still allowed doctors to prescribe normally, "in the course of his professional practice only," and many physicians continued to write opioid prescriptions for people with addiction—whether they were shady "scrip doctors" who sold opioids by the pound or conscientious providers who carefully prescribed consistent, regulated doses. Prohibitionist federal prosecutors conflated these practices, and they wrote new enforcement regulations claiming that all opioid prescriptions for people with addiction were illegal unless part of a plan to wean down to abstinence. Their justification hinged on the question of whether addiction was a disease—their argument was that it was *not*, and so, necessarily, prescribing any opioids to people with addiction was not legitimate medical practice. It was a stunning reinterpretation, one that morphed a law for the orderly regulation of medicines into a total prohibition against prescriptions for addiction, no matter what the physicians said or believed. Individual physicians were no longer able to exercise professional judgment, and the medical profession as a whole no longer got to determine the nature of disease. Federal prosecutors led an all-out assault, pursuing convictions for huge numbers of physicians and patients. Many fought back, but even when the physicians won, the publicity often ruined their careers.

The first case to hit the Supreme Court was Jin Fuey Moy's. The prosecutors targeted both Dr. Moy and one of his patients, to try to make it a crime merely to possess the drug. They failed—the court ruled that Congress had never intended to give prosecutors that much power—and in 1916, Moy and his patient were both exonerated.

The next year, the United States entered World War I, and intolerant nationalism and anti-vice fervor reached its peak, helping to accelerate campaigns for prohibition. Now led by the Anti-Saloon League, an even more aggressive organization than the Women's Christian Temperance Union, the alcohol prohibition movement increased its focus on the idea that alcohol was an enslaving toxin closely associated with the "foreign invasion of undeveloped races." (German Americans, once a powerful force against alcohol prohibition, were essentially sidelined.) Racist and anti-immigrant panics were in fact central motivators throughout all of the temperance movement for alcohol prohibition, from anti-Catholic panics in the 1840s and the stereotypes of drunken Irishmen to the more general anti-immigrant and nativist sentiment of the late nineteenth century to this early-twentieth-century alcohol prohibition movement—which not only was supported by the KKK but actually helped to revive the Klan.

The war also brought the 1918 influenza pandemic. As the fatal disease spread from town to town, local officials told the public not to worry, but people watched as their friends and family members died horrible deaths. It was a fearful time in America. At the close of the war, Americans were terrified by the success of the Russian Revolution, and at home in the States, during the first "Red Scare," Bolsheviks and anarchists were added to a growing list of threatening minorities. Drug use, already associated with degeneracy and vice, became indefensible— even alcohol prohibition, once a very hard sell, was starting to look feasible.

By 1919, the stage was set for Prohibition. The states ratified a constitutional amendment prohibiting the production, transport, and sale of alcohol throughout the nation, and the government transferred authority for narcotics enforcement to a well-funded home, the Narcotics Division, within the new Prohibition Unit. The United States also finally succeeded in exporting international drug prohibition in a series of drug treaties, just as it had catalyzed an international temperance movement. And a crucial pair of cases about the prescription of opioids to people with addiction reached the Supreme Court. Only three years after *United States v. Jin Fuey Moy,* a very different court decided 5–4 against prescribing opioids to people with addiction. In *Webb et al. v. United States,* the majority opinion wrote curtly that a prescription for morphine not for the "attempted cure of the habit" but simply for "maintaining his customary use" was so obviously a perversion of medical care "that no discussion of the subject is required." In a barely three-page-long opinion, the court had vastly expanded the scope of the Harrison Act and seemingly outlawed an entire domain of medical practice. Jin Fuey Moy, who had never stopped his scrip mill, was once again dragged into the Supreme Court in 1920, this time losing and serving two years in prison.

Prohibition had fully arrived. Would it work? Some people call the American experiment with prohibiting alcohol a success, because it *might* have reduced the rates of consumption and lowered medical complications from alcohol. For years afterward, rates of cirrhosis and other liver diseases did drop appreciably, but even the conclusion that Prohibition caused that decrease is disputed, as there was already a downward trend in drinking before its imposition. Prohibition also increased binge drinking and caused widespread injuries from the use of illegal alcohol, as well as injuries caused by poisons that were required to be added to industrial alcohol. Looking at the harms beyond medicine, the cost of Prohibition was high indeed. Crime and violence exploded. Enforcement of Prohibition restrictions was grossly inequitable. People lost respect for the law. Even the Right Reverend Brent had his doubts, and later in his life questioned the wisdom of alcohol prohibition.

The costs of drug prohibition were also high. The black market flourished: numerous poppy fields sprung up in northwest Mexico in the 1920s. On the eve of the enactment of the Harrison Act, drug users panicked and ran out to buy drugs. In major urban centers, the street price of opioids went sky-high. With supply restricted, people turned to potent forms of administration, encouraging drug users to inject intravenously. This is a version of what drug policy activists call the "iron law of prohibition": as law enforcement gets more intense, people will naturally gravitate toward stronger forms of the drug ("the harder the enforcement, the harder the drugs"). The examples of this law are legion. Earlier in the current opioid epidemic, clamping down on access to prescription opioids pushed people to heroin, and then, when law enforcement cracked down on that supply, it encouraged a shift to the even more powerful, easily trafficked, and more deadly fentanyl.

Beyond the immediate effects of drug prohibition, the Harrison Act also created something entirely new: a fundamental legal division between different types of psychoactive drugs. It reflected, reinforced, and intensified the racially driven division between the right and wrong kinds of users, and thus created a novel, formal division between the right and wrong kinds of drugs. It effectively prohibited "narcotics" (i.e., non-medical opioids and cocaine, drugs associated with minorities and the poor) while allowing for a regulated market of "medicines" (i.e., substances associated with white, middle-class users). In time, this would prove to be an enormously significant division. In the meantime, a crucial question remained about the use of these drugs, and who exactly got access to them.

Even into the 1920s, serious questions remained about the legality of prescribing opioids to people with addiction. The practice was outlawed for regular medical providers, but physicians sympathetic to the treatment of addiction hoped that organized, public "maintenance treatment" might be allowed to take its place. The U.S. Public Health Service had recommended this measure, and soon cities and towns from New Orleans to the Eastern Seaboard set up roughly one dozen "narcotic clinics" to dispense opioids to people with addiction. A significant public backlash ensued: magazines were full of sensationalistic accounts of vice districts springing up around the clinics, with peddlers roaming adjacent streets and patients using drugs in nearby parks. In New York, patients had to queue up in long lines outside the clinic, and they were regularly harassed by the blaring megaphones of sightseeing buses chock-full of tourists. Officials in the Narcotics Division went after the clinics with a combination of inspections, legal pressure, and outright threats, and many of the clinics caved. (This meant a crackdown on urban users, of course, not those in the white, less urban areas, where a gray market of morphine thrived.) It was essentially the death of community-based addiction treatment in the United States. From the 1910s to 1938, more than 25,000 physicians were reported, 2,000 paid substantial fines, and 3,000 went to prison—and not all of those were bad "scrip doctors."

The hovering threat of law enforcement imbued the clinical encounter around addiction with a sense of mutual distrust that has persisted to this day. Prescribing opioids such as buprenorphine or methadone for addiction is labeled "maintenance," implying something that is not quite therapeutic. Physicians are subject to extra scrutiny and law enforcement surveillance of those prescriptions. Any other kind of improper prescribing can of course be regulated—such as benzodiazepines like Xanax or stimulants like Adderall—but to this day, opioids stand apart.

At that point in the early 1920s, despite all the prohibitionist prosecutorial pressure, the legal status of addiction treatment was still hazy. In one 1922 case, the Supreme Court decided that "maintenance" treatment with high doses was illegal on its face, because relying on the patient's own "weakened and perverted will" to manage his medications could only result in "gratification of a diseased appetite for these pernicious drugs." But in a 1925 case, *Linder v. United States*, the court decided instead that it was acceptable to give someone with addiction "moderate amounts" of medications in order to relieve the symptoms of addiction, as long as it was part of regulated and careful professional practice. This was an extraordinarily important ruling, and one that was deliberately overlooked for years. Prescribing opioids for people with addiction wasn't truly illegal, but prosecutors just continued acting as if it was, effectively banning it through misinformation and brute force.

The medical profession might have done more to fight for maintenance treatment, or generally for a therapeutic approach to addiction, but physicians themselves were taking a harsher view of the problem. They had long been undecided—back in 1876, the American Medical Association had passed a resolution saying inebriety was both a disease and a vice, and likewise, a Treasury Department survey from 1919 found that physicians were almost evenly split on whether addiction was a "disease" or a "vice." Even those who treated people with addiction were divided on whether indefinite maintenance treatment was appropriate practice. In 1920, though, the AMA took the "vice" side of the debate and opposed maintenance treatment. By the end of the 1920s, it was publishing the names of physicians convicted for providing such treatment. The association's Committee on the Narcotic Drug Situation issued a report that "emphatically condemned" maintenance treatment, and in a follow-up article that drips with sarcasm and mockery, one of the committee's members declared, "The shallow pretense that drug addiction is 'a disease' which the specialist must be allowed to 'treat,' which pretended treatment consists in supplying its victims with the drug that has caused their physical and moral debauchery . . . has been asserted and urged in volumes of 'literature' by self-styled 'specialists.'"

Medical views on the core problem of addiction were in disarray, and overly reductionist explanations hurt more than they helped. A massive review of theories about opioid addiction published in 1928, *The Opium Problem*, summarized four thousand competing studies, ranging from hormone abnormalities to psychological and psychoanalytic ideas to "crystals in blood." As the authors themselves identified, when it came to the medical understanding of addiction, there was a "chaos of contradictory opinion."

In the absence of any medical consensus, crushing stigma rushed in to take its place. The dominant cultural opinion was expressed in the 1928 bestseller *Dope: The Story of the Living Dead*, which described drug addiction as "a wasting, loathsome, hideous, cruel disease" and people with addictions as "carriers" of a disease "worse than smallpox, and more terrible than leprosy." It uncannily echoes the rhetoric of an 1832 fire-and-brimstone tirade against drunkenness: "He stalks about like a moral pestilence, scattering his vile contagion with every breath. He is a walking plague, a living death. He caters for hell." One century later, that disparaging portrait was the prevalent view, and even today, almost two centuries later, the same language about drug use is easy to find. In this light, the word "stigma" seems weak and insufficient. A better word would be "oppression."

By the end of the Progressive Era's drive toward prohibition, the dominant stereotype of drug users was profoundly negative, and society was left with no compassion for people with addiction. They were "demons," "villains," "scourges," "plagues"—everything at once, subhuman, contagious, and possessed, yet all by choice. Just as recent reports have described people with addiction scavenging failed construction sites for drug money, by the 1920s urban addicts were known to pick through city dumps looking for scrap metal, which they sold to illicit dealers to fund their drug use. They were known as "junkmen"—later, "junkies"—and like any nickname that sticks, the label worked on many levels, evoking not just how these people survived but also the way respectable America viewed them: as human trash.

America had seemed so close to a compassionate, therapeutic response to addiction, but it was lost, not to be rediscovered for decades.

PART THREE

THE ROOTS OF
MODERN ADDICTION

Seven

THE MODERN
ALCOHOLISM MOVEMENT

Hundreds of elegant passengers poured off the *Queen Mary*, the enormous luxury liner, and down to the docks of 1936 New York City. Among the jostling crowds, Marty Mann's mother and sister craned their necks, eager to catch a glimpse of Marty. They wondered: how had their brilliant debutante changed after six years in Europe, hobnobbing with the likes of Virginia Woolf and others in the famous Bloomsbury Group?

The stream of passengers thinned out. Where was she? Finally, some crew members emerged at the top of the gangway, hauling a stretcher with a woman sprawled across it. It was Marty, unconscious, reeking of alcohol.

What her family didn't know was that Mann had needed to borrow money to book passage home. Once a successful advertising executive and glittering socialite, her drinking had long been out of control. She had already attempted suicide twice. She had meant to sober up on the trip home so she could disembark with a clear head and finally get her life together, but by the time land came into sight, Mann was passed out at the *Queen Mary*'s sumptuous art deco bar.

Her mother immediately found a place for her to be hospitalized, and for the next several years Mann's life would be consumed by one question: What, exactly, was wrong with her?

Mann bounced from psychiatrist to psychiatrist, seeing more than half a dozen doctors, but most psychoanalysts of the time didn't consider addiction a proper subject for psychiatric treatment, and no one would take on her case. Soon she was homeless, living from couch to couch, blackout to blackout, drink to drink, with no relief in sight.

Imagine the terror of suffering from alcoholism in the 1930s—having the sense that something was wrong, but not quite understanding what. The profusion of theories, explanations, and cures, none of which seemed to work. The confusion and despair. This was a dark time for patients with addiction, the pessimistic attitudes captured well in the original 1937 version of the film *A Star Is Born*: Norman Maine's alcoholism is a death sentence, one that compels him to walk into the Pacific Ocean to relieve the burden on his wife.

Eventually, and only through the influence of some well-connected friends, Mann managed to be admitted to Bellevue Hospital's neurological ward, then gain admission as a charity case to Blythewood, an upscale mental health facility on a fifty-acre estate in Connecticut. Mann threw herself into psychotherapy, meeting with her psychiatrist Harry Tiebout an hour each day, but even then she struggled. She was given weekend passes to visit the city, each time confidently ready to test her resolve not to drink. She'd have a string of successful visits, but before long she would return drunk, ashamed, and most of all baffled. After months of treatment, a defeated Tiebout told her that if something didn't change, he'd have to discharge her.

Then, one day in early 1939, Tiebout excitedly called Mann to his house and showed her a prepublication draft of a new book, one written by a small group of alcoholics who had founded their own new program: Alcoholics Anonymous. Flipping through the pages, Mann felt hopeful. She was skeptical about the religious language she saw in the book, but the prospect of relief that the group promised—through a method entirely outside the medical profession—seemed worth investigating. Tiebout put her on a train to New York City once more. This time, Mann was cautiously optimistic, wondering what she might find at her first "meeting."

Alcoholics Anonymous was a tiny, scrappy, informal fellowship in those early days. Of course, it would soon become the most significant and enduring social movement in the history of addiction, one that has defined our national understanding of substance problems—arguably exerting an even greater influence than that of the medical profession.

Less widely appreciated is the role of Margaret "Marty" Mann in this history. Mann was a brilliant strategist and a public relations genius who played a crucial role in midcentury alcoholism advocacy. Today she is largely forgotten, even to many of the most ardent AA devotees, despite the fact that she might have been more important to the rise of AA's popularity than founder Bill Wilson himself.

Bill Wilson, Mann's "sponsor" in AA, is inextricable from the fellowship he created. It's Wilson's own story, after all, that forms the first chapter of *Alcoholics Anonymous*—the "Big Book," its "bible," which Mann read in draft form—and it was Wilson's Brooklyn home that Mann traveled to that day in 1939.

For more than a decade before Wilson got sober, his house in Brooklyn was less a refuge than ground zero for his battles with alcohol. During the Prohibition era, he brewed dandelion wine in the bathtub upstairs and, too impatient to wait for it to fully mature, drank it raw and became violently ill. To his long-suffering wife, Lois, he made countless solemn promises that he would stop, even writing out pledges in their family Bible, but he always broke them sooner or later. On one occasion, Lois found him passed out in the entryway, bleeding heavily from a scalp wound. Later, when his drinking had become worse and he was paranoid and suicidal, Lois dragged a mattress downstairs to the living room so he could sleep there and not be tempted to jump from their upper-story window.

Like Mann, Wilson had bounced from doctor to doctor but found no relief—one simply prescribed more willpower and sent him on his way. Lois's wealthy brother paid for multiple stays in the Charles B. Towns Hospital, a stately private facility on Central Park West where well-to-do alcoholics received an "unpoisoning" treatment of "purging and puking" based on Towns's own "cure" formula. Towns, like many providers of his day, was committed to the reductionist notion of a biological cure for addiction, a dream inspired in part by advances in other branches of medical science. In 1910, the "magic bullet" anti-syphilis medication Salvarsan, the first modern antimicrobial medication, was introduced to the world, and researchers dreamed of "antitoxic" treatments for addiction, too. Inspired by pioneers like Emil von Behring, who won the Nobel Prize in 1901 for discovering how to produce diphtheria antitoxin serum by the bucket from horse blood, one group of San Francisco researchers claimed to have discovered anti-alcohol antibodies. They purified a supposed antitoxin serum from the blood of horses that had been fed high doses of alcohol, but trials in humans, of course, fell flat. This didn't stop entrepreneurial hucksters from marketing other "antitoxic" addiction treatments with a random mix of fats, proteins, and vitamins (which, not surprisingly, caused a number of deaths).

There were often other dimensions to these treatment efforts. Leslie Keeley's "Gold Cure" was a farce, but it got people in the door of his institutes, where, aside from regular injections, people participated in patient-run societies called the Keeley Leagues, and upon discharge were encouraged to stay connected. These mutual-help efforts may have been the most helpful and influential element of the treatment experience, spreading clubhouses and meetings that eventually formed 370 chapters across the United States. Yes, the "cure" framing and the leagues themselves were marketing tools, but at the turn of the twentieth century, the Keeley Institutes also promoted interest in both therapeutic and mutual-help approaches to addiction at a time that prohibitionist stigma dominated public attitudes.

Towns's hospital lacked such mutual-help efforts, but it provided other treatments to patients like Wilson: chiefly a sort of intensive psychotherapy organized around the notion of willpower. Towns himself—profiled as a "giant of will" who lifted weights two hours a day—taught patients about his method of detailed scheduling ("time control") and other exercises to strengthen the will. This all spoke to Wilson, a Protestant, libertarian-leaning New Englander who had always put great stock in personal grit. He underwent a major shift in his thinking during one of his several stays at Towns: a physician there, William Silkworth, finally convinced Wilson that he was fundamentally different from other men and could never drink again safely. But even though Wilson left the hospital resolved to abstain, and despite the advertised 95 percent "cure rate" of the Towns treatments, he relapsed soon after each of his discharges. Against his supposedly strengthened will, he watched himself walking toward a bar, repeating desperately to himself, "I won't go in. I won't"—all the while knowing that he would.

One day in 1934, Wilson was paid a visit by Ebby Thacher, an old boarding school friend and drinking buddy, who arrived with the shocking news that he had given up alcohol and joined the Oxford Group, a prominent evangelical Christian organization at the time. For hours, Thacher described to the Wilsons how he had been saved by faith. Thacher seemed "a little cracked" to Wilson, who had long been skeptical of organized religion, but he was also desperate enough to give this route a try. Wilson had long talks with Thacher and tried throwing himself into the Oxford Group, which put a strong focus on spiritual practices like small-group discussions and frequent confession. Still, he couldn't stop drinking. Once again, he set off for Towns Hospital for what he hoped would be his last detox.

Back at Towns, Wilson fell into a deep depression. Nothing was working. Years of striving had failed. The Towns treatments had failed.

Religion had failed. In his hospital room, desperate, he cried out to the God he didn't even fully believe in: "If there be a God, let him show himself! I am ready to do anything."

Suddenly, as Wilson later recounted, the room filled with a blazing white light, then he was standing on the summit of a mountain. A great wind blew through him, and a voice told him, "You are a free man."

Wilson wasn't sure what to make of this. Was it really a religious experience, or was he just hallucinating? After all, he was in the midst of alcohol withdrawal and loaded up on powerful psychoactive substances such as belladonna (deadly nightshade) and hyoscyamus (henbane). The next day, Ebby brought him a copy of William James's *The Varieties of Religious Experience*, which recounts the mystical insights of spiritual practitioners across different traditions and, notably, includes descriptions of drunkards who reformed through epiphanic conversion. Wilson was captivated by one passage in particular: "The only radical remedy I know for dipsomania is religiomania." James's approach, which he later developed as the philosophical school of pragmatism, was to judge religion not by some standard of metaphysical truth but by its effects alone: "You must all be ready now to judge the religious life by its results exclusively." James offered a broad definition of religion as "the belief that there is an unseen order, and that our supreme good lies in harmoniously adjusting ourselves thereto." Later, in the book *Alcoholics Anonymous*, Wilson approvingly cited this pragmatic and flexible approach to religion to underscore the point that AA was a spiritual program only in the sense that it insisted on some sense of the divine or transcendent, not adherence to any particular dogma or religious practices, and the only requirement for a "higher power" was to "turn it over" to something other than one's self.

Wilson threw himself into the Oxford Group, and he stayed sober for a few months more, but this new religious practice wasn't enough for him. One day, on a business trip to Akron, Ohio, he found himself beset by cravings in a lonely hotel lobby. He started panicking, then thought that perhaps if he connected with another alcoholic he could stay sober. He reached out through his Oxford Group connections and eventually met a surgeon named Bob Smith (later described affectionately as Dr. Bob), and the two had an instant chemistry, talking and drinking coffee for the next five hours.

The point of alcoholism, for Wilson and Dr. Bob, was that it was a hybrid condition, made of physical, mental, and spiritual elements— what Wilson later called the "threefold nature" of alcoholism. As they worked together to create their own "twelve-step" program for alcoholics, they merged three important ideas. First was the medical insight that Wilson had received at Towns Hospital: that a true alcoholic could never again drink safely (later formulated as step one of the twelve-step program: accepting one's powerlessness). Second, tempering the first, was the spiritual lesson that the shift in perspective required was actually the *opposite* of willpower: to recover from alcoholism, it was necessary to let go and trust in some form of pragmatic spirituality greater than the self (steps two and three: believing in a "Power greater than ourselves," and allowing for a personal definition of "God as we understood Him"). Third was the ongoing work to change: full-on identity reconstruction and service to others, all strongly inspired by the Oxford Group's practices (the rest of the steps). This framework speaks to why only the first step mentions alcohol. Forsaking alcohol was necessary but not sufficient, and ongoing health required a program of complete personal change—a process that would soon come to be known as "recovery."

As many critics have noted, AA was created by and for those in power—namely, white, Protestant, middle-aged, professional men—and it wasn't easy for women in AA in those early days. Around that time, the prevailing stereotypes of female alcoholics were legion: sexually promiscuous, neglectful mothers, sicker than men, and harder

to cure. Dr. Bob in Akron was particularly notorious for distrusting female alcoholics. Generally, many men in AA referred alcoholic women
to their wives rather than trying to help the women themselves, worried
that the presence of women in meetings would be too tempting—a
common saying of the era warned members, "Under every skirt there's
a slip." A 1945 article in *Grapevine*, an official AA publication, outlined
all the reasons why most women weren't well suited for AA: they talked
too much, they didn't like other women, they demanded too much attention, their feelings were too easily hurt, they wanted to run things,
and eventually a "woman-on-the-make" would get into a group looking
for phone numbers and dates. To this day, men outnumber women in
AA by nearly two to one. Subsequent female pioneers in AA fought
those ideas, and others created alternatives. For example, in 1975, the
feminist sociologist Jean Kirkpatrick founded Women for Sobriety, an
abstinence-based group that crafted "Thirteen Statements of Acceptance" emphasizing empowerment, assertiveness, competence, responsibility, and positive thinking.

At the time, Mann had no such alternatives. Arriving in Manhattan
on that chilly April evening in 1939, she rode a clattering subway down
to Wilson's home in Brooklyn Heights. Initially nervous, she hid upstairs until Lois coaxed her down to join the group in the living room.
She immediately felt an unmistakable rightness to it all: "I could finish
their sentences! They could finish my sentences! We talked each other's
language! It was not a room of strangers. These were my people."

For Mann, even more skeptical of religion than Wilson, the greatest
appeal was identifying with people, having a community, a tribe. Contemporary research on AA has affirmed the role of community in the
group's success: the strongest evidence for the mechanism by which it
helps people maintain sobriety is the communal ties and healthier
opportunities for socialization. Mann was outwardly different from
other AA members. She was a lesbian, and her partner, Priscilla Peck,
later joined AA—they were among the first women to be long-term

members, and certainly among the very first LGBTQ+ people. Nevertheless, she found enormous strength in the mutual identity of an alcoholic. As Mann would write, in her own story printed in a later version of the Big Book, "There is another meaning for the Hebrew word that in the King James version of the Bible is translated 'salvation.' It is: 'to come home.' I had found my salvation. I wasn't alone any more."

Mann became Wilson's sponsee and threw herself into the nascent fellowship, which grew slowly from there. Later in 1939, Bill and Lois Wilson, Mann, and a few others drove to Cleveland to help establish a new meeting. In front of the crowd, Mann quipped, "Wouldn't it be wonderful if some day we could travel across the country and find an AA meeting in every town?" It was a joke, and the hundred or so people collapsed in laughter. For Mann, though, it was only a half joke. In their own circle, people were relapsing, even dying. Surely there was more they could do.

One long year after graduating from medical school, I began my first rotation as a full-fledged psychiatry resident. I was on the service for consultation-liaison psychiatry, a subspecialty that cares for people hospitalized for other medical and surgical reasons. Every day, I entered through the familiar revolving glass doors into the antiseptically cool hospital lobby, the same main hospital where I had spent my intern year. But instead of having to make my way to some windowless conference room to get sign-out from last night's intern, or rushing to do some urgent blood draw or thoracentesis or some other awful splattering-body-fluid procedure, I was finally practicing my chosen field, in charge of my own list of patients and free to rove around the hospital taking care of them as I saw fit.

It was thrilling to finally be a psychiatrist, stepping into the role of the expert consultant and learning skills I imagined drawing on for the rest of my career. Up to the general medical floors, where I'd try to calm the anxious breathing of a pulmonary patient with end-stage emphysema, all the muscles of her neck and chest visibly straining to suck in any last cubic centimeter of air. Then down to the surgical floor for a capacity consult: a pre-op patient with schizophrenia who didn't seem to understand why he needed an amputation. I made medication adjustments for patients with severe depression, and I started courses of psychotherapy in the hospital, right at the bedside.

I loved it, but I still couldn't fully function. It was deeply confusing and terrifying, but, more so, surreal. Even though the chief resident had warned me that my poor intern-year performance had been noticed, I somehow still struggled to control my drinking. I'd blink and it would be 4 a.m., the bar closing down. Or I'd just drink alone in my apartment, bingeing TV. I was supposed to arrive at the hospital by 9 a.m. I resolved to get in by 8 to be safe. More often than not I was rushing in, barely arriving in time for 9:45 a.m. rounds.

It was only a matter of weeks before I got the message I'd been dreading. Sandra, our program director, a fierce woman who kept a megaphone on a ledge near her office desk, wanted to see me right away. As I made my way to her office, I tried to remember if I had showered that morning, and even so, if the scent of alcohol still wafted off of me. As I walked in, my heart dropped. Sandra was there, but so were her assistant director and the chief resident. My thoughts went immediately to the addiction interventions on television shows: dramatic scenes of confrontation and severe consequences.

Thinking back on that conversation now, what I remember most is their careful, straightforward concern. *It's clear you're struggling,* they said, *but don't worry. You're not in trouble, and there's lots of help available*—a confidential house staff counseling service, any referrals I needed. Nothing of the consequences I had dreamed up—no random urine test, certainly no summary firing. But inside, I was still panicking. It felt like the oxygen had been sucked out of the air. I flailed about for an excuse.

I had the feeling that the rest of my life hinged on that moment. The only way I can explain it is that it felt like I would die if I was found out. There was nothing beyond that.

"I know what this looks like, and I'm sure you're wondering if I have a problem with drugs or alcohol, but that's really not it," I said. I told them that I recognized I had been irresponsible and immature, I was sorry, and I was working on it. I spun every possible lie I could think of to try to wriggle out from under their attention, not realizing that doing so wasn't freeing me of my troubles but binding me to them even tighter.

Denial is a profound obstacle to treating addiction—of all the people who have a substance use disorder and are not getting help, fewer than 5 percent think they need treatment—yet, as the philosopher Hanna Pickard has observed, denial is glaringly absent from most modern definitions of addiction. (For example, in the nearly 1,800-page *ASAM Principles of Addiction Medicine,* denial gets only two measly pages in a chapter about ethical issues, tucked away in the back of the book.) Partly this reflects a certain allergy to the concept of denial as an outdated Freudian holdover, but it is hard to deny that denial factors into addiction. Some people deny they have a problem all the way to the face of death, telling themselves that even after this hospitalization for withdrawal, or after this overdose reversal, they'll be fine. Evolutionary biologist Robert Trivers has theorized that our human tendency toward self-deception is not a bug but a feature of our psychology. He argues that it has been selected over the course of generations because self-deception is actually beneficial in some human interactions: we mislead ourselves because that helps us to deceive others more convincingly. It's a provocative theory, but it rings true to me in the case of addiction.

In that quasi intervention during residency, I summoned up every possible excuse I could think of. I was still sleep-deprived after intern year. I was in therapy, working out the "deeper" issues driving my bad performance, like my issues with authority. None of these things were true, of course, but the extraordinary thing is that, in that moment, I truly believed them.

The meeting in Sandra's office, I think, was the last real turning point when I might have chosen differently and gotten help, and it is depressing and a bit frightening to consider just how entrenched I was, even among people so clearly and nonjudgmentally trying to help me.

Sandra, looking skeptical and a little disappointed, urged me, "Whatever the problem is, get help." They were going to require me to meet with the chief resident once a week and generally keep a closer eye on me. I walked out of the room feeling chastised, but not once did it occur to me to actually *get help*.

It's clear in retrospect that what I was really afraid of was change— the possibility that it wouldn't work, or that it might work and that would be even harder. And, of course, I was afraid of the idea that I was different, that I was mentally ill, an incipient alcoholic. If I could latch on to some alternative explanation and pull myself out of my own mess, that would prove that I was a normal person. To accept help, by contrast, would have also meant accepting that I was sick in some way.

It is exactly this type of entrenched denial that Marty Mann was hoping to overcome with her own "alcoholism movement." To counteract a force so strong, she felt, would take all the intensity she could muster.

I n sobriety, Marty Mann was a dynamo. Brimming with energy, brilliant and polished, yet always speaking from the heart, she captivated audiences at AA meetings. She became known in her social circles as the go-to person for advice and counsel. It was also around this time that she met her partner, Priscilla Peck, an elegant and cosmopolitan artist and writer who would later become art director of *Vogue* magazine. AA was growing, especially after a breathlessly supportive *Saturday Evening Post* article by Jack Alexander in 1941 (reporting, among other things, that "fifty percent of the alcoholics taken in hand recover almost immediately" and "twenty-five percent get well after suffering a relapse or two"). The group opened a spacious office near Grand Central Station and was answering a growing volume of correspondence from around the country and, soon, the world. The informal fellowship, which had barely even mentioned meetings in the Big Book, was growing into an organization with a potentially global reach. Yet Mann hungered for more. There were still legions of people, she thought, who had never heard of their lifesaving program.

World War II was raging, and Mann was working in her new job, producing radio programs on American history. One featured Dorothea Dix, the nineteenth-century crusader who led a national campaign against the inhumane treatment of the mentally ill, and Mann was profoundly moved. What if there was a similar battle to be waged on behalf of alcoholics? Soon afterward, she woke in the middle of the night with an epiphany, ran to her typewriter, and banged out a detailed plan for a national campaign that would convince the public that alcoholism was not a moral but a medical condition. Her plan was to reach not just scientists and medical professionals but the whole of society—including people like the younger me, mired in denial and unwilling to accept help. Her project was medicalization: she wanted to make alcoholism into a disease.

In Mann's time, public health advocacy movements were achieving stunning success in destigmatizing diseases like cancer and tuberculosis. Mann herself had contracted tuberculosis as a child in the late 1910s, and at the time, it was so shameful and associated with the lower classes that her parents had sent her all the way from Chicago to a sanatorium in Los Angeles to get treatment—keeping her diagnosis a secret, even from her. Since then, she herself had seen how the National Tuberculosis Association (today the American Lung Association) had completely revolutionized public attitudes by advocating for research, funding, treatment, and above all public compassion for the condition. To Mann, her alcoholism was a disease just like any other, and it should be recognized and treated as such.

Marty Mann, a bit like Wilson, was more innovator than inventor: both tied together existing threads in the zeitgeist rather than fashioning something entirely novel. In the case of Mann's movement, interest in thinking about alcoholism as a disease was already on the rise. In 1941, the U.S. Public Health Service had issued an important publication framing alcoholism as a public health problem rather than immoral behavior. A group of alcohol scientists had also established a group called the Research Council on Problems of Alcohol, which was attempting to promote a therapeutic approach to alcohol problems: "The alcohol addict should be regarded as a sick person," "just as is one who is suffering from tuberculosis, cancer, heart disease or any other serious chronic disorder." The council later hired the PR professional Dwight Anderson, himself a recovering alcoholic, to help promote this view, and Anderson urged them to take a more active role in shaping public opinion, and specifically to focus on the notion that people with alcoholism are "sick" but able to be helped, and therefore "a responsibility of the healing professions." At Yale University, some researchers involved with the Research Council had already begun conducting studies, engaging in state-level advocacy, and generally promoting a new scientific vision of alcoholism.

Mann connected with these Yale researchers—most fatefully, a brilliant and iconoclastic Hungarian American man named E. M. "Bunky" Jellinek. Even in a field populated by passionate oddballs, Jellinek stands out. Earlier in his life, he had fled Hungary with a warrant out for his arrest after a failed currency-speculation-and-smuggling scheme, then spent brief stints in Sierra Leone and Honduras before fabricating several degrees on his résumé and talking his way into a job as a biostatistician in Massachusetts. He was, in short, a con man, though he was also a brilliant and productive researcher. Today, the most prestigious award in alcohol research is named after him.

Jellinek immediately recognized Mann's gifts. She was a stunningly talented speaker. Her social capital was unmatched, including a firm footing in the growing fellowship of AA. As an attractive, upper-class woman willing to identify herself as an alcoholic in recovery, she shattered the dominant stereotype of the alcoholic as a skid row bum. And she had the freedom to devote her life to her new crusade. In just a couple of months, Mann moved in with the Jellinek family in New Haven and spent the summer studying alcoholism. A few months after that, she was ready.

In October 1944, in the luxurious Biltmore Hotel in New York, Mann held a press conference to announce a new national organization to combat alcoholism. In her dignified, finishing-school accent, like Katharine Hepburn with just a hint of a homey Midwest twang, the "tall, smart looking blonde" (as one outlet later described her) captivated the forty-five newspapers in attendance, especially after she revealed herself as an alcoholic, one who had "been free for five years."

Mann announced that her organization, which in time became known as the National Council on Alcoholism (NCA), would embark on a campaign to convince the public that, first and foremost, "alcoholism is a disease." She also recapitulated several of Dwight Anderson's PR ideas from the Research Council, maintaining that the alcoholic is "a sick person," "can be helped," and "is worth helping," and thus that "alcoholism is a major public health problem."

News items about the press conference appeared for a full two weeks afterward. *Time* published a feature story on Mann that month. In less than a year, she made no fewer than forty-nine speaking appearances around the country, and her visibility only rose from there—in later years, she routinely booked more than two hundred public talks a year, sometimes as many as 250. Everywhere she went, she established and developed local "alcoholism information centers" that launched public education campaigns framing alcoholism as a disease. There was a churning positive feedback loop between grassroots organizing and high-level connections. It was the birth of what scholars have come to

call the "modern alcoholism movement," a vigorous yet loosely organized coalition of advocates for mutual-help and therapeutic approaches.

In the space of little more than a decade, the change was already pal-
pable. AA had grown from slightly more than 10,000 members in 1944 to
just shy of 100,000 members in 1950. Though Mann's advocacy contributed to AA's rising popularity, a good portion of this growth and success
can also be attributed to AA's own maturation. As it grew, its leaders inevitably faced challenging questions from groups around the country
about funding, governance, and membership. In the process of that correspondence, Wilson developed certain principles, eventually codified as the
Twelve Traditions, intended to protect the integrity of the organization
and keep its focus squarely on helping suffering alcoholics (as opposed to
wading into political controversies, as the Washingtonians had done). For
example, the traditions clarified that the only requirement for membership was a desire to stop drinking—some early groups had rigid rules for
AA membership and "blackballed" people who slipped more than once.
AA also adopted a deliberately decentralized organizational structure to
avoid authoritarianism and allow the group to adapt flexibly to local
communities.

Mann's advocacy efforts were soon felt in the medical domain. With
one of her earliest New York City friends, a psychiatrist named Ruth
Fox, Mann helped to establish the medical organization that eventually
became today's American Society of Addiction Medicine, the nation's
largest professional organization of its kind. Slowly but surely, these efforts helped to inspire therapeutic approaches to addiction, as community hospitals began establishing specialized alcoholism treatment units.
In 1956, the American Medical Association adopted a resolution recognizing "alcoholism as a medical problem." A year later, the American
Hospital Association passed its own resolution urging general hospitals
to develop programs for treating alcoholics.

A significant cultural shift was underway. Between the smash hit *The*

Lost Weekend, in 1945, and *Days of Wine and Roses,* in 1962, at least thirty-four Hollywood films presented alcoholics as main characters. Some films were Freudian, and some were defeatist (including, perhaps most notably, 1954's *A Star Is Born,* a remake of the 1937 version), but increasingly, films drew upon the ideas of AA—or perhaps more accurately, the ideas of Marty Mann and her organization—presenting the disease concept of alcoholism as a sort of character unto itself. Indeed, starting with *Smash-Up* (1947), AA and NCA members directly consulted on several films about alcoholism. The NCA was not AA, though there was confusing overlap. AA members contributed powerfully to the NCA—most of Mann's initial speaking invitations came from members of local AA groups—and in turn, all the NCA activities, from professional acceptance to public education campaigns, surely boosted AA membership. Yet they were, in fact, different organizations. Mann's unflagging advocacy and willingness to identify herself as a member of AA were part of the reason the organization later adopted a tradition that all members should stay anonymous at the level of mass media. From that point on, Mann and countless other publicly recovering people relied on the tortured syntax of identifying as a recovering alcoholic but not mentioning AA by name. AA took no position on outside issues and didn't engage in any lobbying—but Mann and the NCA certainly did. The fine distinctions between the NCA, AA, and, later, the growing treatment industry would come to be subtle, yet important.

The NCA wasn't the only force driving these changes, but it was often the most visible one. It took out ads to spread the word that the alcoholic was a "sick person" and could be effectively treated, and it lobbied American corporations to increasingly provide treatment rather than summary terminations for people with alcoholism. Mann leaned on her connections with politicians, such as President Lyndon B. Johnson, once a member of the Texas NCA. In 1966, he announced a new program in a special health message to Congress, declaring that

alcoholism was "a disease which will yield eventually to scientific research and adequate treatment." LBJ wasn't the NCA's only ally in the
halls of power. Two years later, Mann and the NCA rejoiced when Harold Hughes, an AA member and an openly recovering alcoholic, was
elected to the Senate, where he proceeded to work for federal legislation
on alcoholism and arranged for both Mann and an anonymous Bill W.
to testify before Congress. In 1970, Congress passed a comprehensive
alcoholism act, known as the Hughes Act. Richard Nixon almost let the
bill die in a pocket veto, but at the last minute Mann's wealthy Republican allies put some backdoor political pressure on the president, who
finally signed the bill into law on the last day of 1970. It was the first
significant federal legislation on alcoholism. Not only did it create the
National Institute on Alcohol Abuse and Alcoholism (NIAAA), but it
laid the groundwork for today's system of addiction treatment and, to
Mann, marked an even more fundamental victory at the level of changing hearts and minds.

Soon after the Hughes Act was passed, Mann gave a speech declaring an end to "America's 150-year war" of alcohol versus alcoholism.
Since the very first days of our nation, she explained, the moralistic
forces of temperance, the "drys," had railed against the evils of alcohol.
The supposed evil of demon rum had attached itself to alcoholics; this
was "the origin of stigma, that smothering blanket which so effectively
prevented alcoholics or their families from recognizing, admitting, or
seeking help for their illness." But then her NCA had brought together
two important countervailing forces: scientists (in the form of the Yale
researchers) and the alcoholics (in the form of AA), and through their
combined powers, the alcoholism movement won the day over the forces
of superstition and stigma. The "primary object of concern" was now, as
it should be, the "people in trouble," not "the bottle." In retrospect, it's
hard not to read her triumphant remarks as a little smug, and more than
a little simplistic. Surely there were things to be concerned about "in the
bottle," too?

Prohibition was repealed in the United States in 1933, but the American war over alcohol raged on afterward. There were continuing and vicious battles between "wets" and "drys," the pro- and anti-alcohol forces, and scientists found it was hard to carry out any research on alcohol at all. Later in the thirties, the State of Virginia commissioned two eminent pharmacology professors, J. A. Waddell and H. B. Haag, to write a balanced scientific report about the effects of alcohol. The report attempted to strike a middle ground, cautiously giving moderate drinking (meaning one drink a day) a clean bill of health, but it was too dry for the wets and too wet for the drys. The state legislature voted to destroy its copies of the report, and in April 1938 the remaining one thousand copies were hauled to the basement of the state capitol and thrown in the furnace, where the assistant attorney general and other state officials were photographed stoking the flames.

The Research Council on Problems of Alcohol, the group with which Bunky Jellinek and Marty Mann eventually connected, faced similar challenges. By the close of the 1930s, the group was low on funding, on the brink of financial death. Like the Virginia researchers, they found that their therapeutic inclinations satisfied neither side of the issue, and they struggled to attract private donors. Only one source seemed willing to fund them: the alcohol industry itself.

Some of the scientists balked at the potential conflict of interest, but in the closing months of the decade, after much hand-wringing and some dry members quitting in protest, the Research Council struck a compromise: it would accept the industry money, but it would also stop studying alcohol and make *alcoholism* its single focus, hoping to sidestep the thorny wet-versus-dry debate entirely and focus on the problems of the person, not the bottle. This move might appear neutral, but it wasn't. The focus of scientific investigation can be a powerful force in itself.

The alcohol industry had long assumed a major role in shaping the way people thought about addiction. In his book *Bad Habits,* the historian John Burnham argues that the fall of Prohibition is best understood not as the weakness of reformers but as the strength of the forces they were contending against. One of the most crucial of those forces was the alcohol industry. More broadly, the post-repeal period marked a wholesale shift in American ideas about vice, and now a constellation of other vices such as smoking, gambling, and sex all became acceptable, even respectable. Burnham maintains that industrialism was a main force in this shift—not just the industries themselves, but the mass media and the growth of advertising, playing to an expanding market.

This wasn't some nefarious plot. The alcohol industry, like any other industry that profits off of potentially harmful products, was doing what it could to increase market share. (This, incidentally, is why the notion of industry self-regulation is a total fantasy.) In the absence of a nuanced perspective on addiction, policy responses to drug use tend to swing between extremes of total prohibition and permissive deregulation. There are severe harms to a prohibitionist approach, but the opposite pole of deregulation has clear dangers, too.

Addiction supply industries have powerfully shaped ideas about addiction for at least a hundred years, in the process also shaping national and international policies, directly interceding in cultural norms, and generally trying to influence our core ideas about health and disease. The argument that the problem is located not in the substance but in the person is one of their most time-honored arguments. As they lobbied to repeal Prohibition, an important element of alcohol industry arguments was an extensive focus on personal liberty and responsibility. The vice reformers of the Progressive Era had focused on the broader, environmental causes of social problems, but those arguing for repeal vigorously returned the focus to the individual. For example, they argued that the fact that a small minority of people used a substance incorrectly shouldn't mean that the rest had to be punished. It proved to be an effective plank of the industry's public relations platform.

After the repeal of Prohibition, the industry found, paradoxically, that the idea of alcoholism was useful in opposing restrictions on alcohol sales. The argument was that the responsibility for drinking problems belonged to sick individuals, and the rest of non-disordered drinking was harmless, normal, and nondeviant. In 1947, the president of Licensed Beverage Industries Inc. noted appreciatively that scientists agreed: "the root of the 'problem drinker's disease' lies in the man and not in the bottle." The Research Council was listed among "potentially valuable allies" in a report by a pro-alcohol lobbying group. For decades after repeal, every major conference on alcoholism received some amount of industry funding.

To this day, a central argument of the alcohol industry is that the most significant harms of alcohol are confined to a minority of excessive drinkers. This is specious—superficially correct, perhaps intuitively appealing to those with a personal experience of addiction, but in fact deeply wrong. Alcohol problems exist on a continuum, and numerous studies have found that most of the harmful effects of alcohol can be seen not among the most severe cases but in the much larger population of drinkers at the middle of the consumption bell curve—a group defined as "hazardous" or "at-risk" drinkers. People don't need to be stereotypical alcoholics to drive drunk, get into fights, commit domestic violence, or develop alcohol-related diseases. Hazardous drinkers have fewer of these problems at an individual level, but they make up so much more of the population that they account for the most problems overall.

The alcohol industry has a powerful incentive to obscure this fact. These hazardous drinkers also account for the most revenue—if we were able to successfully limit the consumption of everyone who drank at hazardous levels and above, it would wipe out a huge portion of alcohol sales, up to 60 percent of their revenue by some accounts. So the PR campaign continues. The industry funds front organizations with anodyne names like the International Center for Alcohol Policies—more than thirty of them by one recent count—to influence alcohol regulation and scholarship. Their goal is often to focus attention on specific groups, like "hard core drunk drivers" or pregnant women, rather than the systemic causes of alcohol problems. Around the time that organizations like the WHO publish major reports and surveys, industry-related groups commission their own works and mail them out free of charge to large lists of constituents, trying to crowd out the public health data with their focus on individual-level interventions. For similar reasons, in the 1980s, industry groups funded organizations like Mothers Against Drunk Driving and Students Against Driving Drunk—groups that focused on individual responsibility and advocated retributive legal penalties rather than the systemic change, such as advertising reform, which was being championed by other consumer protection groups.

The size of the alcohol industry and the concentration of its power are staggering—in 2005, the twenty-six largest alcoholic beverage companies in the world boasted a total net revenue of $155 billion and a total operating profit of $26 billion, and some estimates today put the total global alcoholic beverage market at more than $1.5 trillion—and their ability to shape policy should not be underestimated. As addiction supply industries have grown more powerful, they have targeted entire foreign countries, even continents, to open up their markets and relax regulations, creating in the process what scholars have called "industrial epidemics." The most striking recent example of such methods came in the late 2000s, when four countries in sub-Saharan Africa—Malawi, Uganda, Botswana, and Lesotho—all produced new and uncannily similar draft alcohol policies within two years of one another. Looking more closely, a team of Norwegian researchers found that the four documents were virtually the same in wording, structure, and page formatting—despite being from dramatically different cultures with totally different political processes. (The farthest apart, Uganda and Lesotho, are separated by about two thousand miles.) With a little more digging, the researchers were able to determine that the policy documents had originated with the International Center for Alcohol Policies, an alcohol-industry-funded organization, and SABMiller, the world's second-largest brewer. Four sovereign nations with a combined population of nearly fifty million people had their alcohol policies written by one of the very multinational corporations that those policies were supposed to regulate. The policies, I perhaps shouldn't have to mention, generally ignored the proven and most effective interventions for reducing the harms of alcohol, such as limiting availability and restricting advertising, in favor of an individualistic approach that promoted soft strategies like "consumer education."

Another legacy of the Prohibition era's massive cultural changes was the stark divide between alcohol and tobacco, on the one hand, and other drugs. In the early decades of the twentieth century, the alcohol and tobacco industries paid for millions of dollars in advertising to defend and normalize their products, especially to differentiate them from "drugs." (These industries were in fact important catalysts for the development of advertising as a persuasive technology in the 1920s and '30s, a time when American ads turned from information-dense communications to ones more carefully designed for emotional manipulation and persuasion.) In one dramatically engineered public display, in 1929, the PR pioneer Edward Bernays arranged for a group of women marching in the Easter Parade in New York City to light up cigarettes—or as he called them, "torches of freedom"—as part of a campaign to make it more acceptable for women to smoke. Industry was not solely responsible for the growing acceptability of cigarettes and alcohol, of course, but it was an important player, and the result was a profound divide that continues to this day.

At the turn of the twentieth century, no distinction existed between the conditions of alcoholism and addiction; all forms of addiction were united under the umbrella of inebriety. Decades later, and continuing to this day, there is not only a rift between alcohol and tobacco and other drugs; there is a rift between alcoholism and other forms of addiction, one that not only impairs a nuanced and pluralistic perspective on

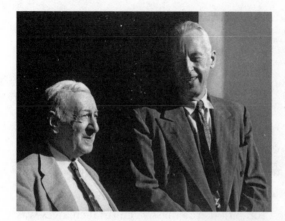

Dr. E. M. ("Bunky") Jellinek (left) and Bill Wilson, 11th Annual Conference of North American Association of Alcoholism Programs, Banff, Alberta, Canada, September 25–30, 1960.

Marty Mann presents AA with a National Council on Alcoholism award in October 1959. Bill W. (Wilson) accepts anonymously on behalf of AA Images courtesy of Stepping Stones. All rights reserved.

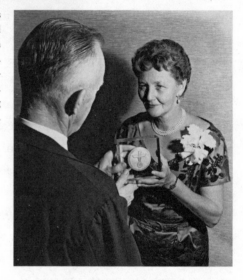

addiction but also continues to enable massive inequities in treatment and the continued use of drug criminalization as a weapon.

As the months after the end of her husband's presidency dragged on, former First Lady Betty Ford was feeling aimless, lonely, and angry—resentful of the country that had voted her husband out of office. While Jerry Ford was traveling around the country lecturing and serving on corporate boards, she was living alone in a leased house in

Rancho Mirage, not far from Palm Springs, writing her autobiography. At least she was supposed to be writing—most days she'd stay in bed until well into the afternoon, drinking and taking increasing doses of pain pills and sedatives. When her family saw her at Christmas in 1977, they were appalled. She had lost a shocking amount of weight, and though she had once danced with Martha Graham, she now shuffled clumsily around the house, her voice slurred to the point of incoherence.

Her family members tried to intercede, as did her doctor, who was a recovering alcoholic himself, but Betty wouldn't listen. So the family began planning for an intervention—at that time a relatively new practice, popularized by the Episcopal priest Vernon Johnson in his 1973 book *I'll Quit Tomorrow*. They summoned a Navy addiction specialist, and Jerry Ford had Henry Kissinger take over his speaking engagements so he could fly back home. Early in the morning of April 1, 1978, with the desert sunlight streaming down and Betty still in her bathrobe, sobbing on the couch while Jerry held her, they all staged an intervention. Betty, reluctantly, told her family she would go to treatment.

Betty entered treatment at the Long Beach Naval Hospital, where, after a second intervention, she released a statement saying that she was addicted to medications and alcohol. In subsequent years, she devoted herself to twelve-step recovery. In 1982, she opened her own treatment center in Rancho Mirage, not far from where she had sat in tears four years earlier, and from that point onward she was a vocal and tireless advocate. It was a watershed moment in the cultural understanding of addiction, when the popular image of the alcoholic shifted from a skid row drunk to, well, anyone. Betty Ford showed that all people could be struck by addiction: friends, family, or co-workers, no matter how successful they seemed.

The popularity and visibility of twelve-step mutual-help programs skyrocketed. Liza Minnelli, Mary Tyler Moore, Tony Curtis, and Johnny Cash all were treated at the Betty Ford Center, with much fanfare. Elizabeth Taylor went public as an alcoholic in recovery (after being encouraged by Betty Ford herself), and she was profiled in a long 1985 piece in *The New York Times,* where she repeated the center's claimed "cure rate" of 75 percent. It was fashionable, not just acceptable, to be an alcoholic. TV shows and movies widely featured stories of people achieving triumphant redemption in twelve-step recovery, such as the 1988 Ron Howard film *Clean and Sober,* starring Michael Keaton. AA membership in the United States and Canada grew from fewer than 200,000 people in 1970 to almost half a million in 1980, then almost one million in 1990. To its most fervent adherents, twelve-step recovery was a utopian movement that was going to change the world. As one recovery magazine put it, "We have been given the privilege of participating in the birth of an exciting change in mindset at a time of world crisis. The 12-Step programs, with their emphasis on a spiritual way of life, on process not product, and on equality, not hierarchy, are our best hope for healing ourselves and our planet." None of this frenzy for recovery would have been possible without Marty Mann.

After the Hughes Act was passed in 1970, Mann continued her tireless work and punishing speaking schedule up until her death, in 1980. Two years later, a Gallup poll recorded the highest-ever number of Americans who thought alcoholism was a disease: approximately 80 percent (up from roughly 20 percent in the late 1940s and early '50s). Yet the relationship of disease language to Marty Mann's therapeutic and mutual-help advocacy was complicated.

Mann herself didn't take credit for introducing the language of disease to alcoholism, but instead attributed the notion of disease to AA. In her telling, she was hit with the revelation the first time she read that early edition of the book *Alcoholics Anonymous*: "I wasn't the only person in the world who felt and behaved like this! I wasn't mad or vicious—I was a sick person. I was suffering from an actual disease that had a name and symptoms like diabetes or cancer or tuberculosis—and a disease was respectable, not a moral stigma." Yet this account has an air of revisionist history about it. The main text of the AA Big Book, the edition she was reading back in 1939, uses the word "disease" only once, and it's in reference to the concept of a "spiritual disease." There is other somewhat medical language like "sickness" and "illness" scattered throughout the text, but the physical is always tempered with, if not wholly subordinated to, the numinous: for example, alcoholism is "an illness which only a spiritual experience will conquer." The whole point of AA's conception of alcoholism was that it was a pragmatic hybrid, a flexible balance between physical, mental, and spiritual elements—what Wilson called the "threefold nature" of alcoholism. Mutual-help approaches often present addiction as just one manifestation of a broader malaise—a common expression in meetings is "I came for my drinking and stayed for my thinking"—and at the core, AA's writings worked hard to present its concepts as ones that were open to personal interpretation, avoiding giving too much weight to any single explanation for alcoholism.

As one of Wilson's biographers put it, AA is built on "finessing the relationship between the sacred and the secular," and Wilson himself made conscious and deliberate choices about balancing those two elements. While the Big Book does insist that people find a "higher power," it generally downplays religion's contributions to AA. Wilson de-emphasized his "white light" experience in it and didn't even identify the Oxford Group by name, instead focusing on the intellectual debt that movement owed to the likes of William James and Carl Jung. Tellingly, he also avoids fully medicalizing alcoholism. AA writings skirt the question of disease, instead calling alcoholism an "illness" or "malady." Wilson later explained, in a 1960 speech, his hesitancy to label alcoholism as one singular entity: "We AAs have never called alcoholism a disease because, technically speaking, it is not a disease entity. For example, there is no such thing as heart disease. Instead, there are many separate heart ailments or combinations of them. It is something like that with alcoholism."

By contrast, Mann insisted that alcoholism was a clear, known, and singular scientific entity (a fairly bold claim that we cannot and do not confidently make more than seventy years later). She emphasized this argument by making analogies to diseases—she often compared alcoholism to tuberculosis, diabetes, and cancer—and the specific examples are telling. Tuberculosis seems closer to her meaning: it's caused by a known bacterium, results in a recognized set of symptoms distinctly different from normal functioning, and is treated with a widely accepted therapy. This is the commonsense idea of disease, a microbiological model of a singular malady with clear causes and cures: you have it or you don't. Today, however, we understand that most diseases are not so straightforward. Diabetes is caused by variable contributions from diet, obesity, genetics, and autoimmune dysfunction. The boundary between diabetic and healthy is not inherently obvious—in fact, that boundary needs to be set by committees, which argue over the proper cutoff for blood glucose levels and other biomarkers. Similarly, cancer arises at the intersection of many different molecular and genetic pathways, and our bodies are in a constant dance of detecting abnormal growths and clearing away pre-cancers. The more we learn about modern diseases, the less they look like the commonsense infection model—a discrete and bounded entity or thing—and the more they look like functional, complex, interacting systems. But for Mann, alcoholism-as-entity was the root of her identity; it was the AA principle that took hold most powerfully for her, the basis for her tribal identification among her new people. Her movement, at least as she originally conceived it, had no real space for pluralism.

The odd thing about Mann's disease language is that it seems that in her own private views, or at least the ones she shared with certain fellow AA members, she was more skeptical of the disease analogy, to the point that she doubted whether medicine could help much at all. In 1945, just after she started the organization that would become the NCA, a local organizer and AA member wrote to her, objecting that her campaign was too focused on medicine, not in tune enough with the spiritual dimensions of AA. She replied, "Not that I, as a dyed-in-the-wool AA, believe that clinics, or any other medical or psychiatric means can straighten out very many 'alkies' (although I know it can in some instances, here and there) but I do believe that the average individual will more readily go into a clinic to find out what to do for what ails them than they will investigate a layman's organization such as ours. And also I believe that the very presence of a clinic will emphasize and advertise to the uninitiated that alcoholism is a disease which is to be treated, not hidden or punished."

For Mann, disease language was a way of communicating hope about addiction, getting people on the road to recovery, and, perhaps above all, reshaping the narrative. The NCA's alcoholism information centers were supposed to "penetrate deep into hostile territory, infiltrating through combat lines of prejudice, to establish this bridgehead of hope for the captive people behind those lines: alcoholics and their families." Her overriding concern was to build a bridge across "an impassable swamp: a No Man's Land of ignorance, fear, superstition, and stigma."

Yet there's something funny about expecting disease language to reduce stigma, considering how often diseases are heavily moralized. Consider the many stigmatized portrayals of tuberculosis, from the Romantic Era to *The Magic Mountain*—not for nothing did Akira Kurosawa, in his 1948 film *Drunken Angel*, use tuberculosis and alcoholism as dual markers of the taint of the American occupation of Japan. Modern research also questions whether a disease framing alleviates stigma. Several studies have found that a binary disease-model view of alcoholism, as opposed to a continuum model, makes it harder for people to recognize their own harmful drinking. In another study, the most potent predictor of relapse was belief in the disease model of addiction. Disease language is often a centerpiece of "anti-stigma campaigns" for addiction and other mental health conditions, such as the national "A Disease Like Any Other" campaign for mental illness—but subsequent research found it to be disappointingly ineffective and even counterproductive, actually increasing stigma by some measures. When I asked Keith Humphreys, a psychologist and senior policy adviser for the Obama administration's drug policy, about stigma reduction campaigns, he flatly declared them a "failure."

Ideas about addiction are life-and-death. The idea that she was an alcoholic and could never drink again saved Marty Mann's life, at least in her estimation. Countless others in her time were told that they could be cured of their drinking problems, build up their willpower, and learn to drink like gentlemen—before relapsing with unimaginable consequences. When I attended the American Society of Addiction Medicine (ASAM) conference in 2019, I heard the writer and addiction advocate David Sheff, author of *Beautiful Boy*, speak about how a disease model of addiction helped him to drop the sense of blame he had toward his son, Nic, and get him the right medical treatment, just as prior generations of advocates had hoped.

But around the time I was born, in the early years of the 1980s recovery craze, both of my parents went to traditional outpatient alcoholism treatment, and they were turned off by it—they weren't willing to accept that they had a medical problem. My mother, in particular, hated it. It wasn't who she was. She was the chairperson of her university department. She had established a Ph.D. program from the ground up. Even as a young boy, I could appreciate that all was not well with her—the drunken driving, the passing out at odd times, the erratic moods. Yet as I grew older and began to challenge her about her drinking problems, I could never get past her most basic belief: "I'm not an alcoholic—look at your father!" He was the one with the disease. She was different.

Eight

GOOD DRUGS
AND BAD DRUGS

William Burroughs was getting desperate. His Harvard pol-
ish was wearing thin under the constant friction of opioid
addiction, and not a single doctor in New York City would
write him a prescription anymore. He tried forging scripts, but he was
quickly busted and caught a low-level charge. He tried stealing from
passed-out drunks on the subways, but he was a small, thin, unathletic
man—since his boarding school days, more given to reading Baudelaire
by candlelight than playing sports—and after barely escaping a beating,
he gave that up. He tried kicking the habit, but he kept relapsing on
heroin. He tried dealing to support his own supply, but the federal
agents were closing in quickly.

It was New York City in 1947, and it was, if such a thing is possible,
a particularly bad time to be addicted to heroin. From roughly the 1920s
to the 1960s, the country was dominated by an anti-drug, prohibitionist
fervor: strict enforcement, draconian punishments, and almost no treatment options. Just days after the Harrison Act went into effect in 1915,
Burroughs's uncle Horace, a narcotics user, killed himself with a piece
of broken glass in a rooming house in Detroit, reportedly because he
foresaw how people like him were about to be bereft of their supply,

hunted down, and jailed. Now, a few decades later, William Burroughs's own heroin addiction was reaching a breaking point, and he was running out of options. So, one cold January day in 1948, he drove his car from New York to Cincinnati, then hopped the southbound train to Lexington, Kentucky, to check into the United States Narcotic Farm, or "Narco."

Narco was a massive prison hospital built on a thousand acres of sprawling Kentucky bluegrass. Even people who had been to Rikers Island or Sing Sing were flabbergasted by its size. On the drive in, you'd pass miles and miles of cow pastures, pigpens, and crops and orchards, then the enormous main building would come into view, sprawling over twelve acres by itself, a central tower rising like an art deco ziggurat, multi-story wings stretching into the distance and wrapping around quads large enough to contain tennis courts and softball fields.

Burroughs didn't stay long—he just wanted a break from law enforcement and a few days of detox. Once they stopped giving him drugs for withdrawal, he took a cab to Lexington, caught a train back up to Cincinnati, and started buying up paregoric (an over-the-counter opium tincture). But for many others, Narco was a humane refuge, an oasis in the middle of a country obsessed with harsh punishments for drug crimes. It was also a sanctuary for doctors and researchers who believed in more compassionate treatment for addiction, and it was a meeting place, both for those few professionals and for their ideas—where the new sciences of neurophysiology and behaviorism were brought to bear on addiction. Researchers and clinicians got to know their patients with addiction, learning that they weren't broken or vicious but often well-meaning, with rich inner lives.

In many ways, though, the work of this era only served to heighten the division between good and bad drugs—and good and bad drug users. An overly reductionist perspective on addiction, one heavily influenced by the biases and prejudices of the time, blinded society to the dangers on both sides of that divide. The result was to further entrench

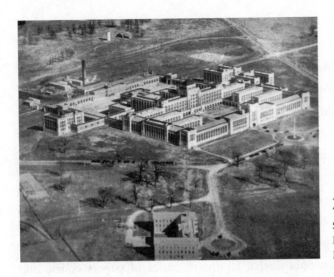

Aerial view of "Narco," the United States Narcotic Farm at Lexington, Kentucky, c. 1935.

the separate and unequal system that failed people with addiction across the whole spectrum, from the most marginalized to the most privileged.

The first head of Narco was Lawrence Kolb, a public-health-minded psychiatrist who had carried out crucial research on the "antitoxin" theory of drug addiction at the National Hygienic Laboratory, in Washington, DC (the precursor of the National Institutes of Health). That antitoxin theory, popularized in part by Charles Towns, had postulated that the root cause of addiction was an immunological reaction in the blood, in line with the idea that addiction was nothing more than a physically determined disorder, but Kolb conducted the definitive studies disproving this theory.[*]

Kolb was not just a brilliant and unconventional thinker; he was a self-made man with an immense work ethic. Despite being born into poverty to a family of fifteen children and never finishing high school, he fought his way through medical school, at first almost failing out, but

---

[*] For example, he showed that if you took serum from humans with addiction and injected it into mice, that wouldn't protect the rodents from morphine overdose.

ultimately graduating third in his class. So when the national Public Health Service brought him to Washington, DC, and charged him with investigating addiction, the laboratory work was only the start. He soon threw himself into an enormous series of real-world studies, traveling from Maine to Alabama to interview people with addiction, their families, and their doctors. At a time when the dominant stereotype was one of "junkies," Kolb was astounded to learn that many of the people he met were doing well, even flourishing—as long as they received regulated, reliable prescriptions of maintenance opioids like morphine and opium. Kolb also recognized that drug use served purposes such as sensation-seeking and relief for emotional problems.

In 1925, Kolb published a landmark series of papers concluding that addiction was caused by underlying psychological issues and not some kind of physiological enslavement by a menacing drug. Specifically, he thought, people with addiction were driven to use drugs because of long-standing personality problems. The language he used sounds harsh today—people with addiction were said to have a "twisted personality" driving their drug use, or to be "inferiors who are striving to appear like normal men," or simply "psychopaths"—but during a time of severe narcotic control, Kolb's model was intended to be compassionate. His fundamental argument was that people became addicted not by choice or because they are sinners or criminal menaces, but because of underlying problems in their psychology.

Today we know that there is no singular "addictive personality." Decades of research have shown that there is no consistent set of personality dimensions or defensive structures that separate people with addiction from the rest of society. Boldness and impulsivity can predispose people to addiction, but so can the opposite tendencies, like anxiety and inhibition. Certain personality types might have a greater risk of addiction, but there is no one personality type for people with addiction.

By focusing on personality, Kolb was following an important trend in psychological science in the earlier part of the twentieth century. Kolb began his career screening immigrants on Ellis Island and studying at the New York State Psychiatric Institute, at a time of great interest in applying intelligence testing and other psychological measurements to immigration screening. However, that research, as well as similar psychological testing on World War I recruits, had revealed that simply measuring intelligence was not enough to screen out mental disorders. Instead, researchers like Kolb searched for other ways of defining stable, long-term mental traits, and the emergent notion of personality became their organizing principle. As Kolb's laboratory studies also showed, the search for a biological cause for addiction had failed, lending support to this approach, and accordingly, many other medical thinkers during the 1920s and '30s proposed theories of addiction as a personality problem.

Kolb's work earned him the job of director of Narco, which at its opening in 1935 was hailed as a "New Deal for the drug addict." Kolb worked tirelessly to shape Narco into a therapeutic facility governed by compassion, starting with his insistence that incarcerated people with addiction be called "patients" rather than "prisoners." Group psychotherapy was an element of the program, but Narco's main treatment philosophy was to put patients into a wholesome environment. Some patients rose before dawn to milk cows, butcher pigs, bale hay, and tend to fields of kale and tomatoes, while others sewed uniforms, cleaned, or were apprenticed to tradesmen like X-ray technicians and electricians. There was a bowling alley, billiards room, and volleyball courts. Patients took courses in creative writing, painting, and jazz. In the 1955 film *The Man with the Golden Arm*, Frank Sinatra's character, "Frankie Machine," returns after six months in Narco with nothing but praise: "Greatest place you've ever seen. Ball games, great food, I even learned how to play the drums." One patient who had been transferred there from a normal prison enthused in a newspaper interview that it was "too good to be true." Other reports derided it as a "country-club prison" and a "multi-million dollar flophouse for junkies."

Narco was a special place for doctors and researchers, too. Well into the 1960s, essentially all the top American addiction researchers got their start at Narco, and nearly all the major midcentury scientific and medical contributions to the study of addiction can be traced back to it: the discovery of opioid receptors, the use of methadone and buprenorphine for addiction treatment, and the characterization of opioid antagonists like naloxone (the active ingredient in the overdose-reversal agent Narcan). During this harshly prohibitionist period, however, the key force in drug policy was not medicine but law enforcement, particularly the Federal Bureau of Narcotics (FBN), which was headed by the domineering Harry Anslinger for thirty-two years, beginning in 1930. He was both a cosmopolitan and charming former diplomat and an angry, thick-necked, unsmiling, and uncompromising enemy of drugs. Later in life, he noted admiringly that "the Nazi regime bore down heavily on the addict, and had the situation pretty well in hand."

Anslinger's tenacity was matched only by his political acumen. When he took control of the FBN, he didn't consider cannabis a high priority, but he quickly noted that there was a powerful prohibitionist movement afoot against that drug, one boosted by powerful anti-Mexican racism. Starting in the 1910s, refugees had fled from the violence of the Mexican Revolution to the United States, only to be doused with gasoline and have their clothes fumigated with Zyklon B at immigration stations like El Paso, then be met with lynching and widespread xenophobia throughout the States. The public associated Mexican laborers with cannabis, and amid the growing anti-Mexican sentiment, prohibition-inclined doctors and western and southern police authorities began agitating for tighter controls on the drug. When Anslinger realized the potential in these twinned narratives of foreignness and drugs, he capitalized on them to greatly expand the powers of his office. From that point forward, he slyly emphasized an association between substance use and racial stereotypes as he relentlessly associated drugs with violence and deviance.

Anslinger was an expert at telling horror stories about how drugs caused uncontrollable addiction, crime, and violence. Not only did he relentlessly cultivate politicians and shape policy; he also took a direct hand in public relations work, writing and placing sensationalistic articles and books, strong-arming and suppressing any media stories not originating from his office, and pushing script ideas about dangerous drugs to Hollywood directors. This was the era of absurd anti-drug films, such as 1936's *Tell Your Children,* made famous decades later under the title *Reefer Madness,* which showcases a lurid string of consequences after high schoolers try cannabis, including hallucinations, a car accident, suicide, rape, and murder.

Most galling to Kolb and other medical professionals, Anslinger readily co-opted scientific language to tell those horror stories about addiction. (For example, he claimed that cannabis made users "develop a delirious rage after its administration during which they are temporarily, at least, irresponsible and prone to commit violent crimes.") Drawing on Kolb's theories, he called people with addiction "psychopaths," who were "created by infectious contact with persons already drug-conditioned." Anslinger insisted that addiction was the unstoppable combination of a fundamentally twisted person with a fundamentally dangerous drug, so addiction could not be dealt with by the medical establishment alone. Prohibition and police power were the only "cure": "Whenever you find severe penalties, addiction disappears." "The best cure for addiction?" Anslinger asked. "Never let it happen."

Throughout his life, Kolb was a forceful advocate for a therapeutic approach and increasingly worked to counteract the prevalent fearmongering about the supposed dangers of addiction—such as anti-drug activists warning that addiction was a "moral and physical scourge" threatening "the perpetuation of civilization, the destiny of the world, and the future of the human race." Kolb conducted scientifically rigorous statistical studies to rebut the misinformation of those crusaders, who were producing grossly inflated estimates of the number of people with addiction. But Kolb was also working during a time when public

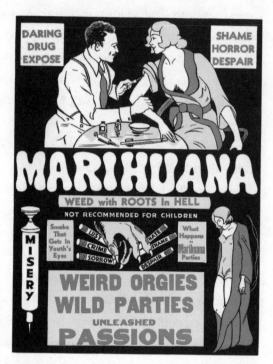

A movie poster for *Marihuana* (1936), one of many anti-cannabis movies from the 1930s.

sentiment had already swung far toward prohibition, and ultimately he was outgunned. Anslinger's views prevailed, and the result was a massive increase in drug arrests and penalties throughout the forties and fifties. In 1940, 682 new patients were admitted to Narco, but that number reached 1,600 in 1949 and surpassed 2,300 in 1950. (Tellingly, Black admissions to Narco rose from roughly 10 percent in 1940 to 30 percent in 1950. Puerto Rican and Mexican admissions soared from 1 percent to more than a quarter of the population by the 1960s.) In time, Kolb left the facility to become the chief of the Mental Hygiene Division of the U.S. Public Health Service, the predecessor of the National Institute of Mental Health, and after he left, Narco became hopelessly overcrowded—and infected with hopelessness and punitive attitudes. A patient from that period recalled, "Nobody got no treatment. We didn't go to no group therapy. We didn't go to no individual therapy. We didn't do nothin' . . . there was no program." In just a few years, what began as a majestic, cutting-edge monument to medical progress had become an authoritarian institution designed for total control.

In 1953, a few years after his stay in Narco, Burroughs published his first book, *Junky*. It was a major milestone in the countercultural reclaiming of the word "junky" (or "junkie")—the drug user identity as a badge of membership and a conscious revolt against bourgeois conformity—but though Burroughs was deeply influenced by Romantics like Coleridge, De Quincey, and Baudelaire, the book was also peppered with surprisingly reductionist views on addiction.

"Junk," he argued, had a way of enslaving the body that was "different from the action of any other drug." "The use of junk causes permanent cellular alteration," leading to "junk-dependent cells." "Junk creates a deficiency so that the body cannot function without more junk at regular intervals. . . . Withdrawal of junk creates a deficiency condition. . . . So far as I know, junk is the only habit forming drug according to this definition." It is this kind of deterministic reasoning that leads Burroughs to one of his most famous conclusions: "Once a junkie, always a junkie."

The upshot, Burroughs insisted, was that opioids were uniquely addictive, unlike, for example, cocaine: "There is no tolerance with C . . . one shot creates an urgent desire for another shot to maintain the high. But once the C is out of your system, you forget about it. There is no habit to C."

Burroughs was following the biases of the top researchers of the time, who dismissed problems with cocaine and other stimulants as only "psychic addiction." Two leading scientists, for example, noted that "without abstinence symptoms on withdrawal, a drug can scarcely be considered to produce true addiction," and Lawrence Kolb himself wrote an influential paper arguing that stimulants were not truly addictive. The dominant assumptions about good drugs and bad drugs were readily reflected in a narrow and biology-based explanation for addiction.

Tucked within the enormity of Narco, there was a tiny laboratory— the only one in the world entirely devoted to the study of drug addiction. By the time Narco opened, years of searching for the biological causes of addiction had failed—all the cleansing, purging, puking, patent cures, and injections were clearly a wash, too—but even so, Narco's scientific program was established on a reductionistic ideal, as it was charged directly by Congress with finding a scientific cure for addiction. Specifically, its first goal was a corollary to the prevailing law-and-order approach to addiction: to find a "non-addictive" pain medication. If there were an alternative to heroin or morphine, the thinking went, with all of the painkilling properties but none of the euphoria or addicting tendencies, law enforcement could step in and eradicate dangerous opioids entirely. But how could researchers define, let alone measure, the "addictiveness" of a drug in the first place?

Neuroscience was advancing by leaps and bounds. The early decades of the twentieth century saw tremendous progress in the field, starting with Golgi and Cajal's 1906 Nobel Prize for elucidating the underlying cellular structure of the nervous system; subsequent research revealed the mechanisms by which nerve impulses traveled down the cell and other mechanical workings of the brain. At the systems level, the world's first brain-imaging scientists had just developed the electroencephalograph (EEG, which uses electrodes on the surface of the scalp to record the summed electrical activity of the brain), and one of those early EEG scientists was brought to Narco to "find out what's going on in the brains of these addicts." The rudimentary tools available in the 1930s weren't powerful enough to provide a satisfying answer, though, so researchers turned to a different methodology: the new psychological discipline of behaviorism.

"First psychology lost its soul, then it lost its mind, then it lost consciousness; it still has behavior, of a kind." Written in 1921, these words mark the falling away of the humanistic psychology of William James in favor of behaviorism, an outright rejection of the tradition of subjectivity in psychology. Behaviorists like John B. Watson promised a "scientific psychology" that would reduce humans to outwardly observable stimuli and responses that followed simple mechanical laws. Behaviorism was immensely popular through the earlier twentieth century, and it still has a powerful influence on a certain strain of psychological research, particularly in addiction research, which has long sought clockwork mechanisms of stimuli, response, and reward that determine habitual drug use.

The scientists in Narco's research lab needed a simple behaviorist measure of a complex phenomenon, a way to explain why drugs were so addictive. They quickly decided that opioid withdrawal—the "cold turkey" experience of sweating, craving, and generally miserable discomfort—would be the best scientific marker for the addictiveness of a drug, the "sine qua non of addiction." The first lab director at Narco noted that "it immediately struck me that this was a very, very dependable kind of illness, that things happen almost by the clock."

Narco patients were enticed into studies by the promise of free drugs—not only were they administered drugs during the studies, they were paid in extra morphine at the end of the trials. In a series of experiments that would make today's ethicists blanch, researchers gave the patients opioids until they developed tolerance, then plunged them into withdrawal by stopping the drugs (or later by giving them opioid-blocking medications). As the patients groaned, the researchers stood by with clipboards, dutifully tracking all the objective signs of drug use and withdrawal to the minute: heart rate, yawning, sweating, muscle twitches, goose bumps, diarrhea, even spontaneous orgasms. To measure pain and suffering, scientists put hot metal on the subjects' skin or administered electric shocks to their teeth, asking them to quantify the results.

The result of all this gruesome research was in some ways useful, because it clarified that opioid withdrawal was a real physical phenomenon—well into the 1940s, people were still debating whether opioid withdrawal was psychogenic (all in the head). However, many clinicians and lay observers alike took the Narco formulation of the "opioid withdrawal syndrome" too far and equated physical dependence with addiction, full stop. In those retellings, all of addiction was explained by the mere presence of tolerance and withdrawal, and nothing more—the complex and multifaceted experience of addiction reduced to the deterministic kinetics of the human body, stripped of any subjectivity.

It's overly reductionist to explain all of addictive behavior in terms of tolerance and withdrawal. Yes, withdrawal can be extraordinarily uncomfortable, even a significant risk factor for relapse, but it's only one of many factors. Most people need more than detox to overcome addiction—in fact, detoxification without further treatment can increase the risk of overdose death more than if the person had simply continued using. It is misleading to draw a boundary between "physical" and "psychological" addiction, especially because that notion has long been used to suggest that a so-called psychological addiction is not a "real" addiction, often to the benefit of market interests and people in power.

Nevertheless, in the 1950s and '60s, researchers, the criminal legal system, and the general public quickly latched on to the notion of tolerance and withdrawal as the defining characteristic of addiction. Police gave people arrested on suspicion of drug use a "challenge" dose of the opioid-blocking medication Nalline, and if they were thrown into withdrawal, that was equated with being addicted. For decades to come—well into the 1970s, at least—research and clinical practice were burdened by this framework; as recently as 1976, the American Society of Addiction Medicine defined the characteristics of alcoholism as "tolerance and physical dependency or pathologic organ changes, or both."

From Burroughs's counterculture to the laboratory of Narco, opioids were the archetype of addiction, leading to the assumption that the physical characteristics of opioid use captured all that was scientifically meaningful about the condition. It was a dangerous assumption, because it prompted clinicians, policymakers, and the general public to overlook the real harms of other substances. This narrow-mindedness was especially shortsighted, considering the recent history of cocaine.

In April 1884, Sigmund Freud was still a junior neuroanatomist in Vienna, studying the nerve cells of crayfish and struggling to climb the academic ladder, when he stumbled across a new "magical substance": cocaine. He took the drug liberally to fuel his own writing, but, more significantly, he used it in an attempt to treat the morphine addiction of his close friend Ernst von Fleischl-Marxow. Fleischl-Marxow loved it, and after finding himself able to reduce his morphine dose for the first time in ages, he urged Freud to publish as soon as possible. Freud rushed out *Über Coca* ("On Cocaine"), his first major scientific paper, a confident account of cocaine's history, pharmacology, animal research, and effects on healthy humans.

Otherwise lucid and readable, *Über Coca* goes off the rails in its last section, where Freud suggests cocaine should be used as a therapy for digestive disorders, asthma, loss of sexual potency, hysteria, hypochondria, and melancholy and, of course, as a "cure" for morphine addiction. Freud was denounced by the German-speaking medical world for his naivete about the risks of addiction. (The eminent German physician Friedrich Erlenmeyer said that trying to cure morphine addiction with cocaine was like trying to cast out Satan with Beelzebub.) Sure enough, in just three months, Fleischl-Marxow became terribly addicted to cocaine, taking more than a gram at a time, which often left him floridly psychotic and hallucinating—plus he had resumed taking high doses of morphine, resulting in some of the world's first "speedballs." After seven years of this torture, he died in 1891 at age forty-five. A guilty Freud hung a photo of his dead friend on the wall of his study for the rest of his life, next to a picture of Alexander III of Macedon and a proverb Fleischl-Marxow had given him, attributed to Saint Augustine: "When in doubt, abstain."

In the coming years, in Europe and the United States, medical doctors repeatedly came to the realization that cocaine was not a magical drug but one with serious addictive potential. Yet it continued to be used as a pharmaceutical treatment for several years, and Freud's story also illustrates how defining a substance as a treatment can falsely insulate it from scrutiny and obscure its harms. Freud himself continued using cocaine heavily through the 1890s, which he justified to himself as a treatment for severe headaches and "dysgraphia" (disinclination to write). Writing to his friend Wilhelm Fliess that he was struggling to control his consumption, he confessed, "I need a lot of cocaine. . . . The torment, most of the time, is superhuman."

I tried to be more cautious after the quasi intervention from my program director. I actually did get to bed earlier. I cut down on drinking for a time. But I wasn't quite sure what to do with myself. Drinking had become a core part of my identity. It had provided structure and regularity to my days and nights and predictability to my mental states.

To fill the void, I piled on research projects and commitments—I figured I could addict myself to academic success as a substitute. In the meantime, I was also starting to worry about money—I had blown my budget to live in the trendy West Village of Manhattan—so I took on a part-time job editing journal articles. Before long I was waking up at 5 a.m. to try to write, then dragging myself through a day of seeing patients, but that still didn't quiet the voice inside. I couldn't escape the feeling that I wasn't enough. I wasn't really on track to become a respected academician. I was broke, writing obscure bioethics papers, and barely squeaking by in my residency. The harder I tried, the more I seemed to fall short. I needed to work harder, to be someone better, to find a way to be special.

It was around this time that I started using more Adderall to get by. Some part of me realized that I was being sucked into unhealthy levels of busyness, that perhaps I shouldn't have to pump myself full of amphetamines just to cope with the life I had created, but I used the drug as directed, and the prescription never ran out early, so I told myself it wasn't really a problem.

My drinking crept back in, but as it did, I found that the Adderall helped me to manage. If I went out drinking during the week, an Adderall the next morning would dampen the hangover and compensate for my mental sluggishness. I'd wake up, take a pill, have a quick nap, then wake up for good. If I started flagging in the evening, another pill would set me right. It was a harrowing balancing act.

Still, I managed to get by in residency until my vacation that fall, a precious and rare two weeks off. I had planned a road trip down the Eastern Seaboard to visit friends. (I christened it "Bender November" ahead of time, which speaks to just how little awareness I had of my problems.) I applied the same mechanistic logic about balancing stimulants and drinking—a little Adderall here and there to keep the party going, a few more shots if it felt too speedy. By the time I reached Delaware, I was coming apart. Even my body was accumulating physical evidence that was getting hard to deny. I passed out in a hot tub with no one else around, then I lost my key, figured it was in the pool, and dove and dove again, feeling across the enormous white bottom for the white key, scraping my face until there was a weeping abrasion on my nose. I eventually found *a* key, and got into *a* room after trying every door on multiple hallways—thankfully, no one was there. Later, in North Carolina, I realized I had a deep gash down my back from who knows where. I was no longer using the Adderall for focus at work, as it was prescribed, but I was still only using one or two a day—at least that's what I thought; I wasn't keeping close track anymore—so I figured: How bad could it be?

Despite more than a week of partying and vanishingly little sleep, I began waking up spontaneously at 6 a.m. with way too much energy. I impulsively bought a same-day flight back from North Carolina to New York that I couldn't afford. A cautious part of me recognized that something was wrong. I was too impulsive, too oddly ebullient. But that part was losing ground, and another part of me decided that I was having a spiritual awakening. On the clattering E train back into the city from LaGuardia Airport, I gazed benevolently around the subway car, giving some poor woman a big, weird smile.

In the mid-1940s, Allen Ginsberg paired up Burroughs with Joan Vollmer, a streetwise and brilliant Beat author from their Greenwich Village days who would become Burroughs's wife. Her tastes in drugs ran in a different direction: she favored amphetamine, introduced to her by Jack Kerouac and readily available in those days over the counter as Benzedrine. In 1946, she received the dubious honor of being Bellevue Hospital's first female case of amphetamine psychosis, arriving covered in sores, beset by delusions about atomic testing and worms tunneling through her skin. Just a year later, in an attempt to avoid Burroughs's narcotic charges, they fled for Texas with their young son, Billy Jr. Visitors arrived to find an infant Billy naked and defecating on the floor, while Vollmer compulsively chewed on the crook of her left arm and raked little lizards out of the trees. Yet while Burroughs Sr. was struggling with heroin—they soon had to flee the country entirely to escape narcotic charges yet again—Vollmer just had to drive to a Houston pharmacy to get her drug of choice.

They were in the middle of a decades-long enthusiasm for stimulants like amphetamine, and in general the country was enamored of new pharmaceutical medications. For a huge swath of the midcentury—and, in a way, continuing to this day—multiple waves of novel prescription drugs were sold to the populace as safe, only to quickly backfire. Throughout, the country missed the obvious dangers, a blind spot that was partly the result of prejudices about the "junkie" paradigm of opioid addiction, partly the intended effect of concerted marketing efforts, and partly the "honeymoon" period that has struck again and again when a society has warmed to a new compound. But at a more fundamental level, this attitude was the harmful product of a deepening perceptual division between good drugs and bad drugs.

Even though cocaine's honeymoon period had only recently passed, new stimulant drugs quickly emerged to take its place, as the historian Nicolas Rasmussen has documented in his superb and wide-ranging history *On Speed*. In the 1920s, there was a brief craze for purified hormone medications such as ephedrine and adrenaline, but the real eureka moment came in 1929, when a young chemist named Gordon Alles self-experimented with a series of new, chemically related synthetic molecules. Alles eventually happened upon a mystery molecule that raised his blood pressure, cleared his nose, and resulted in a "rather sleepless night." He had discovered amphetamine. Amphetamine was quickly and successfully adopted by the pharmaceutical firm Smith, Kline & French (SKF), first as the Benzedrine Inhaler for congestion, then later in pill form for a range of indications, including depression, alcoholism, and dieting and weight control.

Some early observers tried to call attention to the addiction risks of amphetamine use. In early 1938, a high-profile article in the *Journal of the American Medical Association* cautioned against using amphetamine for dieting, because patients seemed to be having trouble getting off the drug. Another report described that amphetamine "effectively" cured alcoholism but then became the new drug of choice for patients. Reports accumulated of the Benzedrine Inhaler being used non-medically— people could buy it over the counter and take a heavy whiff to get high. In those days, before Charlie Parker picked up heroin, he was using

Benzedrine Inhalers heavily; after a night of playing music, one observer recalled, the white plastic empties piled up on the floor like snow.

All the while, though, the medical field remained obsessed with opioids as the paradigm for addiction—as Lawrence Kolb himself had implied, stimulants were just "mentally addicting." So, rather than being reined in, the stimulant trade only grew. And then it received its greatest boost yet: World War II.

Drug use has been closely associated with warfare for centuries. Mesopotamian soldiers were paid in beer rations, the ancient Greeks made wine the drink of fighting men, Benjamin Rush bemoaned how much rum soldiers were being given, and Bavarian soldiers were issued pure cocaine in the late nineteenth century. But World War II was the first war involving widespread use of *synthetic* drugs, which were being mass-produced on almost the same scale as planes and battleships. The Germans pioneered amphetamine use to fuel their Blitzkrieg ("lightning war") tactics and help Stuka dive-bombers tolerate ten-thousand-plus-foot drops without blacking out. German forces consumed 35 million methamphetamine tablets in just three months at the peak of the Blitz. After investigators discovered the pills in the wreckage of downed German airplanes in the fields of southern England, the Allied forces themselves quickly adopted stimulants. Soon, the U.S. Army was issuing amphetamine as a regular part of combat first aid kits. Though some soldiers hallucinated and battled unseen enemies, American troops returned home with their enthusiasm for these new drugs, to a postwar culture that idealized energy, hustle, and drive—in 1940s lingo, "pep."

Oddly, the Americans used amphetamines at much higher levels than other forces on both sides of the conflict. The Germans and the British were much quicker to appreciate the dangers of addiction—as early as mid-1941, the Germans put amphetamines under special prescription control and issued a stark declaration that the drugs were dangerously addictive, and the British issued similar controls soon afterward.

The Americans, though, showed no such caution. The uniquely American enthusiasm for marketing and consumerism, and its effect on notions of addiction, is part of the reason why.

From the first warnings about addiction and amphetamine, Smith, Kline & French began deploying increasingly sophisticated advertising and marketing efforts to counteract the concerns. It was almost as though SKF were writing the playbook for how to create a prescription drug epidemic. First, use aggressive advertising to broaden your consumer base. (SKF kicked off the Benzedrine craze by marketing it as an easy way for general practitioners to treat depression, pain, alcoholism, and obesity.) Second, when regulators and the public start to get concerned, manufacture ostensibly abuse-deterrent formulations to placate them. (SKF added dye and the irritant capsaicin to Benzedrine Inhalers, which didn't work to stop non-medical use but did help to get legislators off their backs.) Third, and most significantly, fund scientists and clinicians to argue that your drug isn't really addictive. (Pharma-funded doctors argued that any so-called stimulant addiction was the fault of the individual's psychology, not "any pharmacologic action of the drugs themselves.") Using the prevailing model of addiction as physical dependence, they claimed the drugs weren't truly addictive because they didn't produce withdrawal. The result: Benzedrine became one of the first blockbuster drugs.

More blockbusters were soon to arrive. The postwar era was an age of affluence for the United States, with an expanding middle class streaming out to the suburbs and filling up their homes with dishwashers, radios, televisions, and all the other trappings of their newfound wealth. Just as consumer spending was framed as an act of citizenship, prescription medications were framed as a consumer good. Pharmaceutical marketers sent "detail men" into doctors' offices in droves. By the 1950s, as many as 95 percent of doctor visits culminated in a prescription, and total drug sales rose from $300 million to $2.3 billion in the space of just two decades. These developments provided the foundation for the Purdue Pharma empire. Well before OxyContin, in the 1960s, Arthur Sackler pushed pharmaceutical marketing to the limit for the new "minor tranquilizers" Librium and Valium (benzodiazepines, like the later Xanax). Sackler pioneered momentous innovations such as bestowing extravagant payments on researchers who voiced opinions favorable to the company, twisting research findings for marketing purposes, and funding both front publications and purportedly independent interest groups.

Pharmaceutical marketing strategies offer a through line that takes us all the way up to today's dominant medical practice, particularly in psychiatry, which heavily prioritizes treatment with medications. Medications are tactile, substantial, and clear; they promise a carefully calibrated and titrated control of the unruly body. There is a recurrent and selective amnesia that the greatest drug harms—including addiction—are almost always caused by legal products: morphine and cocaine in the nineteenth century, stimulants and sedatives in the mid-twentieth century, opioids more recently, and, throughout and always, alcohol and tobacco.

Amphetamines evaded tighter controls in part because they were so dissimilar to opioids—playing off the overly reductionist fixation on withdrawal as the sine qua non of addiction—but at least that distinction had some reason to it, misguided as it was. As time went on, and as the asymmetrical power of the addiction supply industries kept working to widen the division between good and bad, addictive versus benign, the justifications became nearly absurd—and dangerous.

In the summer of 1951, a middle-aged physician came to Narco for help with addiction. At first he seemed fine—he said that he had already tapered down his codeine dose—but just one hour after being admitted, he threw up and became soaked with sweat. Before long he was hallucinating, his heart was hammering, his blood pressure

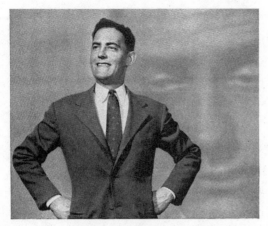

"...if the individual is depressed..."

"... . if the individual is depressed or anhedonic . . . you can change his attitude . . . by physical means just as surely as you can change his digestion by distressing thought . . . *In other words, drugs and physical therapeutics are just as much psychic agents as good advice and analysis* and must be used together with these latter agents of cure."

Myerson, A.—*Anhedonia*—
Am. J. Psychiat., July, 1922.

When this was written—in 1922—the only stimulant drugs employed in the treatment of simple depression were of limited effectiveness.

Only in the last decade has there been available—in Benzedrine Sulfate—a therapeutic weapon capable of alleviating depression, overcoming "chronic fatigue" and breaking the vicious circle of anhedonia.

BENZEDRINE SULFATE TABLETS

(racemic amphetamine sulfate)

SMITH, KLINE & FRENCH LABORATORIES, PHILADELPHIA, PA.

XIII

An advertisement for the amphetamine Benzedrine for the treatment of depression, 1945.

destabilized, and his temperature soared to 107. The doctors, dumb-founded, threw everything they had at him—wet packs, ephedrine, in-sulin, penicillin, sedatives—but nothing helped for long. Six hellish, sleepless days later, he died of an apparent heart attack. It was only later that the doctor's wife was able to tell the team the real story: he had been secretly addicted to secobarbital (Seconal) and was taking up to fifty capsules of the powerful barbiturate daily.

Barbiturates were another blockbuster of the day, a powerful seda-tive that seemed purpose-built for what W. H. Auden called the "Age of Anxiety": the cold war, fears of the atomic bomb, and a vogue for psychoanalysis, all promoting awareness of anxiety as a phenomenon. According to one study from around that time, half of city dwellers reported clinically significant anxiety. In this environment, barbiturates—a class of medications that carry a high risk of overdose and death—became immensely popular. By the late 1940s, enough barbiturates were being manufactured and consumed for twenty-four doses per person every year. There were some concerns about barbiturate addiction in medical journals and the popular press, but, given that it was a product primarily available to white and well-off consumers, most researchers and regulators wrote off barbiturate problems as "habituation" rather than true addiction.

Thus, barbiturates had long evaded attempts at tighter regulations, which was a striking example of the illogic of the good drugs/bad drugs divide, especially in light of the opioid withdrawal model for addiction. Like opioids, barbiturates do cause clear physical tolerance and withdrawal, but, even worse than opioids, that withdrawal can be fatal, as that physician patient at Narco demonstrated. Some scientists had already been trying to raise awareness of this fact and highlight the addiction risks of barbiturates. The Narco clinical team had missed the true cause of that physician's death, but Harris Isbell, the director of the Narco research lab at that time, had already published a paper on barbiturate addiction one year earlier, insisting in its first sentence that "chronic intoxication with barbiturates represents a true addiction—no matter how addiction is defined." Some reformers accordingly began pushing for tighter controls on barbiturates—assigning them to the same category as morphine, for example—and in 1955 Congress held extensive hearings on the subject. Senators were shown disturbing movies of Narco patients in violent, psychotic withdrawal from barbiturates. The assistant surgeon general echoed Isbell when he proclaimed that barbiturate addiction was worse than "narcotic" addiction and more difficult to treat.

Still, Congress declined to take significant action. The reason why could be found in the comments of one unlikely opponent of regulation: Harry Anslinger. Anslinger was usually in favor of enacting tighter drug controls, but in this case he said that regulating barbiturates would cause hardship to all the people using them for tension—namely, middle-class white people. It also bears noting that he was supported in this effort by pharmaceutical companies, because nearly every medical, druggist, and pharmaceutical industry trade group powerfully opposed the congressional interest in regulating barbiturates. In the end, a blunter meaning of "addiction" prevailed: it was a term for "junkies" and generally the wrong sort of people, and therefore, problems with pharmaceuticals must be fundamentally different.

By this point, the separate-and-unequal system of good drugs versus bad drugs was too entrenched to overcome. Some drugs, deemed "pharmaceuticals," were treated as therapeutic goods, and their potential dangers were overlooked. Other drugs were called "drugs"—at this point, the term predominantly meant opioids, cocaine, and cannabis—and treated as if they were universally addicting; accordingly, they were met with prohibition. The historian David Herzberg has called this line of reasoning an example of a problematic "therapeutic entitlement." The racist panics of the early twentieth century had intensified the false dichotomy between addictive drugs and therapeutic medicines, a division that was formalized by the Harrison Act. One class of substances casually called "drugs" was prohibited, while a regulated market of others, called "pharmaceuticals," was allowed to continue as social entitlement preferentially available to middle-class whites. But this was a double-edged sword, causing great harm on both sides of the divide: destructive and ineffective drug wars on one side and lax pharmaceutical regulations on the other. A rational drug policy focused on actual harms would find a balance between these oversimplified extremes—ironically, Anslinger's FBN did a fairly good job of reining in legal opioid use in white markets through the mid-twentieth century, keeping sales relatively stable—but we have rarely occupied that space, nor have we dwelled there for long.

Instead, to this day, our inconsistent responses to drug policy reflect distorted and different understandings of addiction: certain substances are illegal, others are tolerated, and alcohol and tobacco are barely considered drugs at all. By this measure, Herzberg argues, the mass incarceration and the opioid crisis of the early twenty-first century were simply two sides of the same coin—the system was operating exactly as designed, preserving access to pharmaceuticals as an entitlement on one side and using drug crimes as a way of controlling minorities on the other.

One grim Chicago winter in 1955, Sonny Rollins, the great jazz saxophonist, hopped the train from Chicago to Lexington and checked himself into Narco. Like many young musicians, he had first tried heroin because he was emulating his idol, Charlie "Bird" Parker, but Sonny, the young man once heralded as Parker's heir apparent, didn't even own a saxophone anymore. Rollins stayed in Narco for months, eager to get better. The Kentucky weather turned to spring and blossoms appeared on the hillside, and one day he learned that his friend and idol Bird had died back in New York City. Parker's body was so ravaged by the complications from his drug use that the coroner estimated his age at fifty-five or sixty. He was thirty-four.

Rollins, Bird, and countless others were part of a massive postwar heroin crisis, which struck the jazz world with particular force. Billie Holiday, Miles Davis, John Coltrane, and many others famously struggled with opioids—one historian has estimated that as many as 75 percent of 1940s and '50s bebop musicians experimented with heroin. Gerry Mulligan, a baritone saxophonist and arranger who appeared on Davis's *Birth of the Cool*, summed it up simply: "In the end, the carnage was immense."

In contrast to the lax approach to pharmaceuticals, the government's response to this heroin epidemic was a prohibitionist crackdown. Anslinger called for ramping up prosecution, which directly suppressed early efforts to establish mutual-help approaches to drug problems—these were the early years of Narcotics Anonymous, and their efforts to organize were hampered by the presence of police surveillance and even undercover agents at the meetings. Anslinger helped to engineer the 1951 Boggs Act and the Narcotic Control Act of 1956, together perhaps the apex of harsh drug prohibition, requiring extraordinarily long mandatory minimum sentences for drug offenses and even the death penalty in some cases. For example, a first cannabis offense would *start* at a sentence of two to five years and a fine of thousands of dollars.

The crackdown only fueled the socioeconomic drivers of the epidemic. In the postwar Second Great Migration, millions of Black Americans had sought a better life, leaving the South in search of relief from Jim Crow and better jobs, but, from Los Angeles to Chicago to New York, Black people were systematically excluded from America's "age of affluence." Racially restrictive housing policies crowded people of color into "redlined" and underserved city neighborhoods—soon to be known as "inner cities," a term born during that era. Black veterans were prevented from taking advantage of the education and housing provisions of the G.I. Bill, and other discriminatory policies were rife in housing, rising to the level of the Federal Housing Administration. The "inner city" was marred by poverty and unemployment, creating a perfect, concentrated population for heroin markets. After the war, as trade routes reopened, heroin use surged, and it soon became a staple in the otherwise limited inner-city economy. Anslinger himself described these factors with racist language suggesting that Black families were at fault: "The increase is practically 100% among Negro people in police precincts with the lowest economic and social standards. . . . There is no drug addiction if the child comes from a good family, with the church, the home, and the school all integrated." Of course, his only answer was escalating the drug war.

In the meantime, entitlement to pharmaceuticals was also causing harm among white markets. While the crackdown focused on the dangers of cannabis and heroin, pharmaceutical use was booming. By the late 1940s, barbiturates were already the leading cause of death from accidental poisoning, involved in roughly one-fourth of all poisonings in hospitals, and the deaths kept coming through the 1950s and '60s. Marilyn Monroe died in 1962 of a widely publicized barbiturate overdose, an early loss in a torrent of barbiturate-related celebrity poisonings and suicides: Judy Garland, Charles Jackson, Mark Rothko, Malcolm Lowry, Diane Arbus, Edie Sedgwick, and Jimi Hendrix. Around the same time, amphetamine use was skyrocketing. By the late 1960s, one in twenty American adults were using amphetamine prescriptions, and at least half as many were using it non-medically, in a bellwether of the coming epidemic of "crank" (methamphetamine transported in the crankcases of Harley-Davidsons). Other sedatives followed soon after, and by the early 1970s, 5 percent of all Americans (ten million people) were using the Purdue-marketed Valium regularly—meaning daily for months or more—and the figure was twice that for women.

Reinvesting in the pharmaceutical/drug divide had only exacerbated the public health crises on both sides. Not only were pharmaceutical markets dangerously under-regulated, but informal heroin markets grew further—the prohibitionist crackdown was a boon to organized crime, just as alcohol Prohibition was in the 1920s—and that dangerously deregulated market of impure heroin plus the punitive policing further devastated communities of color.

The reality is, as Burroughs's life shows, we cannot keep these spheres of psychoactive drugs separate, as villainizing drug users will naturally undercut therapeutic options for all. One night in 1951 in Mexico City, during a drunken William Tell–type act for some houseguests, Burroughs shot his wife, Joan Vollmer, in the face, and she was dead on arrival at the hospital. Their young son, Billy, was sent to live with his grandparents in St. Louis, then later to South Florida, but the trauma haunted him for the rest of his life. He began using white-market drugs to dull the pain: drinking alcohol, yes, but also gravitating to the natural choice for an affluent white suburbanite in the 1960s, a drug that was also the title of his own first book: *Speed*. Eventually Billy got in trouble with the law, and in 1967 his father returned from abroad to help him get treatment. Burroughs Sr. brought Billy back to Narco, almost exactly twenty years after his own admission there. But by this time, under the onslaught of decades of prohibitionist drug policies, Narco's decline had been precipitous, and it had become a chaotic and hopeless mess. Billy found it "the most useless such establishment (by its own standards) that I have ever seen. I wasn't there two weeks before I was approached with a connection for Dilaudid."

In the end, it was the mixed amphetamines of Adderall that tipped me over the edge into a complete breakdown. I had accessed the drug easily, because it was an entitlement for a white and privileged user like me. I got it through medical channels, paid for it with medical insurance, and, most of the time, used it in a relatively sanctioned way. It is the kind of drug that preserves and supports the existing social order; stimulants get you to work, after all. Not long after it was in my hands, though, I began using Adderall dangerously, and the combination of alcohol, amphetamine, and days of sleeplessness combined to put me into a drug-induced manic episode.

At first, it was glorious. I felt the total dissolution of my ego and a lucid clarity, a taste of an imminent and transcendent mystical experience. Then the delusions set in. I understood that I had gotten wrapped up in a spiritual war of good versus evil. I had neglected my spiritual practice, and I had to meditate more to escape from the confusing feelings. At times I did wonder whether the drugs had caused a psychotic mania, but I could no longer identify reality, as all those thoughts and feelings and fears came rushing in at once. We describe mental illness like it's an entity, a clearly demarcated state, or at least a state with some sort of checkpoint or transition, but I passed no such gate. I felt like I was straddling the gap between sanity and insanity, or, perhaps better put, inhabiting the quantum uncertainty of both at the same time, multiple states of being flashing through my disordered mind.

I had an alcohol withdrawal seizure that brought me to the hospital, where I thought the team of doctors were evil beings sent to persecute me. They told me that a finding on my electrocardiogram suggested an electrical conduction problem with my heart. I might be at risk of sudden cardiac death, and they urged me to stay in the hospital overnight for continuous monitoring. But they also told me they had called an addiction medicine consult for my obvious drug problem, and I knew that this whole chain of events was likely to get back to my residency program, and that I'd have to get treatment. Even when I was delusional, I felt a simultaneous and coldly rational urge to hide my addiction so that I wouldn't have to face reality. So, keeping it all bottled up inside—the delusions and the worries about addiction too—I signed out against medical advice and went back to my apartment, alone.

A few days later, I knew I was not thinking clearly, and it was getting harder to deny to myself how bad things had gotten, but in my mind I still protested. I started whispering the same phrase over and over to myself: "I know what crazy is, and this is not it. I know what crazy is, and this is not it." For just one precious moment, I saw just how wrong I was, and, realizing that I couldn't do it myself, I screamed out for help. My neighbor called the police—reporting an "emotionally disturbed person," thank goodness, or they might have come in guns blazing rather than how they did, which was actually quite carefully and compassionately. The notes from the hospital say they called a SWAT team to get in, but I just remember seeing my doorknob being dismantled from the outside, then a little mechanical arm coming through the hole to unlock it. A chipper young officer with a buzz cut and wearing a heavy Kevlar vest stepped slowly into the room, calmly holding out his hands, and he soothingly asked, "All right, buddy, are you going to come along nicely?"

Even in that moment, I knew I couldn't trust myself.

"Probably not!"

They shot me with a Taser, and the darts flew across the room and fastened themselves right under my left nipple, dangerously near the peak of my heart.

PART FOUR

ADDICTION ON TRIAL

Nine

REHABILITATION

O ne cold February night in central Los Angeles, an old car full of young Black people was pulled over by two plainclothes policemen. Lawrence Robinson, a twenty-five-year-old Army veteran, was sitting in the back with his girlfriend. As his friend Charles Banks stepped out of the driver's seat, Robinson, despite the chill, was sweating. It was partly withdrawal—he was a heroin user and hadn't had a fix in a while—but it was also fear of the law, even though they weren't carrying drugs or any paraphernalia. In California in 1960, it was a crime just to be addicted.

Sure enough, once the officers found a fresh needle mark on Banks's arm, they promptly arrested him. Robinson and the others were ordered out of the car and up against a nearby building. By this point, Robinson was in a full-on flop sweat. The officers made him take off his coat and roll up his sleeves, finding an unmistakable constellation of scabs and splotchy bruises up and down the crooks of both his elbows. He was arrested and taken to the police station, where an LAPD narcotics expert grilled him further and took photos of his arms as evidence.

To fight the charges, Robinson secured Samuel Carter McMorris, an energetic young Black attorney who had recently won a case in front of the U.S. Supreme Court. At first, Robinson and McMorris objected on grounds that might be obvious today: the group had been "driving while Black," and the pretext for the traffic stop in the first place was pretty flimsy (supposedly, their license plate wasn't properly illuminated). But they lost the trial.

McMorris scrambled to appeal, probing for a deeper issue to contest. He challenged the police procedure of the traffic stop, and disputed several other elements of the case, but he also took a crucial step further and went after the law criminalizing addiction itself, arguing that it was unconstitutional to punish addiction as a crime. Robinson's crime wasn't an action at all, but the status of being addicted to narcotics. He sent off the appeal to the superior court, and he waited.

In the intervening months, the country continued a historic turn toward social reform. John F. Kennedy, a young, telegenic senator from Massachusetts, took the Democratic nomination from Lyndon B. Johnson and went on to defeat Richard Nixon. JFK and LBJ would hold the presidency for most of the next decade, commanders in chief of a new war against poverty and disease. McMorris's appeal, meanwhile, was shot down in California. He refined his arguments and appealed to the Supreme Court, arguing that it was cruel and unusual to punish addiction as a crime. The California statute was in fact a holdover from drug laws written in 1929, during the harsh era of narcotic control. Now, McMorris argued, people recognized that addiction was not a crime but a disease; it belonged in not the legal but the medical domain. The court took Robinson's case, and McMorris, barely forty years old, soon found himself again before the old white men of the Supreme Court.

Today, many of the cases that reach the Supreme Court are the products of long-term planning more akin to a rocket launch or military invasion than legal proceedings. Advocacy groups spend years combing the country for the perfect test case, the right combination of a sympathetic defendant and the ideal facts, and, of course, a star attorney. Not so in this case. McMorris was a true underdog, fighting what seemed to be a hopeless fight. When he appeared before the Supreme Court for oral arguments, he fearfully stuttered his way through the justices' questions. On the face of it, he seemed woefully overmatched—but he had a gift, it seemed, for sniffing out the bigger philosophical issues that mattered to the court.

Addiction itself was on trial. The attorney for Los Angeles argued that addicts were responsible for their own addiction: Robinson was not some helpless victim, but someone who "willfully and voluntarily" chose to put "foreign fire into his veins." The justices didn't take too kindly to this notion at oral arguments. What about cigarettes, they asked pointedly, or people who have surgeries and then get addicted to pain pills? Would it really be fair for the state to punish all cases of addiction? Even by the end of the questioning, it seemed clear that Robinson and McMorris had found a sympathetic audience.

Sure enough, the court handed down a sternly worded 6–2 decision exonerating Robinson, proclaiming that "even one day in prison would be a cruel and unusual punishment for the 'crime' of having a common cold." Justice William O. Douglas compared the law criminalizing addiction to medieval times, when the criminally insane were "burned at the stake or hanged; and the pauper insane often roamed the countryside as wild men and from time to time were pilloried, whipped, and jailed." At bottom, they agreed that addiction was a matter for medicine, not the law: "the addict is a sick person," and it would be "barbarous" if the law "allowed sickness to be made a crime and permitted sick people to be punished for being sick."

The decision in *Robinson v. California* was more than a tweak in the criminal code. It marked the decline of the old, prohibitionist approach and the rise of a more widespread acceptance of addiction as a medical problem. Harsh enforcement hadn't worked. The biological research wasn't leading anywhere—there was no scientific fix to addiction, no nonaddictive painkiller after all. The cycle of reform had turned again, and a new, revolutionary, rehabilitative ideal was on the rise: that addiction could be dealt with as a therapeutic matter.

The medical profession was finally speaking out against harsh drug laws and enforcement. The New York Academy of Medicine advocated for restarting opioid maintenance clinics—the strategy quashed by the Federal Bureau of Narcotics in the twenties. From his semi-retirement in California, Lawrence Kolb fired off a blistering rebuke of federal policy in a 1956 *Saturday Evening Post* article in which he also supported the plan for maintenance treatment. The rising prominence of social science scholarship also bolstered this movement, and the sociologist Alfred Lindesmith was especially influential in criticizing federal drug policy. Lindesmith's research argued against simplistic explanations by questioning the line between so-called normal people and those with addiction, and by describing addiction as a learning process beyond simple physical dependence. In 1958, Lindesmith edited a widely read interim report of the American Bar Association and the American Medical Association that critiqued the punitive regime, doubting "whether drug addicts can be deterred from using drugs by threats of jail or prison sentences" and recommending experiments in maintenance treatment (inspired in part by the "British System" that had been providing controlled prescriptions of morphine and heroin to people with addiction since the 1920s). Harry Anslinger was livid. He mounted a sustained and vitriolic attack against the report, even trying to suppress it entirely, but he wound up looking desperate and out of touch. On one side was a respected coalition of physicians and attorneys, headed by an eminent academic who had spent years calling out the illogic of the punitive regime. On the other was the architect of that failed regime. The ABA/AMA issued their full report in 1961. Anslinger, chastened and now in his early seventies, retired the following year, the same year the *Robinson v. California* decision was handed down.

Consensus was growing: treatment would no longer be confined to the basements of AA or the rarefied laboratories of Narco. No longer would we try to arrest our way out of the problem. And yet there was still great uncertainty about how exactly to help. People with addiction often denied that they had a problem and resisted treatment. Wasn't there a point beyond which there was a need for some (hopefully benevolent) coercion? The dissenting opinions in the Robinson case highlighted exactly this tension. The justices who disagreed argued that addiction is complex, and that perhaps the law could be therapeutic by getting people off the streets who wouldn't make that choice otherwise, committing them to a program of rehabilitation and cure. Perhaps, they argued, the goal wasn't to control people but to catch them in early-stage addiction and head off their problems before they progressed.

The court didn't know it at the time, but when McMorris argued Robinson's case before the Supreme Court, he was hiding one crucial piece of information about his client. Robinson himself had long since died of an overdose; ten months earlier, he had been found dead in a Los Angeles alleyway. Who knows whether Robinson would have been safer in jail than on the streets, but one thing was clear: despite the fact that people were finally ready to try to treat addiction, it was not yet clear how exactly to help.

After they tased me, the NYPD forcibly removed me from my apartment. I remember it in pieces: the handcuffs, the straps on the stretcher, the dizzying angle of descent as the seeming dozens of officers navigated the narrow hallway of my five-story walkup, smiling and joking with one another now that the adrenaline rush of breaching my door and subduing me had passed. I felt ashamed as they hauled me down the stairs, thinking to myself that this wasn't right, there wasn't anything that wrong with me, they shouldn't have to carry me like this. They took me to the psychiatric emergency room at Bellevue, the preferred destination in New York City for "emotionally disturbed persons." There, in the fishbowl of the ER, this time on the other side of the plate glass windows, I remained terrified, disoriented, and delusional. There were moments of lucidity, but for most of the time I believed I had been captured by shadowy forces and imprisoned in a fake ER, surrounded by fake patients. Or I had died and gone to purgatory, or some other in-between bardo state.

The delusions began to recede as the antipsychotics kicked in, and by the time I was taken up to the dual diagnosis unit, my mind became clearer. I was not in the afterlife, or some holy war. There were still flashes here and there—I spied a dragon tattoo on the inside of an aide's wrist and had a brief moment of panic, wondering if it was a mystical sign of membership in some sinister organization—but for the most part I was starting to contend with a different, subtler challenge to my reality.

My attending physician, Dr. Goldman, was a relatively young, awkward guy in glasses, someone I might have seen as a friendly senior colleague at a different time. There was a reassuring honesty behind his stiff nerdiness, and for the first time, I started to feel comfortable opening up about the true extent of my drinking. I broke down, telling Dr. Goldman and his colleagues that I was an alcoholic. But soon afterward, I felt riven by doubt and fearful uncertainty, calling my friends and buttonholing the other patients to talk about whether I was a "real" alcoholic, my mind changing back and forth in the course of a single day. I was willing to admit that I was deeply, profoundly sick, much more than I had even come close to realizing. Still, I wasn't sure how to understand what had happened to me.

At some point during my time in the ER, a resident had put a grainy, photocopied trifold pamphlet into my hands and said I should contact a physician advocacy organization: New York State's "physician health program," a part of the medical society that helped doctors with addictions and other mental health problems get back to work safely. From the hallway payphone on the dual diagnosis unit, I called their offices in Albany and asked for their help, scribbling notes on that pamphlet in crayon, the phone cradled in the crook of my neck. I learned that I was not in trouble with the state licensing board, which was good—the licensing board's investigations are notoriously punitive, whereas the physician health program is more focused on treatment. But though I was not quite mandated to treatment, it was muddy. My case manager at the physician health program wanted me to go to their preferred rehab and get an extended evaluation. In the coming days, as I got more restless, I wondered if I couldn't just leave the hospital and go to outpatient treatment. I knew I wouldn't drink again. For the first time in my life, I was actually ready to go to AA. But when I asked the case manager if that was possible, she told me that if I did outpatient treatment rather than inpatient rehab, it would probably take half a year before I was cleared to work. Frustrated, I asked why I couldn't just go my own way entirely, seeing as I was supposedly coming into the program voluntarily, and she replied that if I went entirely off the map, after I had called them and detailed my problems, they would be obligated to report my case to the licensing board.

I had seen these types of interactions dozens of times from the other side, and yet I felt like I'd been thrown into a game partway through without knowing the rules. I was in an uneasy space between voluntary and involuntary treatment, and though I wanted to be compliant, before I even realized it I had wandered into the role of the wayward patient. I worried that simply by voicing my preferences, I had already given her too much evidence of my poor judgment. I knew how this was supposed to go. The psychiatric patient must acknowledge his problems. He must be disturbed by what has happened to him. A blithe dismissal of the events bringing him into the ER was not good coping, but cause for alarm. So I decided to go to the rehab, of course, even though by that point I wasn't sure if I wanted their help anymore.

Dr. Goldman escorted me down to the ground floor and out through the chaotic halls of Bellevue. I had first passed through those hallways as a residency applicant to NYU's program. This time, I had entered in handcuffs.

We stepped out onto First Avenue on a clear, frigid December day. A car waited at the curb to take me to the rehab.

At a sparse, fluorescently lit nurses' station, I met a lanky, stoop-shouldered counselor. He watched as I peed in a cup, then gave me a thorough pat-down as he told me about the time he found kilos of cocaine in a new patient's prosthetic leg. Next, a grumpy nurse in scrubs had me sign some forms, then led me to a back room where she combed through my luggage and confiscated all my reading material, raising her eyebrows at the novels and folders stuffed full of journal articles on moral psychology. (I was hoping to catch up on some pleasure reading and get some work done.) She cut off my flimsy Bellevue ID bracelet to attach a thick, rigid band, apparently—and ominously—designed for weeks of wear.

My spirits fell as the counselor led me around. The place was drab, depressing, institutional. In the empty dining hall, a kitchen worker emerged from the back and passed an enormous plate of buttered noodles across the top of the sneeze guard—like what you give a child who refuses to eat anything else. I ate it alone, looking out over the dark, wooded backyard, then retired to the detox unit, a thin curtain separating me from the constant groans of withdrawal.

The next morning, after signing a few forms at the business office, I was ceremoniously handed a copy of the Big Book of Alcoholics Anonymous from one of the hundreds lining the shelves. I met my orientation buddy Amit, a spry, birdlike anesthesiologist who had already been there for several weeks for a serious opioid problem. I told him I was hoping to be discharged to an outpatient program after the weeklong evaluation. He laughed, and my stomach twisted. He didn't want to be there, either, but the idea of an evaluation was just a formality, he said. People always stayed. I just had to do my time like everyone else. He suggested that I keep my head down and not cause any trouble. They scrutinized your every move, he said—even the cleaning staff was watching.

The schedule was absurdly packed with group meetings, talks, and activities. We made our way to the lecture hall, where a wiry older man with a stern, weather-beaten face was telling his own addiction story: stealing opioids from the hospital, getting shot at by his ex-wife, and slamming fentanyl in the bathtub until his heart stopped. "People say rehab is like brainwashing," the man said. "Well, sure, back then my brain could use some washing." Amit whispered that this was the medical director of the rehab, Dr. Summers.

By this point I had decided that I needed to get out of rehab as soon as possible, and I fixated on how I could possibly be discharged after the evaluation, despite Amit's warning. Throughout the day, I rehearsed my story to the other doctor-patients. I was only here because I'd had a manic episode. My drinking hadn't been the healthiest, but I didn't need rehab; I was ready for outpatient treatment. Some seemed convinced. Most thought I was full of it.

The following day, I was summoned to meet Dr. Summers in his office for my intake interview. I had heard that he probably had final say over my case, and I had been watching him closely as he stalked the hallways with an impatient, kinetic energy. This I could work with. I had spent my entire career sucking up to older doctors.

As soon as I sat down in his office, though, he scowled and began to interrogate me: How much had I been drinking, exactly? What else was I using? Was I sure? My hopes withered, but I tried to stay positive and calmly presented my case: young man with binge drinking exacerbated by Adderall and occasional cocaine, in the context of overwork and burnout. Far from healthy but now highly motivated. I could really do this as an outpatient. I had learned my lesson and wanted to get better.

I watched his face for any signs of an opening. Instead, after a long pause, he leaned across the table and told me that he'd be testing my hair for drugs.

"Tell me now," he asked portentously, "what will we find?"

At first, I was confused—I had just told him everything I'd been taking—but then the realization landed: I wasn't a colleague or a trainee anymore, not to him. I was an addicted physician, the worst kind of patient, perfectly equipped to massage my story and maintain my denial. In Bellevue I had also been a patient, but treated with respect, even like a colleague. Here, though, I was just a liar, and apparently I had to be broken down and reformed.

Summers asked me again: Weed? Meth? PCP? Surely there was something else.

My throat tightened with panic as I struggled to reply. I tried one last time to plead my case, but Summers cut me off.

"I'm a doctor, like you, and I'm boarded in Addiction Medicine, but my real specialty is Trouble. And you, son, are Trouble. You're going to have to be here for a long time. Try to get on board. It might save your life."

Paul Morantz, exhausted, breathed a sigh of relief as he pulled up to his little house in Pacific Palisades, tucked away in the canyons of Northwest L.A. Morantz was a Los Angeles attorney who had recently sued Synanon, an unconventional addiction treatment program that had been founded in the fifties as a ramshackle drug treatment commune but soon grew into a full-blown cult. (Synanon maintained its own "Imperial Marines," who beat a former member until they fractured his skull and put him in a coma.) His client was a woman who, upon being admitted to a Synanon program, had had her head shaved and was kept against her will for ninety days. He won, but in the process became a target of Synanon's harassment, and he hoped he could finally unwind that night—it was the first game of the 1978 World Series. On the way in, he absentmindedly checked his mailbox. From its depths, a four-and-a-half-foot rattlesnake—with its rattle cut off for stealth—shot out and drove its fangs deep into his hand. Morantz screamed to his neighbors, "It's Synanon! Synanon got me!"

The rattlesnake had indeed been planted by Synanon, and the story was national news. Morantz was taken to the hospital just in time; it took eighteen vials of antivenom to save his life. Two months later, the Los Angeles prosecutor raided Synanon's $1 million compound to arrest its leader, Charles Dederich, for conspiracy to murder Morantz. Dederich, who twenty years earlier had declared himself cured of alcoholism and done with AA, was found so drunk on Chivas Regal that he had to be carried to jail on a stretcher.

Dederich was a failed salesman who had become a devoted AA member in 1956, and at first, it was his life. He loved speaking at AA meetings, and with his unforgettable presence—he was an enormous man with a booming voice, his right eye permanently half-closed from an old bout of meningitis, and a penchant for expounding on philosophy and mysticism—he soon attracted a crew of younger and impressionable types to his side, some of whom called him Dad.

In time, though, Dederich decided that AA was too parochial—back then, meetings generally refused to accept people with other drug problems—and ultimately too soft. In the process of writing the Big Book, Bill Wilson and his collaborators had rigorously framed everything about their program as a suggestion, to avoid being prescriptive, and, accordingly, an important tradition for meetings was to keep one's focus rigorously on one's own experience and avoid advice-giving or any direct confrontation, otherwise known as "cross-talk." In contrast, Dederich believed his younger charges needed to be shocked and shaken out of their addictions, so he developed his own form of extreme group therapy intended to break down the ego and inspire a quasi-psychedelic experience: marathon confrontation sessions, lasting hours or even days, which he held three times weekly at his seedy Santa Monica apartment. This twisted group exercise—called "The Game," in which participants screamed their frustrations and complaints at each other—became a keystone of the Synanon method. Critics charged the group with brain-washing, but Dederich retorted that most people needed to have their "brains washed out" every so often.

Dederich turned out to be a pretty good salesman—he popularized the catchphrase "Today is the first day of the rest of your life"—and he ably captured both media attention and more recruits. Money trickled in, then poured in. From a run-down storefront in Santa Monica, Synanon grew into a palatial former hotel on the beachfront, then a proper empire with a network of complexes from Marin County to Lake Havasu. There were celebrity testimonials, corporate sponsors, and close alliances with California politicians who rewrote state laws to enable them to operate as a drug treatment facility.

Synanon also catalyzed a movement, spawning hundreds of copycat treatment programs across the country: "therapeutic communities," or "TCs," a form of long-term residential treatment for alcohol and drug problems that continues to exert a powerful influence on addiction treatment today.* Many other therapeutic communities didn't go nearly as far as Synanon, but they did build their programs on the same confrontational foundation: highly structured and hierarchical roles, with former patients working as staff members, and severe discipline for months or even years of inpatient treatment. You may not have heard of "therapeutic communities"—I hadn't until well after residency—but they are ubiquitous and still widely used, treating thousands upon thousands of patients each year, often people on Medicaid or referred by the criminal legal system. Today, many therapeutic communities are still confrontational, but this is not a feature exclusive to those programs. Synanon merely exemplified and helped to promote a notion found across all of addiction treatment: that people with addiction have to be broken down and their character has to be reshaped by any means necessary.

Therapeutic communities became popular partly because of the

---

* Confusingly, there is a different lineage of therapeutic communities, arising out of British psychiatry, for general mental health problems, though it had little influence on Dederich.

medical profession's long neglect of people with addiction. Back in the 1920s, the profession had largely retreated from addiction treatment, leaving therapeutic approaches largely confined to Narco and only a handful of other providers. Even in 1965, in the midst of a rising rehabilitative interest and increasing acceptance of addiction as a medical problem, many states still had no treatment facilities for addiction. Therapeutic communities filled this void. They were both financially and politically attractive—all the unpaid patient labor made for low operating costs, and "tough love" always seems to play well as a talking point. But therapeutic communities never would have taken hold in the first place if people with addiction hadn't been treated so badly in the general medical system, a reality that had driven the earlier development of an even larger alternative treatment system.

In May 1949, a small group of AA members in Minnesota had founded a retreat called Hazelden for what they called "professionals"— upstanding men who had fallen on hard times. Hazelden began simply as a three-week course of lectures on the twelve steps (later expanded to four weeks, thus the prevalence of today's twenty-eight-day model), plus general instructions to "make your bed, comport yourself as a gentleman, and while sitting around, talk with one another." The attendance in early days was sparse; one of the first Christmases there, the sole counselor cooked a meal for two and sat down with his only resident. It grew steadily, though, and in the 1960s, as receptiveness to therapeutic approaches for addiction grew, Hazelden took a page from nearby Willmar State Hospital and began a formal training process for people in AA-based recovery to become counselors, thus marking a turn from a "retreat" model to a more professionalized system. This model of a structured curriculum, plus a system for turning former patients into counselors, proved easy to replicate, and the leaders of Hazelden were driven to share it. It spread through the country as the twelve-step-based "Minnesota Model" of rehab, and it is unquestionably the dominant treatment program for addiction to this day.

Both therapeutic communities and the Minnesota Model created a curious amalgam of mutual-help and therapeutic approaches, and they took hold in the 1960s largely because they were filling the void left by neglect. Marty Mann's advocacy had helped to spur some medical systems to treat alcoholism and to garner supportive statements from medical organizations, and of course AA was becoming more popular every year, but still, few proper treatment programs were available, especially for drug problems. It was the heyday of psychoanalysis, and most psychiatrists still eschewed treating people with addiction. To this day, attempts to get family physicians or psychiatrists to deal with alcohol and drug issues regularly fail because of stigma, limited training, and a lack of institutional and structural support—reflecting and reinforcing the structural stigma of a separate system.

In this context, the Minnesota Model struggled to meet the needs of all its patients. Like AA itself, the model was designed around the idea of the powerless alcoholic voluntarily seeking treatment, but as the sixties rolled on, the patient populations in treatment programs became more diverse—fewer older professional men with alcohol problems, more younger patients with severe drug addictions, who proved more difficult to treat—and in this context, rehabs absorbed some of Synanon's approach. In 1967, some of the Hazelden staff visited a hospital that had deliberately emulated Synanon's confrontational techniques, and soon after that Hazelden instituted such strategies itself, such as putting someone in a "hot seat" in group therapy while other patients critiqued their behavior and attitudes, using a sheet of more than twenty "character defects," like "resentful" and "prideful."

Today, harsh confrontation is used not only in many rehab facilities but also (and especially) in many prison-based programs, boot-camp-like wilderness programs, and the troubled-teen industry. Therapeutic communities, meanwhile, are diverse, and not all are confrontational. Many established therapeutic communities have disavowed the use of extreme and humiliating tactics, and the national and international associations of therapeutic communities have formally opposed "abusive" techniques—though a tradition of intense confrontation continues. The sociologist Kerwin Kaye recently studied a New York City therapeutic community that was supposed to be among the "softer" and more compassionate options, but, embedding in the community for eight months, he watched in horror as staff regularly berated clients, humiliated people in front of groups, and called them names like "dope fiends." In the worst example, after one disciplinary infraction, the staff ransacked all the residents' rooms, overturning mattresses and dumping out their possessions, then made them clean it all up—according to the facility's usual militaristic, spotless standard—until well after midnight.

After decades of study, there's little evidence that such confrontational practices work to promote good substance treatment outcomes—in fact, they are often counterproductive, provoking more resistance. There is also no strong evidence that the months- or even yearslong stays in therapeutic communities provide an advantage over less intense treatments: a 2006 Cochrane review—the highest standard for evaluating medical research today—found little evidence to show that therapeutic communities were better than any other treatments on measures such as abstinence rates. Therapeutic communities may be inexpensive and politically appealing, but according to the best evidence today, the shorter and often less extreme therapies, like twenty-eight-day rehabs or outpatient programs, offer equivalent results.

Yet droves of people attribute tremendous changes in their lives to these types of settings, claiming that the intensive treatment does something to help unravel the deep, personal identification with addiction as a lifestyle. It is not so much the abusive confrontation, but the opportunity to reconfigure ideas about the self, they claim, that lies at the heart of the method. This is often the explicit target of addiction treatment:

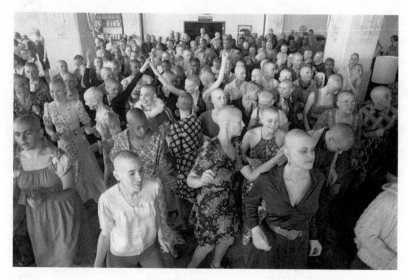

Women with shaved heads dance at Synanon press
conference in Oakland, California, 1975.

not simply remediating pathology, but a sweeping and much more challenging project of reshaping one's very identity.

I n the coming days at rehab, between the group therapy, the skills worksheets, the cutting-and-pasting collages at rec therapy, and the constant strategizing with any sympathetic ear, I still felt torn between acceptance and denial. I went through massive mood swings and sobbed into my bed, finally alone and experiencing the overwhelming fear I had been stuffing down since the manic episode. I started to admit to myself that I had a real problem. I resolved to stop minimizing my actual drug and alcohol intake, which I had been doing since admission in the hope that I could be discharged to an outpatient program. But usually, right after moments like these, I reversed course and convinced myself that these people were idiots, and I just needed to stick to my story and get out as soon as possible. I wasn't sure what was real.

I saw things in the rehab's approach that seemed wrong, if not

downright harmful, which fed my resistance. A sense of fear and surveillance permeated the health professionals' group. A flirtatious surgeon was "therapeutically discharged," not because of any drug or
alcohol problem but because he wouldn't stop talking to female patients;
he was transferred to a long-term care program in Mississippi that
would, we were told, break down the entrenched personality issues
standing in the way of his recovery. In a regular group exercise, "Responsible Concerns," we called out other people for troubling behavior,
such as expressing any doubts about treatment or AA. An older, gentle,
but quietly and awkwardly obstinate family practice physician refused
to stop pointing out the elements of AA that he thought were illogical,
so he was given a pamphlet titled "King Baby" that described how his
resistance was just a symptom of his own immaturity. It all felt crazy to
me. The targets of their interventions were sweeping—people's very
personality and character—and in psychiatry, we would never set out to
engineer a fundamental character reconstruction in the space of a few
weeks or months.

My mother visited me in those early days of the rehab program.
Since my episode, she'd joined me in insisting that everything I was
being put through—the state monitoring program, the monthslong specialized program for doctors—was overkill. She hated, and rejected, the
idea that I was an alcoholic, and she hated AA—after all, she had fought
against its vision of her own drinking problems for most of her life. But
then she surprised me. In that somber dining room, surrounded by
other subdued families visiting their wayward relatives, she looked at
me with resignation and said the time for fighting was over. I just had
to let go and go with it. I felt something like a hint of relief in my body,
and I started to think she might be right.

A week after I arrived, I met with all the counselors together, who
told me that they'd be recommending that I stay for the full course of
inpatient treatment. They insisted I couldn't just go through the mo-
tions; I had to really participate. Most importantly, though, the choice

would be mine. No one would keep me there, and I could walk anytime I wanted. It might take a long time, and jumping through a lot of hoops, if I wanted to practice medicine again, but I could always leave.

The choice should have been easy. Why did it feel so hard? I asked the other doctor-patients what they thought. Some agreed that it was ridiculous that I was being asked to stay; others kept talking about how I had to "surrender." I talked myself in circles.

It was this very conflict, the fearful attachment to who I thought I was and what I wanted, that helped me let go and accept the help being offered, even if that help was imperfect. I watched myself spin around, and the spinning felt sick. I saw just how much I was trying to manipulate the situation, even after all I had gone through, and that in itself scared me. I realized that—even if the specific program had its flaws— all the forces converging on me had a kind intention, they were trying to keep me safe and tell me that something was very wrong here, and, above all, my attachment to my own willpower and self-identity was perhaps the most dangerous thing facing me.

The next morning at roll call, I introduced myself not as "Carl, here for an evaluation," as I had insisted on doing for a week, but as "Carl, alcoholic." My face flushed, and I felt like I'd lost a part of myself. But a part of me loosened up, too.

To this day, I am not entirely sure how to think of that rehab program. Was Summers too harsh, or did I need to be challenged? Could I have gotten by with just outpatient treatment? Was all that focus on character and personality rehabilitation overkill? I am convinced that I did need to be coerced, in the sense of being faced with a hard choice. Most people going to addiction treatment are going with some form of coercion—at least informal coercion, from family and friends—and I was there because I had to be, at least if I wanted to practice medicine anytime soon. I am glad that I was coerced in that sense; if I hadn't had the monitoring program in place, I might not have stuck with treatment and entered recovery, and I could have harmed other people, or died myself. Still, I'd like to believe that whatever deeper rehabilitation I experienced had more to do with connection than confrontation. For all of Summers's bluster at the outset, I didn't really need to be broken down, and the most meaningful and transformative experiences were less about the formal treatment and more about being put in a situation where mutual help could take hold and do its work.

Soon after I decided to stick with the rehab program, I learned that all of us had to present a thirty-minute narrative of our "addiction stories" in front of the group for their feedback on our "character defects." I dreaded the notion, and I imagined the other people in the health professionals group lancing into me. But when I eventually sat down to tell my story, the experience was liberating. The counselor left us in the room, and it was the first time I actually spoke honestly and without artifice about just how bad it had been: the breakups, the late nights, the hiding, the shame, the sense of hopelessness—above all, the constant, failed battles to control myself. Around the room, there were chuckles and smiles, some nods, but mostly just kind attention. Afterward, people wrote me feedback letters about my "defects"; I had expected to be eviscerated, but most of them were encouraging and warm. Just like all the other best parts of rehab, it was nothing more than the experience of being around people who understood.

I n 1943, at the height of World War II, Congress finally allowed women physicians to receive commissions in the armed forces, and one year later Marie Nyswander, a brilliant and iconoclastic graduate of Cornell Medical College, jumped at the chance to fulfill her dream of becoming an orthopedic surgeon. But while the Navy had deigned to allow women to serve as doctors, they didn't want female surgeons. Instead, Nyswander was posted to Narco, a place she hated. It was an unlikely beginning to what would become, years later, the medical profession's greatest contribution yet to the treatment of addiction.

When she arrived at Narco and saw the staff treating patients like convicts and referring to Black patients with the worst possible racial slurs, Nyswander was both horrified and inspired to do better. She had always dreamed of medicine as a way of addressing social ills. During her teens, she had been confined for a year to a tuberculosis sanatorium, where the struggles of impoverished patients inspired her to read Karl Marx and Friedrich Engels and join the Young Communist League for a time. When she became disenchanted with political revolution, she turned to medicine instead. Now she was in Narco, a hopeless institution, one designed for control, containment, and quarantine—hardly the reform Nyswander envisioned. She resolved to find a different way.

Once her year of service at Narco was up, Nyswander rushed back to New York and immersed herself in psychiatry. In contrast to the bourgeois craze for psychoanalysis at the time, Nyswander started two clinics: one for intensive psychotherapy for addiction, the other a specialty clinic for jazz musicians addicted to heroin. Witty, cultured, and street-smart, Nyswander was beloved by her patients. They flocked to her office on East 103rd Street, where casual onlookers were flabbergasted to see her voluntarily making the trek so far uptown during the height of the postwar heroin crisis.

When Nyswander wrote her first book, *The Drug Addict as a Patient*, in 1956, she became a national thought leader for compassionate, nuanced care. Reading Nyswander today is still inspiring. Her fierce optimism and respect for the dignity of her patients shine off the page—including recognition of the diversity of psychological and social factors that influence drug use. Casting aside psychoanalytic stereotypes that would reduce all addicts to "masochists" or people seeking a "crude substitute for masturbation," she instead speaks evocatively about the depth and variety of her patients' motivations for using drugs, describing how drug use can serve perfectly understandable functions: "a way of keeping alive whatever life and joy they can feel," or even "a way into a mystical experience," "a clarity of feeling and oneness of perception."

Even so, Nyswander was demoralized by her patients' actual outcomes. It seemed like even the best psychoanalysis in the world wasn't enough to heal her patients; they invariably returned to poor, struggling communities, surrounded by other users and faced with innumerable temptations and few reasons to stay off heroin. She needed something stronger to help them.

Something was gnawing at Vincent Dole. It was 1962, and Dole, an eminent metabolism researcher, was comfortably ensconced at Rockefeller Institute for Medical Research, in New York, but on his commute from a rich suburb in the Hudson River Valley, as he walked down from the 125th Street train station—unbeknownst to him, past Nyswander's office—he could no longer ignore the scope of the opioid epidemic around him. He "had the sense of moving between two highly privileged oases through a truly epidemic sea of misery." He mentioned his concerns to a colleague (the distinguished physician and writer Lewis Thomas, as it turns out), who, about to depart on a sabbatical, gave Dole his position on a crucial New York City committee on narcotics.

Dole became a dedicated student of addiction and, coming across Nyswander's book, he promptly hired her and shifted his research focus to opioids. They began with basic research, admitting people with addiction to their hospital ward and studying the effects of various drugs, and in 1964 they made a curious observation. While most of their subjects quickly became preoccupied with their supply, fixated on when they'd get their next shot of heroin, morphine, or hydromorphone (Dilaudid), the picture was dramatically different when they tried a different drug: methadone.

Methadone, like Nyswander herself, was from the world of Narco without being *of* it. One of many synthetic opioids, it was first synthesized in Germany in the 1930s, and when U.S. intelligence teams discovered the compound in 1946, they promptly shipped it off to Narco for further testing, where it became the preferred drug for treating withdrawal. Methadone is an extremely slow-acting opioid, both because it breaks down into a diversity of longer-acting compounds and because a reservoir of medication builds up when it's taken daily. As a result, methadone sustains its action for well over twenty-four hours, and, crucially, it doesn't produce a euphoric high when administered in regular doses on a consistent, daily basis.

Thus, when Dole and Nyswander switched two opioid-addicted patients to methadone, the subjects not only stopped stressing about the next dose; they became newly invigorated, even "normal." The older generation of Narco scientists were philosophically opposed to opioid maintenance, but Dole and Nyswander, working as they were in a busy city, soon found themselves in the middle of a maintenance experiment at their subjects' own insistence. As Nyswander later recalled, "The older addict began to paint industriously and his paintings were good. The younger started urging us to let him get his high-school-equivalency diploma. We sent them both off to school, outside the hospital grounds, and they continued to live at the hospital. Neither of them—although both of them had every opportunity—copped heroin on the outside. From two slugabeds they turned into dynamos of activity." Nyswander and Dole immediately saw the implications for treatment. They hired another Cornell physician straight out of residency, Mary Jeanne Kreek, and started an experimental program to give methadone to people with addiction.

In 1965, they dropped a bombshell report in *The Journal of the American Medical Association* describing remarkable results. Twenty-two "mainline" heroin users with multiple prior unsuccessful treatments—many with more than half a dozen attempts at traditional rehabilitation at Narco and other hospitals—had been successfully treated with steady doses of methadone. All experienced complete obliteration of any "narcotic hunger" and turned their lives around, returning to school, securing jobs, and reconciling with family members. Four patients did tentative "experiments" in shooting heroin on the street, but methadone "blocked" any euphoric effects: the patients were "astounded at their lack of reaction" and not only immediately stopped any further use but also came back to the research ward and discouraged the other patients from trying.

For the first time in the history of medicine, a simple medication promising an apparently total cure for addiction actually had the evidence to back it up. The title of the paper demonstrates the authors' holistic aspirations: methadone wasn't just "maintenance," but a form of "medical treatment" unto itself. Methadone was a sensation. Walter Cronkite featured Dole on the *CBS Evening News*, announcing that "a new experimental method of treatment offers hope of freedom," and Nyswander was profiled in a sprawling two-part feature in *The New Yorker*, in which she compared their innovative use of methadone to the discovery of the microscope. The two continued to churn out research papers as their cadre of twenty-two patients expanded to 128.

Their work expanded rapidly. The New York City commissioner of hospitals gave Dole carte blanche to start a program on a formerly empty floor in the Manhattan General Hospital, perched over Stuyvesant Square Park at the edge of the East Village, at the time the city's epicenter of social marginalization and ethnic strife. The city's first voluntary methadone clinic followed soon afterward in 1969, in Brooklyn's Bed-Stuy neighborhood, marking methadone's transition from a rarefied experiment to an everyday treatment. Before long, President Richard Nixon would declare that methadone was the "best available answer" to the problem of addiction.

Methadone was just one piece of a "chemotherapeutic revolution" taking the world by storm. The first antipsychotic medication, chlorpromazine, had been discovered in France in 1950 and occasioned remarkable recoveries in asylum-bound patients previously written off as intractable cases. Chlorpromazine came to the United States as Thorazine soon after, and at the same time, lithium, LSD, and the "minor sedative" Miltown were all exploding in popularity. It seemed as if psychiatry had finally cracked the biological code of mental illness and could treat ever-expanding swaths of suffering with simple pills. A huge new range of mental problems were sucked up into the ambit of psychiatric practice. It changed the very scientific model of mental illness: the drugs showed that neurotransmission was chemical, not electrical, as had previously been thought, leading to the increasing belief that the fundamental causes of mental disorders could be found therein.

Still, methadone encountered serious opposition and criticism. Medical professionals channeled the American obsession with abstinence: a leading addiction medicine physician complained to *JAMA* that "these research workers are openly giving addicts narcotics to gratify and perpetuate their addiction." The researcher Harris Isbell, visiting from Narco, refused to believe how well the supposed former addicts were doing and flatly declared to Dole, "Those are not addicts."* There was staunch opposition from Black community leaders, who dismissed it as "a solution given to us by white, middle class America" that failed to address the underlying cause of crime: namely, the concentrated poverty and the deliberate marginalization and neglect of "inner-city" communities. Black community leaders warned that it would be a form of social control: "Some of our officials would just as soon narcotize the whole ghetto population on a cheap synthetic if that would stop crime." However, the strongest opposition came from leaders of therapeutic communities, who believed that addiction required full-on character reconstruction; one declared, "Methadone is insidious. It's immoral. It treats the symptoms but not the disease."

From the outset, Dole and Nyswander themselves did not frame methadone as a simple miracle cure but rather sought to use methadone as one element in a deeper project of rehabilitation, the brain in balance with the social and psychological domains: "Our objective is to

---

* When Isbell left, the patients gleefully reported to Dole that they had all been to Narco, some multiple times, but the methadone program was the only thing that had worked for them.

rehabilitate addicts. We are looking for better ways to remove heroin users from the streets and jails, and return them to their families, to schools, and to jobs." In addition to the medication, their program provided extensive social services—Nyswander had learned from her years of psychotherapeutic work that, while psychosocial efforts alone were often insufficient, those interventions were often necessary. However, at other times, and especially as attacks on the legitimacy of their treatment mounted, Dole and Nyswander slipped into defensive and overly reductionist biological explanations of the nature of addiction. In their influential 1967 article "Heroin Addiction—a Metabolic Disease," they argued that the root of addiction was not an "addictive personality," as generations of Narco physicians had assumed, but a "neurological susceptibility." From the academic press to the evening news, Dole and Nyswander emphasized how methadone flatly abolished the "drug hunger" in treated patients, that it returned patients to "normal," with methadone producing nothing less than a "blockade" against further drug use. This only fanned the flames and prompted further criticism—Dole himself admitted later in life that this deterministic language was a bit of an overreach, one born less out of scientific precision than the perceived need to counter the criticism they were facing. There was no real need for the factionalism, as these various approaches—medications, other therapies, and mutual help—were not really in opposition. Still, very few were open to a truly pluralistic approach to addiction treatment.

There was tremendous enthusiasm for a therapeutic response to addiction, but that energy was dispersed across multiple fields with different understandings of the problem—from therapeutic communities to nascent rehabs to early methadone clinics to the few doctors who actually treated addiction. Was it a physical disease, a character disorder, a spiritual sickness, or something else entirely? Common ground was hard to find, and the whole enterprise was threatened by infighting. In the meantime, the 1960s middle class worried that the drug culture

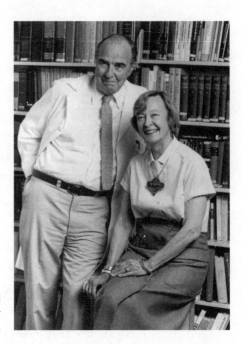

Vincent Dole and
Marie Nyswander
in 1983.

was spinning out of control. Their own kids, born in the baby boom after the war, were now racing toward adolescence and increasingly experimenting with drugs. In 1967, fifty thousand people gathered in San Francisco for the "Human Be-In," flying cannabis-leaf flags and dropping acid in an event that brought the word "psychedelic" to the suburbs. As the Age of Aquarius dawned, that middle class feared that heroin was close behind: *Time* featured the headline "Heroin Hits the Young," *Life* warned parents about the "ghetto malady" of heroin addiction infiltrating small towns, and the newspaper *Newsday* won a Pulitzer for its coverage of the "heroin trail" leading to suburban Long Island.

In 1968, Richard Nixon captured the presidency on a "law and order," "tough on crime" platform that not-so-covertly played on long-simmering racist ideas. Nixon deftly connected an urban drug and crime wave with the racial fears of those who resisted (or actively opposed) civil rights. In the words of his advisers, "The whole problem is really the blacks," and the campaign strategy was "We'll go after the racists" to get their votes. On the surface, it seemed as though Nixon was destined to return to drug prohibition: he was a puritan who detested hedonistic practices like the Woodstock festival of 1969, he ramped up drug enforcement in Mexico (driving small producers out of business and enabling the later development of massive cartels), and later in life he claimed that "the war on drugs is our second civil war."* Yet there was a jarring discrepancy between Nixon's rhetoric and his policy, as he also called for comprehensive programs of education, research, and treatment. As another wave of heroin was surging forward, it remained to be seen which sentiment would prevail, and whether anyone could help at all.

---

* Nixon's anti-drug attitudes are all the more striking considering that he allegedly developed a sedative habit himself while in office.

Ten

ZERO TOLERANCE

J osie strides through the door confidently, a fashionable Puerto Rican woman with a high ponytail, meticulous makeup, and long nails that scrape against my wrist when she gives me a firm handshake. Then we start to discuss her past. The multiple rapes in foster care. The opioids that she learned would quell the intrusive thoughts, and the un-earned guilt and shame that many survivors feel. The dealer who got her to traffic drugs when her money ran out. She gets quiet, glosses over important details, and tries to change the subject, even though she knows that giving me the full story is important to her case.

I am meeting Josie as part of my work in forensic psychiatry: I'm completing an evaluation for the courts to give my opinion on what would be the "appropriate level of care" for her. She's been through the revolving door of the criminal legal treatment system a few times, in-cluding a few confrontational, boot-camp-style treatments, but they all exacerbated her trauma, and if she had a panic attack or an interper-sonal problem, she was usually labeled "hysterical" and discharged. Her current treatment program includes some mild psychiatric medications, but nothing for addiction—certainly not any medications like metha-done or buprenorphine. As of 2014, only one in twenty legally referred people getting treatment for opioid addiction receives these potentially lifesaving medications.

What is the "appropriate level of care" for Josie? It's a disheartening question, given the gap between her reality and the ideal: real psychotherapy for trauma, a stable relationship with a good clinician, and access to the medications that are proven to reduce overdose death. But this is a fantasy for most people in the criminal legal system. If she's lucky, she won't be forced to get off the psychiatric medications she's already on, which she feels are helpful but not sufficient, and she will be allowed to live in a setting that's not run like a boot camp. That's it.

After residency, I devoted a year to training in forensic psychiatry, where I first encountered patients like Josie. I spent a day a week at New York State's maximum-security prison for women, and it seemed as though every patient sent to our psychiatric clinic had both a low-level drug offense and trauma history. Many of them jockeyed to get time off their sentences by going to tough-love boot camps, where their heads were shaved and they did push-ups in the snow while staff screamed at them. I couldn't shake their stories. The injustice of how, if not for an accident of birth, my own story could have been entirely different. The NYPD chose to take me, a white guy living in an upscale Manhattan neighborhood, to a hospital rather than booking me. If I'd been a person of color in a different neighborhood, I could have been imprisoned, like so many of the people who populate our current system of mass incarceration, or even shot and killed.

Approximately fifty years ago, the United States seemed to be on the cusp of a new therapeutic approach to addiction, one that would have abandoned punitive approaches for a kind and compassionate attempt at care. Then, right on the threshold, the country started to lose patience for the idea of rehabilitation altogether, and it began down a path toward prohibitionist responses, which, perversely, made their way into the nascent addiction treatment system itself.

On June 17, 1971, in the midst of another heroin epidemic, Nixon formally declared his "war on drugs." That year, Americans listed heroin addiction as the nation's third-most-pressing problem, behind only the seemingly endless war in Vietnam and the stagnating economy. (By comparison, in 2019, even during the widely publicized opioid overdose crisis, drugs and drug addiction were rated the twelfth-most-important problem facing the nation.) Worsening the panic further, heroin was widespread in the Vietnam War, too—more than a third of all U.S. enlisted personnel had tried heroin. Street peddlers stuffed vials of 95-percent-pure heroin in the pockets of GIs as they strolled around downtown Saigon, and even a congressional commission with a uniformed Army escort was approached several times by dealers.[*] In 1971, two congressmen gave several high-profile press conferences reporting that as many as 10 to 15 percent of servicemen were addicted. In keeping with the ominous mood, in the television broadcast announcing the drug war, Nixon predicted that drugs would destroy the country, and he claimed, falsely, that heroin users were responsible for $2 billion in property crime every year.

However, the amazing thing about Nixon's war, from today's perspective, is how much it was oriented toward a therapeutic response to addiction: when Nixon made his declaration, it was the only time in the history of the war on drugs that the majority of funding went toward treatment rather than law enforcement. Nixon also presented a relatively young psychiatrist named Jerome Jaffe (yet another Narco alumnus) to the country as the first drug czar, and the administration subsequently took control of the entire federal response to drug addiction treatment, pouring massive funding into those efforts. One of

---

[*] It's important to note that heroin was widely available because the CIA had reportedly protected and participated in the opium cultivation businesses of its strategic allies in the "Golden Triangle" of Southeast Asia.

Nixon's advisers called it the "Camelot period of drug policy," and one scholar has even called Nixon "the first therapeutic president."

Yet within the federal government, there remained serious opposition to therapeutic approaches to addiction, especially treatment in the form of methadone. From its Harry Anslinger days, the Federal Bureau of Narcotics (FBN) had opposed maintenance, to the point of flexing its might internationally to prevent it: in the early 1940s, the Mexican government tried to establish legal opioid maintenance, but Anslinger imposed a total embargo on morphine, thus quashing the Mexican experiment within six months. Federal prosecutors had long enforced their own ban against maintenance treatment—never mind that they had created the ban out of sheer force and it had no real basis in law. So when the FBN heard of Vincent Dole and Marie Nyswander's methadone experiments, they were not pleased.

Soon after Dole and Nyswander started their methadone work, the FBN sent an agent to harass Dole, who found the agent arrogant and a little comical as he pounded the table and insisted, "You're breaking the law." Dole knew that was a lie. A savvy, seasoned academic leader, Dole had already secured New York governor Nelson Rockefeller's support. In the process, their attorneys had learned, to their total surprise, that there was never any definitive law or court case prohibiting maintenance treatment. Dole was placid. As he later recalled, he looked back at the incensed agent and calmly suggested, "You ought to take me to court so we can have a determination on this point." The agent's face abruptly changed; Dole had called his bluff.

In the ensuing years, methadone seemed to have won a secure place in the halls of medicine. Though the FBN continued its opposition—including starting a rumor campaign implying that Dole and Nyswander had fabricated their data—money poured into methadone programs. But the money was both a blessing and a curse. Programs expanded so rapidly that they far outstripped what their actual competence allowed. In New York, even the most ardent methadone advocates urged the health department to slow down. There were unscrupulous physicians who ran "pill mills," but more commonly, "gas station" programs did little more than dispense medications, providing none of the wraparound rehabilitative services that Dole and Nyswander included in their original version, such as job training and other social supports. A *New York Times* reporter twice walked into a clinic and, without any evidence of addiction (or even any identification), bought 280 milligrams of methadone for a $30 fee (the usual starting dose is twenty to thirty milligrams). Non-medical use of methadone, including some overdose deaths, increased. Dole and Nyswander, who had worked so hard to establish warm, holistic, rehabilitative programs, looked on in dismay: Dole bemoaned "the stupidity of thinking that just giving methadone will solve a complicated social problem."

Prohibitionists in the federal government used these problems to fuel their opposition to methadone. In addition to their harassment of Dole and Nyswander, they sounded the alarm about black markets for methadone, played on methadone's symbolic association with Black and Brown inner-city drug use, and counterattacked with a flurry of amendments and regulations meant to limit its use. They couldn't kill methadone, but they could hamstring it and turn it into a system of control. In just a matter of years, methadone treatment was transformed into something more like an arm of law enforcement than medicine: private physicians could no longer offer office-based treatment, and only special federally approved and licensed programs could prescribe methadone for addiction treatment (and only under the looming threat of constant scrutiny from federal drug enforcement). In 1981, the former Communist Marie Nyswander wryly noted that she was "sounding like a Republican" in criticizing the extraordinary federal controls on methadone's use. Today, methadone treatment has significant problems, but many of them stem from overzealous regulation with roots in this period: rigid, arbitrary dosing policies, inflexible schedules, exorbitant fees, and inadequate psychotherapy and other recovery services.

Methadone also remains one of the strongest examples we have of the stark racial disparities in the understanding and treatment of addiction. Black and Brown communities have long had to fight for treatment—for example, in the 1970s, Black and Puerto Rican community groups staged numerous sit-ins and protests to force hospitals to open drug treatment facilities. One demonstration had to occupy the community psychiatry division of St. Luke's Hospital in Harlem for four days to obtain drug treatment for teens. Addiction in communities of color, perennially a major problem, is too often explained in a stigmatized way that justifies prohibitionist approaches: portrayed as self-chosen and irresponsible. On a structural level, addiction is explained away as the intractable effect of poverty or other root causes, treated as inevitable and expected, and thus left to the criminal legal system. Meanwhile, other explanations of addiction fuel entirely separate tiers of addiction treatment.

The medication buprenorphine was first proposed as an addiction treatment by Narco researchers in 1975, but it was long sidelined by anti-medication stigma, especially the regulatory restrictions that were built around methadone. As the scholars Samuel Roberts and Helena Hansen have documented, it was only when the opioid epidemic emerged as a supposedly white problem that buprenorphine was made available. In the late 1990s, treatment advocates warned Congress that "narcotic addiction is spreading from urban to suburban areas," and the "current system" of methadone treatment was "a poor fit for the suburban spread of narcotic addiction." Congress accordingly passed legislation that carved out a special regulatory category for buprenorphine as an office-based treatment—a pharmaceutical and clinical intervention rather than a punitive one—but only through specially waivered physicians who were more likely to take only self-pay and private insurance. Sure enough, three years after buprenorphine's approval, roughly 90 percent of U.S. patients taking it were white. (In fact, some of the only opposition to the buprenorphine legislation came from members of

Congress who correctly identified that buprenorphine would be available only to those with financial resources, and lower-income people with addiction would be left in the lurch.) Today, white people are still far more likely to receive buprenorphine, and the medication largely functions as one piece of the entirely separate system for responding to white and upper-class drug use, relegating the majority of socially marginalized patients to the system of control enacted in the 1970s.

Anti-medication stigma has also, ironically, permeated some of the twelve-step communities so central to addiction recovery today, creating an unnecessary tension between therapeutic and mutual-help approaches that need not be in opposition to each other. Early Narcotics Anonymous leaders spoke favorably about methadone, such as Father Daniel Egan, featured widely in the news in the early 1960s as the "Junkie Priest" for his work ministering to people with addiction in New York City. But the crackdown on methadone drove anti-medication attitudes in twelve-step communities to an unhealthy extreme, and in time, methadone patients in NA weren't allowed to hold a service commitment or even speak at meetings. Soon, people on methadone began avoiding NA groups or keeping their methadone treatment a secret. As recently as 1996, NA's board of trustees strongly suggested that people using methadone should not be allowed to be speakers or chair meetings, and to this day, official communications from NA have consistently specified that patients receiving medications for addiction treatment are not "clean."

That same anti-medication stigma bled outward to all psychoactive medications. In part, mutual-help groups and people in recovery were having a reasonable response to the over-prescription of drugs like amphetamines, barbiturates, and benzodiazepines—as early as the 1940s, AA publications recognized sedative addiction as "chewing your booze." Also, it's important to note that the culture of twelve-step communities is dynamic and heterogeneous, and these attitudes vary by group and continue to evolve today. Still, and especially in treatment settings

strongly influenced by twelve-step fundamentalism, people are sometimes pressured to stop psychiatric medications in search of the ever-
elusive ideal of being "drug-free." I've heard of abstinence-based programs
that have refused to accept people on heart medication.

Medications for addiction—especially for opioid addiction—save
lives. Study after study, from carefully controlled clinical trials to massive
investigations of everyday practice, have shown that buprenorphine and
methadone cut the rate of death among opioid-addicted patients by half
or more. A recent, massive study of more than forty thousand patients
has found that among all treatments—medications and therapy alike,
including intensive outpatient and residential rehabs—buprenorphine
and methadone are the only ones that reduce opioid overdoses. (Another,
newer medication for opioid use disorder, extended-release naltrexone, is
also useful, and it suffers from comparatively less anti-medication stigma.)
There are signs of some softening among previously unreceptive communities to allow for medication treatments, but it is slow in coming, and
often incomplete. In 2012, Hazelden announced that it would provide
buprenorphine. But, like many other treatment centers, it does not allow
its clients to use methadone.

The prohibitionist backlash against methadone was just one development in a relatively diverse drug policy landscape. For example,
cannabis policy in the 1970s was remarkably levelheaded and nuanced,
as exemplified by the National Commission on Marihuana and Drug
Abuse, which in 1972 issued a detailed report recommending against
"total prohibition" and called for the decriminalization of cannabis possession for personal use. Nixon, predictably, ignored the report, but
during the Ford and Carter administrations, bipartisan coalitions continued to give thoughtful and nuanced attention to cannabis decriminalization. In 1975, the Ford administration released an important
"white paper" that called for aligning drug control efforts more closely

with the actual harms of substances, arguing that cannabis enforcement should be given a lower priority and instead identifying amphetamines, mixed barbiturates, and heroin as the greatest risks. In the meantime, the new National Institute on Alcohol Abuse and Alcoholism and the National Institute on Drug Abuse continued the forward momentum toward a therapeutic response to addiction.

However, viewed from another perspective, the assault on methadone was a bellwether of a powerful strand of prohibitionist thinking, one that in the coming years would refashion progressive reforms into tools of enforcement. The 1970 Controlled Substances Act, for example, was initially passed as a relatively liberal reform package, doing away with mandatory minimum sentences and providing support for treatment and research. It helped to impose relatively effective new limitations on sedative and stimulant manufacturers to reduce the harms of those white-market drugs without a total crackdown. However, giving the Justice Department authority for "scheduling"—the system of ranks and regulations that forms the basis for restricting drug use—vastly expanded the federal government's role in drug regulation, setting the foundation for a series of increasingly restrictive and punitive measures that only heightened the division between medical and non-medical use. Soon afterward, Nixon created an entirely new federal drug agency and developed a set of powerful new law enforcement tools: no-knock warrants, wiretapping, preventive detention, and more. He ordered the CIA to join the fight against drug trafficking, declaring "total war" and promising that traffickers would be "hunted to the end of the earth."

As the Watergate scandal increasingly threatened Nixon's presidency, the disjunction between his warlike rhetoric and his sensible, balanced policy grew too wide to continue, and he began to invest heavily in prohibitionist approaches. The drug enforcement budget skyrocketed—from $34 million in 1969 to $217 million in 1974—and the treatment budget was slashed for the first time. In 1973, the Nixon administration created the Drug Enforcement Administration, consolidating the host of federal agencies involved in the drug war (including fifty former CIA operatives) into one superagency, a powerful arm of domestic surveillance that Nixon reportedly intended to use against his own enemies. (Also in 1973, Nelson Rockefeller, stunned the New York legislature when he angrily called for draconian drug laws including, among other things, life imprisonment for "pushers.") Later that year, in a major speech, Nixon insisted on even "tougher penalties and stronger weapons" in the war on drugs: a return to harsh mandatory minimums, all the way up to the possibility of life without parole.

Overall, there was a punitive shift afoot in general law enforcement policies, too, and rehabilitative 1960s ideals were steadily losing ground to the criminalization of poverty. In a *New York Times* commentary in 1973, the influential conservative political scientist James Q. Wilson suggested, "Suppose we abandon entirely the rehabilitation theory of sentencing and corrections." In due time, other supposedly reformist measures of the sixties and early seventies were shaped into more enforcement-oriented tools, such as funding for modernizing the police being used to drastically expand supervision and control in low-income urban communities.

Prohibitionist and anti-drug sentiment in the earlier part of the twentieth century had meant, effectively, the end of treatment for addiction. But this time, something was different. In the meantime, the addiction treatment system was developing a zero-tolerance ideology of its own.

Harold Hughes was a giant, both literally and figuratively. Standing six foot three and weighing 245 pounds, Hughes, the senator who had helped Marty Mann push through national legislation at the turn of the 1970s, was famous for his booming bass voice and forceful, evangelistic speaking style. He was a hero to the alcoholism advocacy movement. An openly recovering alcoholic, not only was he the chief architect behind his eponymous national legislation on alcoholism, the Hughes Act, but he had even run for president. When Nixon tried to block federal funding for alcoholism treatment, vetoing bills and impounding funds, Hughes led a congressional charge to fight him, and in May of 1974, within days of the start of formal impeachment hearings against him, Nixon signed a new Hughes bill into law, opening floodgates of federal cash.

So when thousands of treatment professionals gathered in a massive San Francisco conference center later that year, waiting for Senator Hughes to speak, they must have expected some encouragement for their burgeoning movement. Instead, upon taking the stage, Hughes gave them a solemn warning. He said that the addiction treatment field was starting to resemble an "alcohol and drug industrial complex," a rapidly institutionalizing "new civilian army." He worried that the whole enterprise would be corrupted by money and power. Above all, he urged his audience to ask themselves: Were they truly interested in helping people in need, or had addiction treatment become "a device for massaging our egos by regimenting people in the guise of helping them"?

The field was indeed undergoing tremendous growth. The number of alcoholism treatment programs almost quintupled from 1973 to 1977, and drug treatment programs saw similar expansion. In addition to the federal money pouring in, private health insurance also increasingly covered treatment, and new private treatment programs accelerated the trend. The number of people in the United States receiving treatment for alcoholism had risen sharply since 1942—when Marty Mann's "alcoholism movement" was born—from fewer than 100,000 to well over a million people in 1976.

The explosive growth, however, brought with it a harmful shift to a one-size-fits-all ideology that insisted that all substance problems were the same—an ideology that was increasingly intolerant of alternative views. As was the case for methadone programs, rapid expansion proved corrosive to program quality. Desperate for staff, addiction treatment programs recruited their own recent patient graduates, gave them cursory training, and promoted them to "counselor" positions with no real credentialing system, professional standards, or even any basic quality control. Then, bloated on profits, the vast majority of treatment centers had no incentive to innovate. Most settled into an ossified model: they diagnosed everyone with addiction, treated people in the same old twenty-eight-day model, touted AA as the only treatment method, and discharged them at "graduation" with no follow-up care.

The result was, as Hughes had warned, treatment programs that were "regimenting" people to a hardening and warped ideology. No matter the specifics of their issues, nearly everyone arriving in treatment was diagnosed with addiction, regardless of the severity of their problems, and the programs insisted on abstinence for all. As the director of the Betty Ford Center put it bluntly in 1988, "Patients ask how important it is that they go to AA after they're through here. I say, 'I can give you a guarantee. When you leave here, if you *don't* go to AA, you won't make it.'" In the process of conflating all problems into addiction, the programs missed the true diversity of the issue, in favor of a narrow view of addiction that was at odds with the original intent of twelve-step programs. The founders of AA, in developing a program for people voluntarily seeking help, had formulated a capacious and flexible conception of addiction that allowed people to come to their own understanding. Now, as reflected by the treatment industrial complex, that notion of addiction was changing drastically.

This ideological approach to treatment is harmful because, as contemporary research shows, abstinence is not necessarily the best treatment goal for everyone with a drug or alcohol problem. There are many people who do seem to need abstinence to safely recover from addiction, but even after serious substance problems, some others are able to moderate their use, and still more can improve their functioning in life and overall well-being without lowering their use at all. Furthermore, many people are resistant to the idea of abstinence, and pushing the idea too forcefully can backfire. Too rigid a focus on abstinence can cause an "abstinence violation effect": upon resuming substance use after a period of self-imposed abstinence, those who experience guilt, shame, and hopelessness are more likely to return to harmful use. But in the 1970s, as the first scientific studies establishing these findings emerged, they were met with intense controversy.

In the mid-1970s, the RAND Corporation was on the verge of concluding a massive investigation of the forty-five treatment centers established by the National Institute on Alcohol Abuse and Alcoholism (NIAAA)—the institute established by the first Hughes Act, in 1970. It was by far the largest alcoholism treatment study of its time. Preliminary findings began to trickle out, and word got around that the researchers had made a stunning observation: people who returned to moderate drinking after treatment for what was diagnosed as alcoholism did just as well as those who chose to abstain entirely—both groups had the same likelihood of relapse to harmful drinking.

The results of the RAND report flew in the face of the reigning abstinence-only ideology, and the most hard-core of the alcoholism advocacy movement were livid, perhaps no one more so than Thomas Pike, a powerful California oilman and a devoted member of Marty Mann's advocacy organization, the NCA. Pike was one of the most influential Republican power brokers in Southern California. In 1970, he had been instrumental in getting the Hughes Act across the finish line in Washington: when it looked as if Nixon was going to allow the bill to die in a pocket veto, Pike rallied his CEO friends and made a call to Nixon himself, leaning on his clout as a former chair of the Republican Party Finance Committee in California, Nixon's home state, to pressure Nixon to sign the bill into law.

Pike had been sober in AA for more than twenty-five years—when he died, in 1993, his license plate read AA 47 YR—and he felt in his bones that a moderate treatment goal was dangerous. The Big Book of Alcoholics Anonymous called the possibility of controlled drinking the "great obsession of every abnormal drinker," a siren song that had led countless alcoholics to addiction and death. "We are convinced to a man that alcoholics of our type are in the grip of a progressive illness. Over any considerable period we get worse, never better."

Pike, Mann, and other alcoholism activists worked tirelessly to try to sink the RAND report. In his own words, Pike "fought like a tiger with the authors of the report" and finally resigned from the RAND board in protest when they refused to suppress it. As a last resort, they tried to get the head of the NIAAA to quash it, but the director refused.

In 1976, within days of each other, RAND and the NCA held dueling press conferences, rocketing the controversy to the front page of *The New York Times* and countless other outlets. Advocates impugned the character of the RAND researchers and called the report a "slanted polemic," "unethical, unprincipled, and playing Russian roulette with the lives of human beings." One NCA leader said, "My concern is that a lot of people will try to drink again, and a lot of people will die as a result." Enoch Gordis, a future director of the NIAAA, reflected that "the alcoholism field reacted as if heresy had been spoken in church." It was the most divisive ideological battle over the nature of addiction the field had ever seen. The alcoholism advocates might have recognized the heterogeneity of people with drinking problems—the AA Big Book itself recognized a diversity of alcohol problems and that some hard drinkers could stop on their own—but instead they resisted the data in favor of the reigning ideology. The gulf between scientific research on addiction and the popular conception was widening.

In the midst of the ongoing controversy, a husband-and-wife team of research psychologists, Mark and Linda Sobell, new to the study of alcohol problems, was developing a new experimental treatment for controlled drinking on the alcoholism ward of Patton State Hospital, nestled against the foothills of the San Bernardino Mountains in Southern California. The patients on Patton State's alcoholism ward were severe cases, hospital inpatients who had reached the end of their rope, and many of them had been arrested, been divorced, suffered from delirium tremens, or otherwise had their lives ruined. Nevertheless, the Sobells developed a seventeen-session program to see if the patients could be trained to reduce their harmful drinking through behavioral techniques; for example, by having them practice distinguishing the potency of mixed drinks or monitoring them via closed-circuit TV and administering painful electric jolts for gulping their drinks too quickly. Their findings, reached after months of rigorous record gathering, were shocking: compared with the usual group therapy and AA that regular inpatients received, the experimental subjects were unambiguously doing much better. Not only had their drinking improved; their relationships with family and friends and their job performance showed improvement, too. "These findings directly contradict the concept of irreversibility of alcoholic drinking," the Sobells wrote.

Once again, the research findings flew in the face of the dominant paradigm of addiction, and once again, the reaction was outrage. One disillusioned former patient of the Sobells connected with a group of like-minded researchers and clinicians, one of whom was Mary Pendery, who had been a prominent critic of the RAND report and served as spokesperson for the NCA's press conference attacking it. They tracked down the experiment's former patients, conducted their own reanalysis, and published a bombshell refutation of the Sobells' work in the journal *Science* in 1982. They reported that the majority of the "controlled drinking" subjects had relapsed or died from alcohol-related causes, and they further asserted that the Sobells had completely misrepresented their findings. In an interview with *The New York Times*, Irving Maltzman, a psychologist on the study, insisted, "Beyond any reasonable doubt, it's fraud." The story was picked up by the CBS show *60 Minutes,* which—in addition to featuring one heart-wrenching scene at the grave of a patient—portrayed the Sobells as naive, inexperienced researchers playing with the lives of their subjects.

Eventually, no fewer than five investigations, including ones by a panel of federal research agency leaders and a U.S. congressional investigator, completely exonerated the Sobells. They hadn't been claiming that they had discovered the perfect cure for alcoholism, after all. (In fact, several in their experimental group struggled for a while and eventually chose abstinence.) They had only reported that their method performed better than treatment-as-usual, and their findings were in fact supported by the evidence. The problem, for the traditional alcoholism movement's platform, was that those findings complicated the picture of addiction. One key principle of the Sobells' formulation, which since then has been further supported by considerable evidence, was that some people with drinking problems can show real improvements in life functioning and decreases in consequences without total abstinence. Other studies around that time were offering up findings with similar implications: drug use was not driven mindlessly by the biological effects of the substance alone; some people could use drugs like heroin without serious consequences; and generally, people with addiction did not suffer from a binary "loss of control." Psychology researchers were developing new evidence-based treatments for addiction, such as motivational interviewing and relapse prevention therapy. Addiction, through the research of the time, was beginning to demonstrate more variation and nuance, and there was no reason for mutual-help efforts and advocacy to be in opposition to these new therapeutic approaches— there was room for pluralistic paths to recovery. Instead of embracing this, though, the field became further polarized. It was a setup for serious misunderstandings and outright misuses of the idea of addiction, and the consequences were severe.

In the summer of 1976, Marsha Keith Schuchard, an English professor at Emory University, threw a birthday party for her thirteen-year-old daughter at their home in suburban Atlanta. Later in the evening, Schuchard was amazed to see seventh graders stumbling around red-eyed, giggling, hair reeking, and obviously stoned. She and her husband snooped around the backyard after the party, and sure enough, they were appalled to find papers, clips, roaches, and plastic bags with crumbs of cannabis. Schuchard, a self-proclaimed liberal-leaning college professor, soon adopted for herself the unlikely role of anti-drug activist. She organized other local parents into a "Nosy Parents Association," later renamed National Families in Action, the era's first anti-drug parents group. Soon, a coalition of like-minded parents groups began coalescing around the issue, rising to combat what they saw as an increasingly dangerous permissiveness about drugs.

The parents groups lobbied for more restrictions on drugs, but most people in the late seventies didn't consider cannabis much of a threat at all. Policy wonks countered with evidence that cannabis was not as harmful as it was commonly portrayed, and Jimmy Carter snubbed the groups entirely. But social conservatism was on the rise, the economy was in a slump, and the parents were, as it turned out, at the vanguard of a new anti-drug, zero-tolerance ethos. It wouldn't be much longer before the rest of the nation was swept up in that old fantasy of total prohibition: the ideal of a "drug-free America."

Ronald Reagan won the presidency in 1980 at least in part by taking Nixon's strategy of dog-whistle racism to an even further and highly effective extreme, portraying people on public assistance as "welfare queens" and "strapping young bucks." Upon taking office, he cleaned house and replaced the drug policy technocrats with a new crop of advisers who were interested in tackling the "drug problem" as a moral issue. He, and especially his wife, Nancy, fully embraced the parents movements, which had joined forces in 1980 as the National Federation of Parents for Drug Free Youth. Like the policies of Hamilton Wright or Harry Anslinger, Reagan's anti-drug movement was not an invention but merely an innovation, a return to drugs as an effective justification for punitive programs.

The governing idea of addiction of the time became closely

associated with individual and immoral choices. The Reagans derided drugs as a cause of addiction, but the solution was individual responsibility and family values, not funding for treatment. (Margaret Thatcher took the same approach across the pond in the United Kingdom, where government officials praised "self-help, voluntary initiatives" and discredited public services.) Mothers Against Drunk Driving, also founded in 1980, soon raised millions of dollars and attracted endless public attention by focusing exclusively on the individual wrongdoing of drunk drivers, unlike other organizations that also called attention to the effects of alcohol industry marketing. In the meantime, this moralistic view of addiction further widened the pharmaceutical/drug divide, allowing anti-regulatory reformers to slash Food and Drug Administration budgets, weaken FDA oversight of industry, and approve direct-to-consumer pharmaceutical marketing, enabling a resurgence of sedatives, stimulants, and especially opioids—setting the stage, for example, for the 1990s approval and marketing of OxyContin as safe for "long-term use."

As the political winds rapidly shifted toward prohibition, the drug war provided political cover for expanding the role of law enforcement. In June of 1982, standing in the Rose Garden, Reagan (re-)declared a war on drugs, "taking down the surrender flag"—implicitly, one flying over Carter's administration—and "running up a battle flag." This new war on drugs justified the federal government's involvement in street crime, and the budgets of federal agencies grew accordingly. It set in motion a massive expansion in asset forfeiture laws that allowed law enforcement to seize private property without any proof of a crime. When the crack epidemic hit in the mid-1980s, the administration hired staff to publicize the drug's dangers, and the DEA was tasked with actively promoting media attention to the most sensationalistic stories—an easy task, in fact, when even researchers readily repeated the reductionist narrative that crack was "the most addictive drug known to man," one that would cause "almost instantaneous addiction."

In a major speech in 1986, Reagan escalated the drug war rhetoric even further, calling for "a national crusade against drugs—a sustained, relentless effort to rid America of this scourge—by mobilizing every segment of society against drug abuse." That same year, the Reagans doubled down on their Just Say No campaign, and Ronald signed the Anti–Drug Abuse Act: bipartisan legislation that imposed harsh mandatory minimums. The law established radical sentencing disparities between crack, more commonly used by poor people of color, and powder cocaine, more commonly used by wealthy white people: the threshold amount to trigger a mandatory minimum sentence was a hundred times higher for powder cocaine than for crack.

The 1980s war on drugs ultimately had very little to do with addiction. It was a war on people who use drugs, and people of color in general, for which addiction simply served as a pretext. Its leaders used the idea of addiction as a weapon—a deep-rooted strategy in the history of addiction in America. And in particular, it served as an important component of America's developing system of mass incarceration, which has now famously given the United States the largest system of incarceration on earth—with less than 5 percent of the world's population but more than 20 percent of its prisoners. Drug arrests became an even more significant entry point into the criminal legal system, especially for people of color: today, Black people are more than twice as likely as white people to be arrested for drug crimes, even though Black and white Americans use drugs at almost identical rates.

The impact on the cultural understanding of substance use was tremendous, promoting fears of addiction as a dangerous, spreading contagion to be stamped out by any means necessary. Anti-drug sentiment was further intensified by the uncritical media coverage, the DARE (Drug Abuse Resistance Education) program in schools, and anti-drug advertisements on television and in magazines. Workplaces, too, shifted to a "zero tolerance" model—in a bizarre display of the extent of the phenomenon, in August 1986 Reagan, George H. W. Bush, and

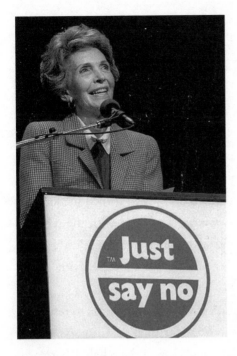

Nancy Reagan speaking
at a "Just Say No" Rally
in Los Angeles, 1987.

seventy-eight other White House officials lined up to urinate in cups for drug tests to "set the example" for the nation, and in the coming months, politicians challenged their rivals to take drug tests.

In his very first Oval Office address, George H. W. Bush outlined his plan for finally achieving "victory over drugs," and he dramatically held up a baggie of crack and announced that you could buy the drug in front of the White House. Bush and his advisers had wanted this visual to show that crack was ubiquitous, but in reality there were no dealers camped out there. The DEA had needed to lure Keith Jackson, a Black teenage boy and low-level dealer, to a park next to the White House just to get the arrest. (In a telling detail about the de facto segregation in cities, Jackson had asked the undercover DEA agent, "Where the fuck is the White House?") Politicians and law enforcement often had to work quite hard to engineer a moral panic about drug use, but it worked. In 1985, fewer than 1 percent of Americans identified drugs as the nation's most important issue, but by September 1989, shortly after Bush's speech, that number was 54 percent.

After a few weeks in rehab, our little group of doctors and other medical professionals started to feel like a community. Weeks of group therapy, nightly check-ins, and our precious half hour of reruns and cereal bars in the TV lounge before bed had brought us together. Others in my cohort were happy to be there, which helped me look for the good in the program. There were real problems with the rehab—the confrontation, the one-size-fits-all approach and exclusive focus on the twelve steps, the lack of medications for people with opioid addiction—but it wasn't all bad.

We health professionals were lucky. Most of us had jobs to return to, but many of the other patients weren't so fortunate. There was a more subdued attitude out in the general population of the rehab, where people were often summarily discharged after their insurance ran out—sometimes while they were still fearfully reporting withdrawal symptoms and powerful cravings. The picture only got bleaker as we advanced to the second phase of our treatment program, which required us to catch rides from community AA members to attend local meetings. The effects of 2008's Great Recession were still ravaging the postindustrial community surrounding our cloistered program. As factory jobs were being offshored at a dizzying rate, we went to meetings in cramped church basements or cavernous, echoing union halls, and people raised their hands and shared their stories of losing work, struggling to support their families, and trying to maintain sobriety amid a creeping hopelessness. Afterward, dozens of people circulated around the rooms with sign-in sheets for parole or other court-ordered programs. The people who gave me rides to meetings all had interlock devices on their car ignitions to measure their blood alcohol levels. Many times, when I started to complain about my situation, I looked at them and realized how good I had it.

I was receiving support, encouragement, and access to treatment from the physician health program. I was part of a system that was looking out for me. Many of the people I met were facing much more serious challenges, yet most of them got only a short detox, court-ordered twelve-step attendance, breathalyzers, drug tests, and no more—and it was called "treatment." It wasn't hard to see that most people in the system were not getting their real needs met, but I didn't appreciate the full extent of why that was until I learned more about how addiction treatment had coevolved with the war on drugs.

Today, the U.S. addiction treatment system is in dire straits—even the word "system" is a bit of a stretch. There are more than fifteen thousand specialized treatment programs serving 3.7 million people a year, at a price tag of $42 billion—but most are woefully under-regulated private organizations, the standards are low, and exploitation is rife. "Body brokers" cruise around rehab hot spots like South Florida to find drug users on the streets and persuade them to go to rehab, earning paid commissions so that treatment centers can collect more insurance funds. Treatment centers rack up charges for unnecessary drug tests; in some centers, managers call their patients "thoroughbreds" because they're just there to urinate. From rehabs to outpatient programs, far too many offer a cobbled-together assortment of therapies organized around a one-size-fits-all model profoundly disconnected from evidence-based practices. These programs often lack licensed medical providers or adequate attention to the other psychiatric problems that so often accompany addiction—and far too many have a blanket ban on lifesaving medications for addiction treatment. Even the more respectable programs are largely built around an acute-care model that treats program "graduation" as if people should be able to manage a perfectly abstinent recovery from that point onward—despite the fact that, depending on the substances involved, between 50 and 70 percent of people will resume substance use in the first year after treatment, up to 35 percent will be readmitted to a treatment program within a year, and nearly 50 percent will be readmitted within two to five years.

The tragedy of our present system has its roots in the harsh prohibition and criminalization of drug use in the 1980s and '90s. The stigma attached to addiction only intensified its status as a separate, relatively deregulated, and often exploitative system, and it was directly and profoundly influenced by the escalating war on drugs. As people flooded into the criminal legal system, more and more were diverted to addiction treatment, and many treatment systems became supported largely, if not entirely, by criminal legal referrals. In the time of MADD, alcohol as well as drug users flowed into treatment: as early as 1983, one of the largest groups of clients was those getting treatment related to drunk driving or other lower-level offenses. To this day, a massive arrest-to-treatment pipeline funnels coerced clients into the treatment industrial complex, and more than a quarter of all clients in publicly funded addiction treatment are referred by the criminal legal system. The coercive approach spread outward to the rest of society: workplaces and schools alike sent people to treatment for any positive result on a drug test, without any indication of addiction or any need for treatment at all.

This tacit alliance with prohibitionist forces changed the character of the treatment system, pulling it toward much harsher confrontation, even for the most privileged. To break down supposed denial and resistance, counselors and interventionists used "tough love" and threats and punishments—for example, one employer-based intervention featured on the front page of *The Wall Street Journal* in 1983 included an executive being told to "shut up and listen" because "alcoholics are liars, so we don't want to hear what you have to say." These approaches were increasingly justified by the popular notion of hitting "rock bottom," a term that, in the original AA program inspired by William James, described a self-defined point of spiritual deflation, but now became a rationalization for escalating punishments as part of treatment, including the still-common practice of terminating treatment when people relapse.

This treatment approach was largely justified in the name of the twelve steps, but it was, ironically, a remarkable departure from that program's original intent. The Minnesota Model, founded on the twelve steps, was built for people who had experienced serious problems and who were voluntarily seeking treatment. However, as treatment programs began to serve a broader spectrum of people, including coerced people who (perhaps rightly) didn't think they had a problem with addiction, they struggled to adapt. In fact, AA never insisted that all problem drinkers should abstain, nor did it ever declare superiority over therapeutic approaches to addiction. In other words, AA was founded to help voluntary, *akratic* addicts—people who had lost the ability to control, struggled, frequently relapsed even with assistance, and in the end chose abstinence for themselves. It never insisted on the language of "disease" and was open to both a heterogeneity of alcohol problems and a variety of ways to recover.

There are people who truly suffer from denial and resistance and need to be challenged, but harsh confrontation is not the way. Psychological research conducted during the 1980s and '90s increasingly showed that clinicians can more effectively increase motivation for change and improve substance use outcomes by supporting people's self-efficacy rather than breaking them down. And the underlying goal of persuading people into abstinence via a twelve-step framework is not appropriate for the full diversity of people with substance use problems. To be sure, abstinence is an excellent treatment goal for many. I frequently recommend abstinence, and abstinence-oriented treatment programs, to my patients. The problem with our treatment system is not its promotion of abstinence as a treatment goal, but the fact that it is often the *only* treatment goal, as if everyone with substance use issues has the exact same problem.

The sad fact of this history is how little has changed since the 1980s. A brief opportunity for a paradigm shift arose when the treatment system crashed in the late eighties and early nineties, due in large part to aggressive gatekeeping by managed-care companies and HMOs. Occupancy rates dropped, and even the poshest rehabs drastically constricted or folded entirely. From 1992 to 2001, insurance spending on addiction treatment services declined by more than 70 percent per covered person. Asked in recent years about the treatment industry, Mark Willenbring, a former researcher at the National Institute on Alcohol Abuse and Alcoholism, said, "What we simply need is a nice bulldozer, so that we could level the entire industry and start from scratch." This crash in treatment thirty years ago was a potential bulldozer moment, when the industry might have reformed. Instead, it limped along until it recovered, largely unchanged.

What can we do for people like Josie, the woman I met who was struggling in this system? A pessimist might think that she must wait for sweeping structural reform before she can hope for better treatment—not just in the treatment industrial complex, but in the legal system as a whole. But another perspective, often called "harm reduction," has attempted to offer an entirely different paradigm for drug problems, one that also has roots in the turbulent 1980s, but in response to a different epidemic.

On April 10, 1983, Larry Kramer—a pugnacious novelist, playwright, and now community organizer—stood in the pouring rain on a New York City sidewalk with a small band of protesters, waiting all morning for the arrival of Mayor Ed Koch. For a year and a half, Koch had been dodging meetings with community leaders, but by this point in the AIDS epidemic, he had little choice but to attend the symposium at Lenox Hill Hospital, tucked away between Park and Lexington avenues on the wealthy Upper East Side. As Koch tried to duck inside, with TV cameras rolling, Kramer pelted the mayor with questions: "When are you going to do something about AIDS? How many people have to die?"

Less than a month later, in cities across the country, activists marched by candlelight to protest political inaction. In San Francisco, the lights stretched for a mile from the Castro down Market Street, a banner at the front declaring, FIGHTING FOR OUR LIVES.

The AIDS rights movement was the most obvious and vigorous example of a power shift in the world of medicine. A new patients' rights movement was sweeping the country, one that had been steadily intensifying through the 1970s and burst into prominence in the 1980s. Cancer patients demanded access to potentially lifesaving drugs. A "consumer movement" of people with mental illness rose up to demand more self-determination in their treatment. Many states adopted their own patients' bills of rights. And though gay men were the most visible organizers in the AIDS rights movement, injection drug users were contracting AIDS and fighting for their lives, too.

Inspired in part by earlier harm reduction pioneers in Western Europe, the first generation of harm reduction activists in the United States began with simple interventions, such as teaching people to clean syringes with bleach and exchanging used syringes for sterile ones, to reduce the transmission of infectious disease during the AIDS epidemic. These programs offered much more than syringes: they were a site for peer education and other ways of promoting general health, as well as a place for community building and support; they are commonly called "syringe service programs" today. Harm reduction was a new way of thinking about drug use, in stark counterpoint to the dominant view of drug criminalization. The primary focus was not stamping out drugs, but decreasing harms and making health and safety the primary objective.

Not surprisingly, given the social and political context of the time, syringe service programs were met with strict opposition from the outset, ostensibly on the grounds that hypodermic syringes were drug paraphernalia, but often with a heavily moralistic undertone. When the New York City health commissioner first proposed distributing sterile needles to drug users in the 1980s, his suggestion was met with outright hostility from prohibitionists like Manhattan's special narcotics prosecutor, who declared, "Drug addicts, in the frenzied and desperate minutes before injecting a needle into their veins, could not care less about contamination," and that "slaves of addiction do not change their daily habits." Mayor Koch rejected the commissioner's recommendation, and it was only after years of advocacy—and after harm reduction activists forced the issue by declaring they'd go ahead no matter what—that the Koch administration grudgingly agreed to move forward and the city and state allowed a clinical trial of the program to proceed. Other activists across the country established underground networks of syringe service programs, as well as aboveground programs, as explicit acts of civil disobedience, but they likewise had to fight long legal and public relations battles to even be allowed to operate.

In the context of the 1980s drug war, harm reduction measures were often derided as tantamount to condoning drug use: Bob Schuster, the director of the National Institute on Drug Abuse (NIDA) under Reagan and Bush Sr., told the scholar Nancy Campbell, "Many people were concerned that if we made it safer for people to use drugs, more people would use drugs. If you used the term 'harm minimization' in the federal government at that time and even now to some extent, you would have to wash your mouth out with soap, if you didn't get fired for it." Federal law banned funding for needle exchange programs in 1988, and despite studies that showed that the programs work to reduce deaths and infections without increasing drug use or crime, the ban remained in place for decades to come.

Now, after years of further innovations, harm reduction includes a wide range of evidence-based practices, including peer education, naloxone (Narcan) distribution for overdose reversal, drug-checking services, and safe consumption facilities. (The last of these approaches is still outlawed in the United States.) On concrete measurements of public health, each of these practices has strong research support showing that they reduce drug harms without increasing drug use or crime. Harm reduction has also been used as an organizing principle for client-centered treatment. Healthcare workers in different contexts have created versions of "harm reduction therapy," using it as an umbrella term for a range of therapies oriented toward improving people's lives without necessarily insisting on abstinence as the initial goal. These approaches are nothing new. History is full of clear antecedents—such as the 1920s physicians who refused to wean people off opioids before they were ready—and a harm reduction treatment orientation is perfectly compatible with abstinence-based approaches. Many addiction physicians follow a "stepped care" model in which a client starts at a lower intensity of treatment, such as basic counseling on substance problems, then escalates to more intensive programs and an increased focus on abstinence if needed. For people like Josie, these concrete practices are simple and pragmatic.

Finally, harm reduction can be stated as a philosophy. While there is no universally accepted articulation, one description would frame it as a social justice movement that advocates for drug user rights, including a transformation of the oppressive systems that create negative consequences of drug use and violate people's rights in the name of drug control. In this sense, a broader view of harm reduction is the opposite of the zero-tolerance, anti-drug dream, and the paradigm is still taking shape today, because we only recently started coming out of the extraordinarily prohibitionist preoccupation that reasserted itself during the Reagan era.

Zero-tolerance ideology was by no means a Republican phenomenon—just as it was not invented by the Reagan administration, it continued for decades after Reagan and was embraced by his followers and opponents alike, as seen by the Democratic Party's commitment to anti-drug and pro-law-enforcement rhetoric in the 1990s. A significant de-escalation of the war on drugs took place only decades after Reagan, during Barack Obama's administration. Obama's first drug czar, Gil Kerlikowske, repeatedly insisted that we "can't arrest our way out" of the opioid overdose crisis and called for an end to the "war" language. When individual states moved toward decriminalization for cannabis, the federal government allowed them to do so (which was by no means a foregone conclusion). And after a long and torturous road, harm reduction practices finally began taking hold. There were increasing investments in naloxone research, service, and supply, and the ban on federal funding for syringe service programs was finally lifted in 2016.

For well over a century in the United States, the idea of addiction has justified prohibitionist policies—from the opium den bans of the late nineteenth century, which portrayed the drug as dangerously infectious, through the separate and unequal pharmaceutical/drug divide that continues today. These policies are not based on the true harms of drugs but rather are reactions to stigmatized views of drug users—driven by the eternal forces of racism and division and visible as early as 1604, when King James I denounced smoking tobacco as a "vile and stinking" custom of the "wilde, godlesse, and slavish Indians." Instead, one of the most important lessons of harm reduction is that policies about drug use need not be policies about addiction. Drug use is not synonymous with addiction, and criminalization is not a rational way to reduce drug harms. In fact, it is often a central driver of those harms. A fundamental shift in our thinking would be the best way to help people like Josie— letting go of the ideal of a "drug-free" world and instead prioritizing policies and treatments that accept the fact that drug use and addiction are facts of life, unlikely to leave us anytime soon.

Eleven

UNDERSTANDING
ADDICTION

One icy day in February, after two months in rehab, I was dropped off at a grungy bus station. It was only a taste of freedom: I was about to catch a Greyhound to New York for my first weekend pass. In the boarding area, where TV screens were suspended from the concrete ceiling, I glanced up to see my high school girlfriend in a glamorous skin-care ad—in the years since we graduated, she had become a successful Hollywood actress. I, on the other hand, was lugging an overnight bag with a detailed schedule outlining my every move for the next seventy-two hours—supposedly a major step for me, a pre-discharge test to see if I had the capacity to take care of myself for a weekend without screwing it all up.

I didn't worry about drinking. The threat of a positive urine test on my return to the rehab, and all the ensuing consequences, made even the thought preposterous. It had been an important transition when I started to calling myself an alcoholic, and I was getting more comfortable accepting that I needed help. By this point I was regularly introducing myself as an alcoholic. The strangeness of the phrase was starting to wear away, and it felt right to me. But as I looked up at my ex-girlfriend's smiling, radiant face, I was horrified at how far I had fallen, and grateful that so few people really knew.

Back in my lonely walkup apartment, I found the Taser wires tangled on the floor, like a loose, copper bird's nest. After a lonely and anxious night's sleep, I checked in with the director of my residency program, afraid of what she might say. I had heard horror stories from other residents about being summarily fired on their first day back from treatment, but despite my sudden disappearance, despite leaving my program with dozens of overnight calls to cover and all the other logistical nightmares that come from losing a doctor from your twelve-person program, she was kind, understanding, even welcoming. They were holding the spot for me, and I had even been paid while I was gone, on my disability policy. I was coming out of the episode surprisingly unscathed, and I didn't feel I deserved it.

Later during that weekend, I met with some friends at a café on the Upper East Side, looking out on bustling Madison Avenue, sipping expensive tea and talking through the events of the past few months. It was helpful to see my friends' reactions. They were shocked at how bad my drinking had gotten—I had hidden it all from them. But they were also shocked at what I now had to do: the monitoring, the mandated treatment, the threat of discipline hanging over me. I had to obsessively ask waitstaff if there was even a hint of alcohol in the food, or else I might have a positive urine test and be back under the program's scrutiny. They asked, was all this really necessary? Did I really think I was an alcoholic?

One of the people there was my ex-girlfriend from my time in Paris. We had drunk together in an unhealthy way. She was fine now; I was clearly not. I thought to myself, What is the difference between us? I knew I had a problem, and a big problem at that. But did I *have* addiction? Was it a thing—something I caught, or that took hold of me—or was it inseparable from who I was, lurking there in my personality or biology or karma for all time? Was it a separate entity that had attached itself to my healthier being, or was my self inclusive of the disorder? And would I have it for the rest of my life, even if I never drank or used again?

In the coming months, I went to treatment and worked on my recovery, but I also wanted to understand. The counselors in rehab had warned me that it could be dangerous to look too closely at the science of addiction—they said my disease could twist that information into a basis for denial—but I still felt drawn to learn more. I wanted to see how the research could help me understand who I was and who I might become.

In the early 1970s, with heroin use widespread among soldiers in Vietnam and a steady drumbeat of news stories about the spreading epidemic, people stateside began to fear that a plague of soldiers with unbreakable drug habits would return home to infect their communities. Preventing the onset of such an epidemic was the first major task for the Nixon White House's new Special Action Office for Drug Abuse Prevention. Its director, Jerome Jaffe, recommended that all returning soldiers receive a urine drug screen, at that point still a relatively new tool in the medical arsenal. Soon a massive effort, mockingly dubbed "Operation Golden Flow," was born: every returning soldier had to pass a urine test or risk a dishonorable discharge. By the fall of 1971, despite the fact that soldiers had sixty days' notice to beat the test and there was a thriving market for urine (one soldier arriving from the States, descending from his plane, was offered heroin in exchange for a sample that would pass the test), hundreds of soldiers were testing positive each month.

Jaffe also wanted to understand the ways in which drug use and addiction were playing out in the lives of these returning soldiers, so he tapped Lee Robins, a psychiatric epidemiologist at Washington University in St. Louis, to study hundreds of soldiers who'd returned from Vietnam after testing positive for heroin use (an enormous study for its time—likely the largest study of heroin users to date). For years, Robins and her team methodically tracked and re-interviewed their cohort and combed through reams of military and hospital records.

Their findings were shocking—a landmark in the scientific understanding of addiction. Just shy of 20 percent of the men had been addicted to heroin in Vietnam, according to their criteria, but only 1 percent were addicted during their first year back. In other words, 95 percent of people addicted to what was supposedly the most powerful drug in the world had simply stopped using. Over a longer time horizon, no more than 12 percent of the people who had been addicted in Vietnam relapsed at any time in the three years after their return. Even more striking, most of the soldiers achieved those dramatic rates of recovery without any treatment, and half of the recovered soldiers resumed occasional heroin use in the States without becoming addicted.

It just didn't make sense. Heroin was supposed to cause an automatic and unbreakable addiction. From the Pentagon to the press, the results were met with incredulity and outright denial. The findings seemed to defy the popular stereotype. Could a condition as supposedly dire and enduring as addiction just go away on its own?

D iagnosis is the art of discernment, of distinguishing one state from another. But how exactly do we define the boundaries of what is normal? This question has dominated the scientific investigation of addiction, and mental illness more generally, for decades.

The Robins study was just one example of a new movement to study questions like these more rigorously. Psychiatry was undergoing a revolutionary shift in the 1970s. The profession long dominated by Freudian psychoanalysis—always idiosyncratic and subjective, with no great interest in, or patience for, standardizing diagnosis—was beginning to experiment with new ways of investigating mental illness as a biology-based science. The Department of Psychiatry at Washington University, Robins's academic home, was the epicenter of this new scientific

approach, one of the few places in the country that eschewed psychoanalysis and instead sought to make psychiatric diagnoses into reliable
and rigorously classified entities.

Robins's Vietnam veterans studies were shocking because they up-
ended an idea closely associated with the traditional disease model of
addiction—specifically, that it was a permanent and progressive condition, like the drunkard narrative of the temperance movement, or Burroughs's "Once a junkie, always a junkie." The findings were in some
ways even more shocking than the RAND report and the Sobells' investigations, which had studied outcomes after treatment, as Robins had
found a high rate of recovery even without treatment. It's important not
to draw simple conclusions from the findings, which are somewhat
complicated by the way that Robins and her team equated physical dependence with addiction—their criteria for diagnosing addiction were
largely based on the frequency of use and the presence of tolerance and
withdrawal—and thus their definition of addiction lumped together
people who had a subjective experience of losing control with those who
merely used drugs frequently in a difficult situation, then stopped when
their context changed. Nevertheless, such nuance was largely overlooked
at the time, as the traditional disease model of addiction held that it was
a discrete and relatively uniform condition.

Older studies had seemingly confirmed the traditional view. E. M.
Jellinek, Marty Mann's close ally from Yale, had done so in a set of studies on alcoholism back in the 1940s and '50s, but huge problems in his
scientific methodology rendered the results relatively useless for understanding the full diversity of addiction. He drew his first set of conclusions from a preexisting survey done by AA itself on its own members,
through the organization's magazine, *Grapevine,* inherently a self-selected
group. Furthermore, the response rate was abysmal, at less than 10 percent, and Jellinek threw out more than a third of the responses, including every questionnaire filled out by a woman. Not surprisingly, Jellinek's
findings were more a reflection of the predominant views of the time

than anything else. He described alcoholism as a relatively uniform disease, one that progressed inexorably through successive "phases" to a severe, "chronic" stage, only after which was the alcoholic amenable to recovery and treatment. In 1952, he published a follow-up study of two thousand people, and though many of the methodological problems were still present, he argued that the results were broadly applicable, "characteristic . . . of the great majority of alcohol addicts"—namely, that alcoholism followed a predictable, permanent, and progressively worsening course. His colleagues ridiculed it as "Bunky's Doodle," but because it fit so well with the traditional disease model, it was widely disseminated and used in treatment programs as a therapeutic tool, especially after his findings were later reconceptualized as a swooping, U-shaped curve, with an upward slope of "rehabilitation" added by the researcher Max Glatt. It perfectly recapitulated the classic temperance tale of the drunkard narrative, a Dantean story of descent and recovery. To this day, the "Jellinek Curve" is featured prominently on the websites of many rehabs and recovery organizations, and one scholar has called it "probably the most widely diffused artifact of the alcoholism movement's disease concept."

The problem with retrospective studies like Jellinek's is that subjects are tested and interviewed at one point in time, which makes them vulnerable to several biases—in this case, the study population was composed only of those people who stuck with AA and cared enough to respond to the survey; it was not representative of the population as a whole. The alternative was the new scientific approach of following people forward in time, *prospectively,* as a way to separate correlation from causation—like Robins's natural history studies, and others that continued to complicate these traditional assumptions about addiction.

Other natural history studies failed to find a clear line separating people with addiction from the "normal" population. George Vaillant, yet another Narco graduate, published *The Natural History of Alcoholism* in 1983, a book-length report of decades of research on hundreds of

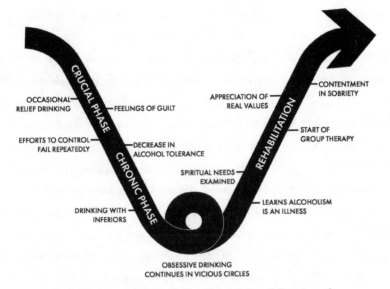

The "Jellinek Curve" (also known as "Bunky's Doodle"), as it was later graphically represented with an upward-swooping curve of "rehabilitation."

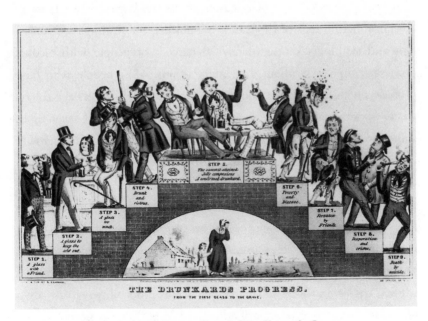

The Drunkards Progress: From the First Glass to the Grave,
Nathaniel Currier, 1846.

Boston-area men, which found no clear division between alcoholics and others, and also found no evidence of any underlying personality problem before the onset of alcoholism. This finding is in line with high rates of comorbidity—the co-occurrence of substance use problems with other psychiatric disorders—which make it still harder to carve out addiction as an issue unto itself. Roughly half of people with substance use disorders also have another psychiatric condition such as depression or bipolar disorder, and in some samples of people seeking treatment for substance use problems, the rate of comorbidity is far higher than that. In fact, there's an astounding rate of comorbidity across all psychiatric disorders—for example, major depressive disorders have comorbidity rates with other disorders approaching 80 percent—casting doubt on the idea that mental disorders are discrete diseases.

Since Robins, the overwhelming majority of large-scale surveys have found that a huge proportion of people with substance use problems spontaneously get better on their own, a phenomenon labeled "natural recovery." Across decades of research, across the largest data sets available, numbering tens of thousands of subjects, the findings are consistent and striking. Approximately 70 percent of people with alcohol problems improve without any interventions. Most people who have problems with illicit drugs stop using them by age thirty. By age thirty-seven, approximately 75 percent of people who have had severe substance problems have no symptoms whatsoever. Even when far narrower criteria are used to restrict the studies to the most impairing and harmful problems, there are still large rates of spontaneous remission.

All this research seemed to challenge central ideas about addiction. For significant numbers of people with substance use problems, it did not seem to be a discrete, permanent, and progressive condition. How, though, can I actually apply these large-scale surveys and observational studies, the proportions and percentages and probabilities, to my own life? Can I actually grow out of addiction? What if I am simply in that percentage who cannot return to safe use? Surely there's a better way to carve nature at its joints? Back in Robins's day, questions like these were inspiring another line of research, one that sought out the very biological roots of disorder.

I'm on the phone with my patient Nicole, who is, unfortunately, drunk. She's in the middle of a monthslong relapse, in fact, which has wrecked her previously thriving relationship and brought her back to her parents' basement. She tells me she really wants to stop drinking and get back on track, go back to work, and generally be independent. In psychotherapy jargon, she is speaking with a fair amount of what is called "change talk," which is a good sign. But when I ask her how confident she is that she could make those changes, she wistfully tells me she will probably drink again anyway. I ask her if she can think of anything she could do to help herself, but even though she was sober in AA for years, and she still has plenty of friends and resources to draw on, she can't come up with anything; she's hopeless. With slurred speech, she says, "It's genetic, right? Alcoholism, I mean. So that means I'll drink no matter what. Right?" It is certainly a rationalization, at least in part, but I also think there is a real fear there—a notion implanted by an overly reductionist narrative that says she is at the mercy of her biology.

In the past fifty years, researchers have made tremendous strides in understanding the biological factors that influence addiction, but as reductionist explanations have made their way into the broader public arena, they are too often exaggerated into the notion that people with addiction are doomed and broken by an underlying, intractable physical abnormality. These stories are just another iteration of stigmatized portrayals of addiction, but in recent decades they have become especially entrenched as more and more captivating technologies have taken hold of the public imagination.

In the early 1970s, the escalations in Nixon's war on drugs also pushed massive funding into drug research, and Jerome Jaffe awarded some of that funding to Solomon Snyder, a researcher at Johns Hopkins, with a mandate to find the opioid receptor in the brain. Former researchers at Narco had hypothesized the existence of such receptors years earlier, but it was far from a foregone conclusion that the task would be successful. It was only in 1970 that the first receptor of any kind was isolated, but only by studying the neurotransmitter acetylcholine in the electric organ of an electric eel, which has one of the densest concentrations of acetylcholine receptors in any animal.

Snyder, along with his colleague and graduate student Candace Pert, were experts in "radio-labeling," a new method of attaching radioactive molecules to other molecules to trace biological processes in the body. After experimenting with various compounds, eventually landing on radio-labeled naloxone, they were able to demonstrate binding to the opioid receptor in rodent brains, and they traced where the receptors were located in different parts of the brain. The publication of their results in 1973 was a major scientific milestone—the first verified receptor in the brain. The excitement was only intensified when, in 1975, the researchers John Hughes and Hans Kosterlitz discovered enkephalins, small molecules produced by the brain itself to fit those receptors.

Further investigations revealed other brain-created opioids, which were coined "endorphins," meaning "the morphine within," and the discoveries kicked off an era of "receptor fever." Researchers spun theories about how receptor abnormalities caused addiction. One idea was that inborn receptor abnormalities determined addiction: that a lifelong defect in the opioid receptors or endorphins made certain people inherently vulnerable to opioid addiction. Another hypothesis was that the frequent use of opioids like heroin damaged the receptor system, causing a lasting and potentially permanent drive to use drugs. In the scientific press, these were ideas to be tested in future studies. In the popular media, they became all-encompassing explanations.

In 1977, *The New York Times* proclaimed from the front page that OPIATE-LIKE SUBSTANCES IN BRAIN MAY HOLD CLUE TO PAIN AND MOOD.

The article speculated that mental disorders as diverse as schizophrenia and addiction may be caused by "biochemical defects" in endorphins. The popular press issued other speculative stories about the role of endorphins, a prominent one being widespread interest in a natural "runner's high." William Burroughs enclosed the *Times* article in a letter to his son Billy's psychiatrist, suggesting that Billy's addiction might stem from a shortage of endorphins and that he should be hospitalized, against his will if necessary, so the psychiatrist could further tease apart the physiological factors at the root of his destabilized mental state.

As it turned out, though, the research failed to find consistent changes in receptors and neurotransmitters that could fully account for even the most basic elements of drug use, such as tolerance and dependence, let alone the more complicated symptoms of addiction, such as cravings. Solomon Snyder wrote that, while he had first assumed that the "conquest of the opiate receptor would resolve the riddles of addiction," he later admitted, "we must plead failure."

Receptor fever was quickly replaced by an overwhelming enthusiasm for genetics. Legitimate scientific advances inspired this shift: a wave of twin and adoption studies through the late 1970s and into the '80s showed that genetic factors increased the risk of developing addiction. But as the work progressed, with each new finding, excited articles in the popular press promised total explanations for alcoholism or addiction. In April 1990, multiple news outlets reported that the "gene for alcoholism" had been discovered by Kenneth Blum and former NIAAA director Ernest Noble. *Time* magazine, for one, proclaimed, "In five years, scientists should have perfected a blood test for the gene, to help spot children at risk. And within a decade, doctors may have in hand a drug that either blocks the gene's action or controls some form of alcoholism by altering the absorption of dopamine." This was an awfully big leap; the gene being described here was a variant of the dopamine D2 receptor, which only slightly increased the risk of alcoholism. Commentators flagged the coverage as a blatant overpromise, but still the news was widely accepted as fact—a 1987 Gallup poll had already found that more than 60 percent of Americans believed alcoholism was inherited.

The treatment industry and popular authors profited off the trend for genetic explanations, using it to explain addiction as an intractable and inescapable disease. Genetics proved to be an effective way to convince potential clients that their brains were fundamentally different from "normal" brains and that they therefore needed treatment. When I went to rehab, one lecturer claimed that genetics was the strongest determinant of developing the disease of addiction, and when I was on the phone with my patient Nicole years later, I wondered if she had picked up her deterministic take from her own stay in rehab a couple of years earlier. But the reality is that no one is foreordained to develop addiction.

This hunger for biological causes is understandable. Addiction is baffling. Many people develop awful problems, or relapse, despite tremendous support in their lives and apparently clear intentions to remain abstinent. It is this terrifying phenomenon that made the metaphor of an "allergy" to alcohol so captivating to Bill Wilson in the 1920s, and to many generations of AA members after him. But it is just a metaphor: there is no allergy, and to date, there is no evidence that addiction is genetically determined, at least not to the extent it's commonly portrayed. Biology does matter, but it is only one of many factors influencing addiction, along with environment and even choice. Genetic research is also not strong enough to explain who gets addiction, or why. The heritability of addiction (meaning the degree of the variation that can be attributed to genetics) ranges from about 25 percent to 70 percent—a significant figure, to be sure, but this finding means that genetic influences are on more or less equal footing with environmental ones: one's prenatal environment, family life, trauma history, social environment, and much more. As one geneticist puts it, "Research into heritability is the best demonstration I know of the importance of the environment."

This lesson applies to brain research as well. The psychologist Keith

Humphreys has argued that the neuroscience of addiction, unexpectedly, only underscores the crucial importance of everything beyond the brain. For example, neuroscience validates just how powerful cue-induced learning can be—advertising campaigns for beer and cigarettes can powerfully trigger cravings, and neuroscience shows us why—but the most effective way to intervene is by enacting thoughtful regulations on the advertising of addiction supply industries. Brain science may explain how certain brain functions work in addiction and substance use, but many of those very same brain findings demonstrate that the most effective and helpful responses will be found elsewhere. No single explanatory framework or set of risk factors influencing addiction will hold all the answers, and only when we search out the interconnections between them is there any hope of charting a path forward.

Was Augustine's addiction the same as Alexander of Macedon's? How about Samson Occom's charges as opposed to Bill Wilson's? Even a pair as similar as De Quincey and Coleridge have important distinctions, not just in their perspectives, but in the factors driving their use.

Since the first days of medical attention to addiction, physicians have suspected that there was not one addiction but many, and that we could divvy up the phenomenon into different subtypes. Carl von Brühl-Cramer, the German doctor practicing in Moscow in 1812, hypothesized five different types of *Trunksucht,* ranging from continuous drinking to paroxysmal attacks after long intervals of abstinence. Another writer, drawing on findings from the Glasgow Lunatic Asylum in the middle of the nineteenth century, reported various "oinomanias," or wine manias.

These types of divisions make sense to most people: a so-called functional alcoholic evokes an entirely different picture from that of an "angry drunk" or a "binge drinker." The idea of subtypes also suggests a way to make sense of research challenging the traditional view of addiction. We cannot pin down one unchanging and essential addiction, but perhaps by looking more closely at the heterogeneity of the phenomenon, we can identify separate categories according to their causes and long-term courses. Proving the hunch scientifically, though, has been challenging.

Later in his career, Jellinek himself was starting to let go of the traditional disease model for this idea of subtypes. In 1960, he wrote a significant book, *The Disease Concept of Alcoholism* (with funding arranged by Marty Mann), but despite the title, Jellinek was actually complicating the disease notion. Rather than a unitary disease, Jellinek hypothesized, alcoholism was made up of different "species" that vary in factors such as the presence of dependence, physical injuries, and certain psychological symptoms. Furthermore, he proposed, these species were strongly influenced by society and culture, emphasizing the multifactorial contributions to the phenomenon. In studies since then, researchers have probed for the presence of subtypes—for example, during the genetic enthusiasm of the 1980s, biological researchers proposed distinctions between different types of addiction based on inherited traits—but it has proved difficult to find clear dividing lines.

More recent studies have delineated a variety of different, powerful influences on addiction, internal and external, biological, psychological, and environmental. Some addictions are closely related to personality traits we'd call anxious-depressive, as Bill Wilson often described himself, while others are more headstrong and impulsive, as both William Burroughs and Alexander of Macedon seem to have been. Some addictions seem intertwined with the need to manage other psychological problems, like the people I met on the dual diagnosis unit at Bellevue. Some addictions are more powerfully driven by nothing more than how rewarding the substance or behavior is—such as the true victims of iatrogenic addiction, from the women receiving morphine injections in the 1870s for "female complaints" to the recipients of all-too-liberal opioid prescriptions in the 1990s and 2000s. Some addictions are almost entirely determined by trauma, whether it be personal, intergenerational, or societal. Still today, none of the research on these factors is strong enough to support clear, stable, and reliable divisions between subtypes of addiction, or otherwise allows for dissecting its fundamental causes. Not only is there no one biological cause; there is no one dominant cause of addiction, or even a set of causes that reliably explains why some people develop addiction.

The best we can say today is that all these variegated influences intersect in a complex and dynamic matrix, changing drastically from person to person, and even changing over the course of an individual's lifetime. It is not that addiction is or is not a brain disease, or a social malady, or a universal response to suffering—it's all of these things and none of them at the same time, because each level has something to add but cannot possibly tell the whole story.

In this way, addiction illustrates a pragmatic and flexible way to make sense of all mental disorders. Psychiatric disorders have commonly been described as categorical, fixed entities, but for all mental disorders, not only is there no natural cut point between disorder and the rest of humanity, but they are dizzyingly multifactorial in their causes. Disorders, in other words, are not ground truths about reality, like chemical elements on the periodic table. Jellinek's word was a good one: they are more like "species" with a general family resemblance—biological species in nature have fuzzy boundaries, and the members of those species are not all the same. We must still make psychiatric diagnoses in order to do research, advocate for insurance payments, or otherwise translate our diagnostic thinking into the real world, but these labels should not be confused with an enduring, unitary, and discrete essence. They need to be tempered with humility.

But for someone in early recovery—someone like me in those months after rehab—wondering whether he truly qualifies as addicted and what that means for his life, all this research and theory can feel hopelessly complicated. What to do, how to think of oneself: addicted or not? There often comes a moment when one has to decide.

I imagined how I could get away with it. Each urine test was able to detect alcohol use only from the prior three days or so. My first vacation, I could kick back, have a few beers, then sober up. It was more about proving a point (to who? To myself, I suppose) that I could keep it under control. That was what I wanted: to be okay, to be in control.

When the time came, though, and I made my way to Boston for a good friend's engagement party, and the groom passed his home-brewed beers around the table, and I looked around and saw that no one who knew my past seemed to be paying attention, I still said no, and went back to my damned seltzer. I wished I could have it. I hated group hangouts in those days—without the heady buzz of alcohol, I felt impossibly awkward. It also felt weird, intensely weird, to say no amid all that quiet social momentum that pushes toward constant low-level intoxication. I urgently did not want to be the weird guy who wasn't drinking.

I had read a fair number of studies about addiction by this point. I understood the scientific arguments against the notion of addiction as a discrete and permanent identity. Addiction seemed contingent, nebulous, probabilistic—more a tendency than a condition. Calling it a disease didn't seem meaningful, and I wasn't even convinced that I was doomed to have serious problems if I drank again. And yet I did not drink, and I have not since.

Of course, a part of my decision was purely practical. Now that I was in the physician health program, I wanted to be honest and to live life without the looming fear of having to hide something. Also, as I had noticed in rehab, there was something that felt unhealthy about the desire to drink in the first place. I wanted to drink, but I also wanted to be free of the urge to drink—someday, if not that day. But even further, I was taking my first tentative steps toward choosing the identity of the recovering alcoholic, despite all the historical baggage attached to that notion. In time, I decided I was the kind of person who should not drink, at least for today.

While there may be no natural cut point between people with addiction and the rest of humanity, the fact of a continuum does not mean we cannot discern one state from another. There is a philosophical problem called the paradox of the heap: If a heap of sand is taken apart one grain at a time, at what point does it stop becoming a heap? There is no natural dividing line in that case, either, and yet we all agree that thousands of grains make a heap and one grain does not. Likewise, I believe we can see addiction as a meaningful description of a real phenomenon, even if it cannot be reduced to a clear and discrete essence. There may be no essential boundary between normal and addicted, yet addiction can still be an awful and life-threatening phenomenon.

I'm still not convinced that I have a specific disease, and I'm not even convinced that I am fundamentally different from the rest of the population—if anything, it seems a matter of degree rather than kind, and addiction is just the place where our universal human vulnerabilities are most clearly on display. Everyone, at some time, will experience a loss of control, a loss of power. Neuroscience research, too, has increasingly found that addiction is not the result of a substance acting on the brain but rather just one facet of ordinary human problems in motivation, reward, and self-regulation. The patterns of brain activations traditionally attributed to the effects of powerful substances have now been shown to be active in a wide swath of reward prediction functions and found in a much broader range of behaviors. For example, brain reward systems show characteristic changes not only in cases of substance addictions but also in obesity and gambling. The elegance of this particular cycle of understanding is that it returns to the original meaning of the word "addiction": not as a thing that happens to you, but a deeply personal phenomenon involving a strong, compelling desire.

In my psychiatry practice, I see "non-addicted" people struggling with food, work, cheating, power, money, or anger all the time. One psychotherapy patient of mine uses compulsive bingeing and purging as a way of managing negative emotions like fear and shame. Another cannot put down his phone or stop checking his email—despite his clear intentions and plans to do so, and despite the fact that it causes real problems in his marriage—because of a crushing need for external validation from his work. I don't insist that they call themselves addicted, and in general I don't assume that the roots of my own addiction are similar to others', or that others need what I have needed to recover. But I also don't see a tremendous division between me and them. We all suffer from a divided self, and we all have too much confidence in our judgment and our ability to exert power over our environments and ourselves. And in that, I think we share a fellowship, too, in that addiction is simultaneously a tremendous problem that causes unthinkable suffering, and something contiguous with all of human suffering.

Likewise, the people I met in rehab were drastically different from me and from one another. Several thought their addictions were just the outward manifestation of a lifelong anxiety. Others felt like they were almost mechanically conditioned to use opioids after receiving legitimate prescriptions for pain. But no matter how varied our circumstances were, even if the causes and conditions pushing us toward that end of the spectrum were impossibly varied, we shared something significant, a common experience that provided a basis for mutual identification: that bewildering state that others have described throughout history. We identified with one another's struggles with self-control, and the remarkably similar existential and social consequences, such as reorganizing our lives around our use and losing what mattered to us, up to and including the loss of our values and purpose. In that way, I think we share a fellowship that runs all the way back to the gambler of the *Rig Veda*, who lost all he held dear—an experience of suffering and a desire to break free.

Conclusion

RECOVERY

Early one morning, I walked down the long, gently sloping sky bridge, high above a twisted five-lane highway interchange, to the New York State Psychiatric Institute. The "PI" building, squatting on its own plot of land next to the Hudson River, is its own self-contained community: a sprawling network of offices, research labs, its own pharmacy, and—tucked away on the very bottom floor—my office in the residents' clinic.

I was roughly one year into recovery, and my days as a patient felt like they were receding behind me. True, I still had plenty to do in the physician health program. I had weekly group therapy for health professionals at a treatment center downtown, I checked in regularly with my own psychiatrist, and I got random urine tests several times a week. Weekdays, I'd get those tests at Columbia, and on weekends I'd go to the apartment of my urine monitor, a gentle older woman way down in the East Village. I'd buzz up, say hello, walk down a narrow hallway into her impeccably clean bathroom, and pee in a cup while she politely but vigilantly watched me to make sure I wasn't smuggling in a bottle of illicit urine. Afterward, I'd pay her $40 cash, we'd exchange some pleasantries about the weather, and I'd go about my day. It was surreal, and sometimes galling, but as time went on, it felt like just another chore, and I focused less on the treatment apparatus around me and more on learning how to become a psychiatrist.

That day, I was headed to my tiny office in PI, which I had received as part of the third year of psychiatric residency. We met with outpatients for therapy and medication management, set our own schedules, and generally worked as if we had our own practices. A supervisor was always a phone call or short walk away, but still it felt like the safety net was gone. With few exceptions, we received real-time feedback only on mornings like this one, when we admitted new potential patients to the clinic, conducting an intake interview, then running the case past a senior clinician.

My new patient that day was a stressed-out graduate student, a sensitive and high-strung guy who felt like he was cracking under the pressure. He told me he had started drinking heavily to manage his stress, up to four or five drinks a night, and he knew it was getting to be a problem because he couldn't cut down. I liked him immediately. He seemed earnest, thoughtful, and sincere, and I imagined that he'd be motivated and ready to work on some concrete strategies for change.

When I presented his case to my supervisor that morning, though, she shook her head grimly and said no. He was drinking too much: cases with such a heavy "substance burden" were just not appropriate for this kind of clinic. I was shocked—in many ways, he seemed healthier than I had been, especially considering that he recognized the problem. I had the sense, even then, that he would have benefited from being connected to care with us, particularly in light of how difficult it is for people to find mental health treatment and reach out for help. We could have tried to work with him, at least, and then made a referral to more intensive treatment if necessary. In fact, strong evidence has since shown that integrating substance use disorder treatment into mainstream healthcare both helps patients and improves the system's overall functioning. Instead, my supervisor told me to send him elsewhere, and we just gave him a list of referrals to other treatment programs. As he left the clinic, clearly disappointed and demoralized, I wondered if we had missed a rare chance to help someone enter recovery on his own terms.

My supervisor that morning was a well-meaning, seasoned clinician. She was a multi-decade veteran of one of the most challenging inpatient units in the institute. For most of her professional life, she had cared for people with severe schizophrenia, suicidal depression, and other debilitating disorders. We regularly worked with people who had those severe mental disorders in our resident clinic, but to her, a substance use disorder was somehow uniquely dangerous or difficult to treat, or, more simply, just not in our job description. I do not believe that she thought substance use disorders made for bad people, but she was reflecting the idea that we were bad patients, or at least inappropriate patients, even at a top training program for treating mental disorders. She was simply following the long tradition of consigning people with substance problems to a completely separate treatment system, segregated not only from the rest of medicine but from psychiatry, too. Stigma is not just one person's negative beliefs and attitudes. It can also take the form of structural stigma at the system level, manifested through policies and practices that exclude people with addiction from opportunities to heal.

Today, the medical system is coming up woefully short in its treatment of addiction. Medicine does not hold all the answers, but we clinicians have a crucial role to play, and we have yet to fully meet the challenge. There are massive barriers to receiving mental health care in general, but the problem is even more pronounced for people with substance use disorders: only about one in ten receive treatment—as compared with roughly 40 percent of those with other mental health conditions—and treatment is often insufficient even for those few.

Medicine could save countless lives if we took simple steps that are known to work. In addition to mainstreaming care for substance use disorders, we could scale up harm reduction measures—like distributing naloxone—which can be delivered in a medical context but don't need to be confined there. We also need to provide more care in the first place: there is an urgent need to expand the workforce of practitioners who can treat addiction and to improve the quality of that care through evidence-based treatments. In particular, we have much further to go in lowering barriers to medications for opioid use disorder. The uptake of lifesaving medications like buprenorphine and methadone is stymied by unnecessary legal obstacles, especially the arcane system of federal regulations severely restricting their use. It is not a rational system: medical residents can prescribe opioids that are more dangerous, like morphine, weeks out of medical school, but physicians cannot prescribe buprenorphine unless they go through an extra licensing step and get a special waiver from the DEA. Today, fewer than 10 percent of eligible medical providers have taken the time to get that waiver. These changes— expanding harm reduction, expanding the workforce and improving the quality of care, and removing unnecessary barriers to medical practice—would be simple, and would save lives.

If any structural changes in addiction treatment are to work, however, the medical profession must also embrace the care of this population, as stigmatized attitudes about addiction themselves will remain a tremendous barrier to care. At the time of this writing, the Biden administration has committed to "lifting burdensome restrictions" on medications for opioid use disorder, but if and when they do, it will only be the first step. Of the physicians who do have the waiver to prescribe buprenorphine, most see only a small handful of patients, and many see none at all—in some samples, up to 25 percent of waivered physicians don't prescribe the medication. In surveys about the barriers preventing them from doing so, doctors report structural concerns, such as lack of reimbursement and institutional support, but they also demonstrate stigma at a more basic and personal level, saying they don't want to be overwhelmed by needy or uncooperative patients. Bear in mind, these are the findings among providers who have actually taken the time and effort to get the waiver to provide addiction treatment, and this is to say nothing of the racialized and separate system of methadone treatment.

The first steps we medical providers need to take as a community are to decide that it is our job to work with addiction and work harder to dismantle stigma from the bottom up.

And yet, there often needs to be some element beyond the boundaries of traditional medical care, too—one that goes beyond saving lives to promoting well-being and flourishing. To truly meet the challenge of addiction, a therapeutic response alone is not enough. For centuries, people have sought out a further step, something more recently called recovery.

In those early years of my own recovery, I felt okay, but not much more than that—I was restless and lonely, liable to binge on snacks or finish a pint of ice cream in one sitting (which, for the record, I still sometimes do). I was still filling up my days with too much academic striving, reaching after status and acclaim by overworking myself on extra research projects. When I rode myself too hard, I'd blow off steam by bingeing preposterous amounts of TV, which was much better than drinking but still left me feeling gross and unfulfilled. Something about it all felt dangerously familiar—I was still going against my own best instincts.

There was a surreal discrepancy between my low-grade discontent and the awful consequences of addiction I saw around me. Friends from rehab had already relapsed. In our group therapy for medical professionals, I saw people struggle with slips or relapses. People were losing their jobs and their livelihoods. In rehab, I had met doctors who were back there for the second or even the third time, who had relapsed, right on schedule, after their own five-year monitoring contracts finished. I had the sense that that could be me—that my own simmering unhappiness, left unchecked, could progress toward the downstream consequences of addiction. I didn't feel close to relapse myself, but how could I really know? Peace felt out of reach.

I was still in the process of figuring out what recovery meant to me. I was comfortable with the AA idea of a "higher power"—I understood that I could arrive at my own conception of what that meant, and it felt reasonable to make it the collective consciousness of the group. I readily accepted that I needed some guidance from outside myself, and I wanted the peace that "turning it over" to a higher power and letting go of my own preferences seemed to offer others. I knew that my previous ways of taking care of myself, and even my previous values—such as prioritizing my own self-fulfillment and achievement—were not serving me. In other words, I had no resistance to this idea of recovery, once I had passed that first hurdle of my resistance to addiction. But I found it challenging to integrate it into my life.

I went to AA meetings, but I felt like I was doing it wrong. In rehab, they had hammered home the need for everyone to complete a "90-in-90" (ninety AA meetings in ninety days), find a home group, and get a sponsor—right out of the gate, no matter what. But in those days, I had trouble finding a meeting that I really liked, and though I tried working with sponsors, one never stuck. In local meetings, I met bright-eyed enthusiasts who credited AA with saving their lives and giving them a newfound measure of peace and contentment, and I felt ashamed, almost as if I was hiding a dirty secret. On paper, I was doing fine: I was not drinking. I was doing well at work. If I were a subject in a clinical trial, I would have been in the successful "remission" category. But it didn't feel like success. The therapist in our health professionals' group said that I could ease up on the idealistic expectations and be more flexible—some weeks, after all, I was working twelve-hour overnight shifts and had no chance of making it to a meeting on those days. But a little voice in the back of my head told me that I was screwing it up.

I didn't really start to let go of that voice until I started working on this book and learned about the wide variety of recovery experiences. For many years, under the strong influence of the multi-billion-dollar treatment industrial complex, the dominant understanding of recovery has been synonymous with the traditional AA pathway: a definition of recovery as total abstinence and a certain type of participation in a twelve-step program. This understanding is so deeply ingrained in our culture that I myself didn't learn about other ways to think about recovery until I had not only started psychiatric training but also been admitted for substance use disorder treatment at a top hospital, participated in a specialized rehab, and done my own research. Indeed, it's only in recent years that clinicians and researchers have started to fully appreciate the diversity of personal approaches to recovery: how it is initiated (alone, through peers, or within the treatment system), the type of recovery (moderation- versus abstinence-based, and abstinence from all substances or just one's primary drug of choice), the role of treatment supports (such as medications and psychotherapy, or not), the framework that one chooses (traditional twelve-step, other mutual-help groups, or no mutual-help groups at all), and so forth. The important point is that amid this wide diversity, there are many paths to wellness, many ways that people change.

In recent years, a growing body of research on recovery outcomes has clearly shown that people overcome addiction in a variety of ways. Approximately 9 percent of people in the United States—more than 22 million adults—self-identify as having resolved a problem with alcohol or other drugs. A little less than half of them identify themselves as "in recovery," and even fewer regularly attend twelve-step groups. Instead, they have overcome their problems by drawing on different resources, such as jobs, families, or religious communities. People go to the increasingly robust mutual-help alternatives to twelve-step groups, such as explicitly atheist groups, groups based in other faith traditions, psychologically informed meetings like SMART Recovery, and programs that focus on moderation rather than abstinence. People frequently resolve their substance use problems without any formal medical treatment or mutual-help group involvement. In the case of alcohol use disorder, about 70 percent improve without interventions, and fewer than 25 percent use alcohol-focused treatment services. (It's important to note, however, that problems with different substances often require different approaches, such as opioid use disorder, which has a greater need for support with medication treatment and perhaps psychosocial support too.) Treatment providers are increasingly coming to appreciate these "multiple pathways of recovery," a fact now visible even in traditional treatment venues; when someone I know relapsed not too long ago, he chose to go to a rehab that was once a flagship for the twelve-step approach, but he was thrilled to find it offered meetings of both the secular alternative SMART Recovery and the Buddhist group Recovery Dharma.

Recovery research is not entirely new but rather a continuation of investigations begun years ago, by researchers like the Sobells and their cohort, who were interested in the full spectrum of ways that people with substance problems get better. This perspective is captured today in a broad definition of recovery: a process of ongoing positive change, rather than simply the absence of pathology. In 1984, in the aftermath of the attacks on their studies, the Sobells noted that the addiction studies field was undergoing a paradigm shift, and such shifts are often accompanied by revolutionary conflict. Now, nearly forty years later, the shift is still underway, but it is gathering momentum, especially as communities of recovery become more comfortable with an inclusive definition of recovery.

The findings from this field are hopeful. Taking this broad definition of recovery—stable improvements in functioning and purpose in life—most people with substance problems will recover, and most do not need medical help to do so. And, according to the largest survey studies we have, the longer people are in recovery, the better their quality of life, family engagement, and functioning. In the first months after entering recovery, happiness and self-esteem tend to drop after an initial period of stability, but after that, general measures of well-being increase exponentially for the first five years and continue to increase in subsequent years.

Intriguingly, these findings are in line with neuroscience research that demonstrates great capacity for change in addiction. For generations, people with addiction have struggled against the stereotype of a "broken brain" that supposedly meant we were fundamentally damaged and irredeemable. Today, any evidence of physical brain changes is commonly taken to mean that addiction is permanent, but this is inaccurate. The brain does change in response to addictive behaviors—sometimes powerfully and in a long-lasting way—but it can change back. It is true that the brain undergoes significant changes in people diagnosed with severe substance use problems; any repeated experience, especially a powerfully rewarding one, will change networks of connections between different brain areas. (After all, how could you ever remember or learn anything if something weren't happening in the brain?) Over time, those changes will be represented in function—the way brain areas work together—and structure; for example, a reduction in the volume of gray matter in certain brain areas. But in at least one study of people in recovery from cocaine addiction, after roughly three years of abstinence, those brain areas had returned to a normal baseline level, and even more compellingly, the gray matter volumes increased even further the more time the person had been abstinent, beyond the "normal" levels. Addiction has a powerful effect on our biology, but we must be careful not to interpret those findings in an overly reductionist way, because so does recovery.

Those findings resonate with me. Once I had stuck with my own recovery long enough, I eventually began to feel better—perhaps not steadily better, but better. Then, in time, I returned to my spiritual practice. Many years earlier, during my brief stay in South Korea after college, I had become devoted to Zen, but I lost my connection with that practice after starting medical school. It was part of the existential loss that addiction had brought about in my life—losing a sense of purpose and values—and only after I finished my psychiatric training did I start going to a nearby Buddhist center more regularly. I found, to my surprise, that the center also hosted addiction recovery meetings in a different mutual-help tradition, which convinced me all the more that it was the right place for me. I have great respect for AA, and I do not think that program is incompatible with the path I'm on now, but in the end, to fully feel grounded in my recovery, I needed to find a different framework than the one initially offered to me. Only then did I get a taste of the relief those AA members had described to me earlier: the feeling of being held by the earth and by something larger than myself, something that could help me make sense of suffering and be of purpose in the world. With a more confident footing in my recovery, I was actually able to re-engage with AA in a way that felt more comfortable to me, and today, though I do not consider it my primary home, I continue to get a lot out of it, and I am grateful for the interconnections and shared experiences in the broader fellowship of recovery.

Years pass, and I don't drink. The monitoring program is still a pain, but it chafes less, and there isn't a doubt in my mind that I will finish successfully in a couple of years. I have a loving partner and a toddler. But just when I think I'm doing well, a major test presents itself: my mother gets lung cancer. She has no one else in her life, so I decide to help her with everything—the insurance hassles, the home health aide, the bags of mail she stuffed behind the couch when she got overwhelmed. I am now an assistant professor in the Division of Law, Ethics, and Psychiatry, which I suppose means I should know something about how the healthcare system works, but for the life of me I cannot navigate the mounting piles of bills and the tangled webs of insurance, and we are stuck with thousands of dollars in medical debt.

Through it all, she drinks. She drinks even though she is old and frail and falls when she drinks, and even after we realize that her drinking suppresses her blood counts and causes her to miss the chemo sessions I have worked so hard to arrange. She says she does not want to die—she is terrified of dying, and she doesn't want to leave her grandson—but still she drinks. It is terrifying and enraging—like it always has been, but worse.

On the drive from Brooklyn to Jersey, I recite to myself that she is suffering and resolve to treat her with compassion, yet every time, I am screaming at her for something—the fact that she sent her aide out for wine, or sent her aide away entirely even though she cannot really care for herself. Then, I am ashamed to see the hurt in her eyes. Back at home, I feel like I am drowning—I am trying to learn how to be a doctor and write a book and enjoy life, and it is too much. One day, during an argument with my partner, I kick in our metal trash can until it is twisted and dented. She tells me that I am not being a very good Buddhist, after all those hours on Saturdays she spends watching our son so I can meditate with my group. It's a little funny, but painfully true. I am not living up to my values, and that means I have more work to do. Anger feels like my addiction now. I see myself venting it on the women in my life, like I have done so many times before, and I am worried.

I reach out to someone I know for recommendations for a psychotherapist. I am ashamed to be doing this—I have been sober for years, and I am supposed to be the one helping people, so I feel like a fraud. The therapist, even worse, practices a technique called Internal Family Systems, which I have barely heard of, and which seems to require a kind of inner-child work I've long dismissed as hokey and soft. She has me lie down on the couch and talk to different "parts" of myself, and I feel like an idiot. But in no time, I start to cry, really cry, and over the course of more sessions, I feel a real change.

I am not a saint from this point on, but therapy helps. I feel like most of my supervisors at Columbia would turn up their noses at it—IFS does not have much of an evidence base, and it has neither the cerebral cachet of psychoanalysis nor the prestige of the more explicitly scientific therapies. But something about it works for me. As I learn to be more compassionate with myself, I am more compassionate with the people around me, especially my mother. It helps me show up for her, while also helping me to set healthy boundaries and let go of what I can't change. This, in itself, feels like a triumph.

What I have seen over and over again—in patients, fellows in recovery, and myself—is that recovery has no endpoint; in fact, it is contingent on a process of ongoing change, of growth past the boundaries of the usual medical outcome of remission. How do people change? There are as many answers as there are people in recovery. The key is to try. I think of my patient Joey, a thickly muscled businessman who came to me for treatment for opioid addiction. A classic Brooklyn tough guy, he insisted from the start that he had just gotten "hooked" and there wasn't any sort of secret psychological pain lurking beneath. He had previously been involved in NA and received buprenorphine from an outpatient clinic, but only a few months later, the clinic thought he would be "cleaner" if he was weaned off the medication, and the rapid reduction led to a relapse. I restarted him on buprenorphine, and he responded well. The people in his NA group gave him some grief at first—asking how long until he got off the medication again, or even questioning whether he should be allowed to help put the chairs away after the meeting—but after people saw his sincerity and stability over the course of many more months, he became one of the pillars of the group.

At this point, Joey was a success story—he would have checked all the boxes in a traditional clinical trial, and his obsession with opioids had lifted—but he was starting to notice addictive behaviors emerging in other ways. Even though the IRS was breathing down his throat, he compulsively shopped for nice things to shore up his self-image. He started dabbling in day trading, a thrilling search for a big payout that would quell his financial fears. He noticed an unhealthy attachment to his weight-lifting regimen and his body image. Without the chaos of opioid addiction, though, we had more space in our sessions to talk about his life in a broad context, and as it turned out, there was more there after all: abuse he'd received at the hand of his alcoholic father and insidious shame from growing up poor. As we explored the history of that pain, he began to see the connections to his behaviors. Frustrated one day, he complained that he was sick in the head after all. I told him the point wasn't that he was sick, but that he was alive, and now he got to go further and work on what helped him to heal and flourish.

Biomedical science has a great deal to offer. I am deeply grateful that there are lifesaving medications for Joey and others like him. There are even newer options available for treating opioid use disorder—injectable and implantable forms of buprenorphine, and a long-acting naltrexone injection, which offer great promise for people who experience vacillating motivations and want to bind themselves, Odysseus-like, to medications that will dampen their ability to get high and lower their risk of overdose. Psychedelic psychotherapy is also immensely promising, and there are even early-stage trials for deep brain stimulation (DBS) surgery for addiction underway, which implants a small electrode in the brain to decrease cravings and urges. But even if our most futuristic therapies prove to be highly successful at saving lives (and even if we are able to implement them in a way that respects patient autonomy, as we must), I suspect that will only be the first step.

Helen Mayberg, the neurologist who pioneered DBS for depression, described to the writer Lone Frank the story of one DBS patient who also had a drinking problem. After the patient had electrodes implanted, she went home and waited for something like the sense of release that alcohol used to give her. The woman felt her depression diminish, but nothing more; disappointed, she returned to Mayberg to ask if there was some further adjustment that could be made. Mayberg replied that this was it—this was life. The procedure had only relieved the disabling depression enough for the person to work on the realities of her life. It was now her responsibility to find something to replace her depression and substance use.

These stories—mine, Joey's, the DBS patient's—all show that even after futuristic therapies save lives, we will still need recovery. Science will help develop new treatments and demonstrate what works and what doesn't, and this is tremendously important, but after that, more work will still be needed. We will still be human beings with intention and agency, and we will need to make decisions about what we choose to value in this one brief life. We will still need to grow and change— not after addiction or beyond addiction, but with it, because addiction is a part of us.

Millions before us have struggled so fiercely and desperately with addiction. When we accept that addiction is a part of life, and that there is no single solution, we give those who are suffering a better chance for relief. We need more quality treatment, but we also need to be wary of quick fixes and simplistic stories, and especially wary of the potential of medicine to be co-opted as a tool of control. We need to let go of the oppressive prohibitionist policies that cause harm and despair, but we still need some small dose of regulation, at least in the form of commonsense oversight of harmful products, especially when they are pushed on us by asymmetrical forces. We need science to help us better understand the phenomenon, but we also need the humility to see that the chief lesson of science is so often the crucial importance of everything beyond the brain. And no matter what technocratic aims we pursue, we will always need the grassroots wisdom of mutual help, in all the forms it takes, from a sponsor passing along what she has learned through the twelve steps of AA to harm reduction activists banding together to save lives in their own way.

Does history give us any hope for this kind of pragmatic and pluralistic perspective? There were brief opportunities for a holistic response to addiction at certain points throughout time, such as the inebriety movement of the late nineteenth century and the therapeutic movements of the 1960s, but those efforts were quickly divided into narrow and ideological factions and eventually overpowered by the crushing stigma attached to drugs and drug users. Today, amid our latest addiction epidemics, we are faced with another precious and rare opportunity for synthesis, and I have hope that we can unite around an inclusive definition of recovery as being any kind of positive change. But in order to do so, we will need to turn to the pain of our shared past, because, as in the case of individual addictions, pain and purpose are so often intertwined, and our despair comes from somewhere. The suffering of addiction is not an individual malady—it also comes from deep, ancestral wounds. We need to face that fact too, in order to fully recover, together.

We have a better sense today of the concrete factors that support recovery from addiction: physical resources like money and housing, personal resources like knowledge and skills, and social resources like family and other relationships. Some researchers have summarized these factors as "recovery capital," and the economic implications of that term suggest what is missing in a response to addiction that focuses only on medical treatment. Far too many people start their recovery process with substantial disadvantages in terms of that "capital," and the research shows that certain groups have more psychological struggles in recovery—in particular, women, mixed racial groups, and former opioid and stimulant users. Not only are the factors driving addiction distributed inequitably, but access to recovery is also inequitable. Poverty, class, racism, sex-based discrimination, and other drivers of inequality powerfully affect people's ability to enter and sustain recovery. In the face of these factors, how far can individually focused treatment alone take us? Instead, what would it mean if we saw the opportunity to recover as a right, and we had the political and moral imagination to confront all the ways that right is routinely denied to so many? To attempt to do so will pay great dividends, because especially in the case of addiction, what happens to one of us affects all of us, and recovery is less an individual journey than a communal experience. We are united by our efforts to meet the profound yet universal challenges of addiction.

This is what the history has been trying to say all along. Addiction is profoundly ordinary: a way of being with the pleasures and pains of life, and just one manifestation of the central human task of working with suffering. If addiction is part of humanity, then, it is not a problem to solve. We will not end addiction, but we must find ways of working with it: ways that are sometimes gentle, and sometimes vigorous, but never warlike, because it is futile to wage a war on our own nature.

Acknowledgments

First and foremost, I am indebted to my patients and their families, as well as all my colleagues, friends, and fellows in addiction recovery. Out of respect for their privacy, I have not written extensively about many of their stories, but make no mistake, every word of this book has benefited from their shining examples of humanity, strength, and hope. Thank you, all.

I must also thank all the professionals who helped me in my own recovery from addiction. Our treatment system—however imperfect it may be—is full of wholehearted workers doing their best to help everyone who crosses their path. I am grateful for the kind efforts of every therapist, clinician, case worker, counselor, and healer along the way.

I was truly blessed when Libby McGuire first encouraged me to write the proposal for this book. Then, I was doubly blessed when the inimitable Alia Hanna Habib took me under her wing—thank you for your friendship, wisdom, and steady and unwavering support. Many thanks, too, to Sophie Pugh-Sellers, Rebecca Gardner, Will Roberts, Ellen Coughtrey, and the rest of the team at The Gernert Company.

Profound gratitude to my extraordinary editor, Emily Cunningham, who devoted countless hours to countless drafts over the course of years, including the tragedy and misery of 2020, without ever flagging in her efforts or wavering in her dedication to this project. I am deeply grateful for your brilliant guidance and your sincere, tangible commitment to this work. Thanks also to Ann Godoff, Scott Moyers, and everyone else at Penguin Press for believing in this book and making it possible. I was lucky to be helped by my wonderful research assistants Henry MacConnel and Stephanie Wykstra. Gratitude, too, to Ethan Corey for his meticulous, excellent fact-checking, and to Will Palmer, who copyedited this book with tremendous skill and insight. I would like to thank Beowulf Sheehan for taking my author photo.

The scholarship in these pages owes incalculable debts to the work of experts across many fields, and I am personally indebted to the many thinkers who generously shared their time and insights and who, in many cases, reviewed my writing prior to publication. I am particularly indebted to Ben Breen, who provided crucial guidance as I began this effort, as well as Robin Room and William White. Srinivas Reddy shared pivotal insights regarding the *Rig Veda*, not to mention his warmhearted love and appreciation for the truths therein. Jon Soske's nuanced and compassionate inquisitiveness about the nature of addiction and recovery was truly refreshing. George Koob was thoughtful and generous with his time (it bears noting that most neuroscientists are often far more humane and sensitive about reductionist narratives than they are given credit for, so I openly acknowledge that credit here). Many others graciously gave of their time and assistance: Rebecca Lemon, Chris Budnick, Kerwin Kaye, David Courtwright, Henry Cowles, Keith Wailoo, Jose Cree, Jessica Warner, Peter Mancall, Caroline Acker, Nancy Campbell, Richard Bonnie, David Herzberg, Scott Taylor, Jonathan Jones, Ron Roizen, Nick Heather, David Armor, John Helzer, William Miller, Maia Szalavitz, Mark and Linda Sobell, Keith Humphreys, Gary Mendell, and David Sheff. Any errors are my own.

I gratefully acknowledge the generous support of the Alfred P. Sloan Foundation's program in the Public Understanding of Science and Technology. During my own early forays into writing for the general public, I benefited greatly from the Kavli Foundation's Scientist-Writer Workshop at NYU, NeuWrite at Columbia University, and the able editorial guidance of Michael Segal. The Jentel Artist Residency Program provided refuge, space, and above all a warm and supportive community, all of which were essential for making sense of the structure of the book—and for strengthening my conviction that it was a story worth telling and that I could do it justice. For archival support, thanks to Olga Nilova at The Rockefeller University and Sally Corbett-Turco at Stepping Stones.

For many years now, Columbia University's Department of Psychiatry has provided an exemplary home for research and scholarship rooted in patient care. More importantly, the good people there personally supported me with great compassion and professionalism during the most trying moments of my life, and for that I will be forever grateful. Thanks especially to the dedicated folks in my residency class who covered my work responsibilities while I was sent to treatment, and the leaders and administrators who welcomed me back afterward—you did not have to do that, as countless other sad examples demonstrate, and for that I thank you from the bottom of my heart. Thanks to all my teachers, supervisors, and mentors along the way, especially Mike Devlin, Jim Spears, Maria Oquendo, Melissa Arbuckle, Lisa Mellman, Holly Lisanby, Ken Hoge, and Paul Appelbaum.

Undying gratitude to all the friends and colleagues who read early drafts and otherwise provided crucial support for both my writing and recovery: Ben Ehrlich, Taylor Beck, Tim Requarth, Marin Sardy, Alex Tilney, Steve Hall, Ferris Jabr, Jaime Green, Olivia Koski, Kevin Griffin, Susannah Cahalan, Brian Patchett, Bevin Campbell, Kristin Polman, Ram Murali, Qusai Hammouri, Pedro Pascal, Ravi Kavasery, Luke White, Marc Manseau, Lauren Osborne, Ben Everett, Richard Brockman, Ellen Vora, Aerin Hyun, Barron Lerner, and the indefatigable Arthur Williams. Kim Jaime, Halley Feiffer, and Lauren O'Conner generously helped me to understand and navigate the publishing industry. Dear friends, thank you: Jeremy, Ron, Bryan, and Wes. Dear sangha, thank you: Ella, Kaishin, Maya, Hank, Kosen Gregory Synder,

Laura O'Loughlin, Teah Strozer, Hyon Gak Su Nim, the Buddhist Recovery Network, and the mahasangha. Thank you to my parents, who gave me life and many moments of joy and love, and who opened up to me and shared their struggles as I wrote this book. My father is now a devoted grandparent, as was my mother before her death from cancer, and I am grateful for our closer relationships in recent years thanks in no small part to their own growth and sincere effort. Immense thanks to the rest of my family—the many years and endless rewrites shifted enormous obligations onto their shoulders, even and especially during the COVID-19 pandemic, and I am forever grateful. Infinite thanks to Beth, Kuza, David, Annie, Liz, Preston, and especially John and Marie, grandparental models of heroic devotion and commitment. Thanks, Gus, my love, for waiting for so much of your life for your dada to finish this book, and for your curiosity, imagination, and tender spirit that inspire me every day. I will never forget you climbing onto my lap to do your "invisible work" as I wrote. Last and biggest thanks to Cat, my love, for your fierce support, joyful humor, invaluable writing and storytelling insights, and inconceivable generosity through it all.

Thank you to the community of people around the world practicing recovery from addiction in your lives, and for your efforts to pass on what you have learned. And thank you, reader, for coming this far with me and engaging with this challenging and often mystifying material. In the words of Mark Kleiman, no doubt, you have disagreed with at least one of my opinions so far, and that is how it should be—this book is a starting point, one small offering in a centuries-old quest to make sense of addiction. If I have prompted you to think just a little more deeply about the phenomenon, or provided a quantum of encouragement or peace, this book will have served its purpose. I believe we are united in our common desire for recovery and flourishing for all beings as we walk this path together.

Notes

Introduction

xii **"theories of addiction":** Robert West and Jamie Brown, *Theory of Addiction*, 2nd ed. (Hoboken, NJ: Wiley-Blackwell, 2013), chaps. 3–6.

xiii **not just the opioid manufacturers:** Ben Goldacre, *Bad Pharma: How Drug Companies Mislead Doctors and Harm Patients* (London: Fourth Estate, 2012); Allen Frances, *Saving Normal: An Insider's Revolt against Out-of-Control Psychiatric Diagnosis, DSM-5, Big Pharma, and the Medicalization of Ordinary Life* (New York: William Morrow, 2013); Allan V. Horwitz and Jerome C. Wakefield, *The Loss of Sadness: How Psychiatry Transformed Normal Sorrow into Depressive Disorder* (New York: Oxford University Press, 2007).

xvi **stigmatized and "odious disease":** Benjamin Rush, *An Inquiry into the Effects of Ardent Spirits* [. . .], 8th ed. (Boston, 1823), 5, https://books.google.com/books?id=-6UoAAAAYAAJ.

Author's Note

xix **real effect on stigma:** Robert D. Ashford, Austin M. Brown, and Brenda Curtis, "'Abusing Addiction': Our Language Still Isn't Good Enough," *Alcohol Treatment Quarterly* 37, no. 2 (2019): 257–72, https://doi.org/10.1080/07347324.2018.1513777.

xix **shifts from era to era:** Michelle L. McClellan, *Lady Lushes: Gender, Alcoholism, and Medicine in Modern America* (New Brunswick, NJ: Rutgers University Press, 2017), 23.

Chapter One

4 **fewer than 5 percent:** Substance Abuse and Mental Health Services Administration, Key Substance Use and Mental Health Indicators in the United States: Results from the 2019 National Survey on Drug Use and Health, HHS Publication PEP20-07-01-001, NSDUH Series H-55 (Rockville, MD: Center for Behavioral Health Statistics and Quality, 2020), 54, https://www.samhsa.gov/data/report /2019-nsduh-annual-national-report. This oft-quoted statistic comes from the NSDUH, and it classifies people as having a "need for treatment" if they had an SUD in the past year or received substance use treatment at a specialty facility in the past year. This classification can be contested.

5 **the word *philopotēs*:** Iain Gately, *Drink: A Cultural History of Alcohol* (New York: Gotham, 2008), chap. 2. Notably, the Greeks had other words with more negative connotations, such as *philoinous* (wine lover, from Plato's *Republic*, 475a), or *akratokothones* (literally "unmixed tankards," referring to people who drank unmixed wine) from Athanaeus, *The Deipnosophists*, 245f–46a.

5 **works describing *shi jiu*:** Edwin Van Bibber-Orr, "Alcoholism and Song Literati," in *Behaving Badly in Early and Medieval China*, ed. N. Harry Rothschild and Leslie V. Wallace (Honolulu: University of Hawai'i Press, 2017), 135.

5 **as old as human civilization:** Peter Ferentzy and Nigel E. Turner, *The History of Problem Gambling: Temperance, Substance Abuse, Medicine, and Metaphors* (New York: Springer, 2013), 1–4.

5 **dates to before 1000 BC:** Stephanie W. Jamison and Joel P. Brereton, trans., *The Rigveda: The Earliest Religious Poetry of India* (New York: Oxford University Press, 2014), 3:1429.

6 **"power over the gambler":** Jamison and Brereton, *The Rigveda*, 10.34.5, 10.34.7.

6 **"Downward they roll":** Ralph T. H. Griffith, trans., *The Rig Veda* (n.p., 1897), 10.34.9, https://en.wikisource.org/wiki/The_Rig_Veda/Mandala_10/Hymn_34. Ancient Indian dicing was a different kind of play than what we think of today, involving pulling small brown (*vibhīdaka*) nuts out of a hollow in the ground.

6 **drastically different translations:** Jamison and Brereton, *The Rigveda*, 1429–30; Jan Gonda, *Vedic Literature (Saṃhitās and Brāhmaṇas)*, vol. 1, *Veda and Upanishads* (Wiesbaden, Germany: Otto Harrassowitz, 1975), 147; Srinivas Reddy, email message to author, May 20, 2020.

7 **"another foe to conquer":** Reddy, email message to author, May 20, 2020.

7 **outside of the historical process:** Joseph Michael Gabriel, "Gods and Monsters: Drugs, Addiction, and the Origin of Narcotic Control in the Nineteenth-Century Urban North" (PhD diss., Rutgers University, 2006), 5; Robin Room, Matilda Hellman, and Kerstin Stenius, "Addiction: The Dance between Concept and Terms," *International Journal of Alcohol and Drug Research* 4, no. 1 (June 2014): 27–29, https://doi.org/10.7895/ijadr.v4i1.199; Robin Room, "The Cultural Framing of Addiction," *Janus Head* 6, no. 2 (2003): 221–34.

7 **free choice versus total compulsion:** Nick Heather and Gabriel Segal, eds., *Addiction and Choice: Rethinking the Relationship* (New York: Oxford University Press, 2017), introduction, chaps. 9, 25.

8 **"weakness of the will":** *Akrasia* has long been a controversial topic in philosophy. I have benefited greatly from many commentaries, including Kent Dunnington, *Addiction and Virtue: Beyond the Models of Disease and Choice* (Downers Grove, IL: InterVarsity Press, 2011), 27–56, 102–5; Nick Heather, "Addiction as a Form of *Akrasia*," in Heather and Segal, *Addiction and Choice*, 133–52; Robert C. Solomon, "Aristotle, the Socratic Principle, and the Problem of Akrasia," *Modern Schoolman* 49, no. 1 (1974): 13–21; Donald Davidson, "How Is Weakness of the Will Possible?," in *Essays on Actions and Events* (New York: Oxford University Press, 2001), 21–42; Richard Kraut, "Alternate Readings of Aristotle on *Akrasia*," in *The Stanford Encyclopedia of Philosophy*, ed. Edward N. Zalta (Palo Alto, CA: Metaphysics Research Lab, 2018), https://plato.stanford.edu/entries/aristotle-ethics/supplement1.html.

8 **often "quarrel inside us":** Plato, *Phaedrus*, trans. Alexander Nehamas and Paul Woodruff (Indianapolis: Hackett, 1995), 237d–38a.

8 **declared in the *Protagoras*:** Plato, *Protagoras*, in *The Collected Dialogues of Plato*, ed. E. Hamilton and H. Cairns (Princeton, NJ: Princeton University Press, 1961), 358b–c.

8 **deeply invested in the idea of akrasia:** Christopher Shields, *The Oxford Handbook of Aristotle* (New York: Oxford University Press, 2012), 593–94, 601–2; Heather, "Addiction as a Form of *Akrasia*," 12–13, 120; Davidson, "How Is Weakness of the Will Possible?," 32.

9 **slice of pie in the fridge:** Alfred R. Mele, *Irrationality: An Essay on Akrasia, Self-Deception, and Self-Control* (New York: Oxford University Press, 1987), 22.

9 **Socrates attributed poor choices:** For more on Socrates regarding addiction, see Brendan de Kenessey, "People Are Dying Because We Misunderstand How Those with Addiction Think," *Vox*, March 16, 2018, https://www.vox.com/the-big-idea/2018/3/5/17080470/addiction-opioids-moral-blame-choices-medication-crutches-philosophy.

9 **the two horses:** Christopher Bobonich, "Plato on Akrasia and Knowing Your Own Mind," in *Akrasia in Greek Philosophy: From Socrates to Plotinus*, ed. Christopher Bobonich and Pierre Destrée (Leiden, Netherlands: Koninklijke Brill, 2007), 41–60; Thomas Gardner, "Socrates and Plato on the Possibility of *Akrasia*," *Southern Journal of Philosophy* 40, no. 2 (Summer 2002): 191–210, https://doi.org/10.1111/j.2041-6962.2002.tb01896.x. Though it is debated whether Plato intended for the divided self to answer specifically to the issue of *akrasia*: Joshua Wilburn, "*Akrasia* and the Rule of Appetite in Plato's *Protagoras* and *Republic*," *Journal of Ancient Philosophy* 8, no. 2 (November 2014): 57–91, http://doi.org/10.11606/issn.1981-9471.v8i2p57-91.

9 **torn between love and duty:** Dan Curley, *Tragedy in Ovid: Theater, Metatheater, and the Transformation of a Genre* (New York: Cambridge University Press, 2013), 182.

9 **psychological feature of "delay discounting":** Warren K. Bickel and Lisa A. Marsch, "Toward a Behavioral Economic Understanding of Drug Dependence: Delay Discounting Processes," *Addiction* 96, no. 1 (January 2001): 73–86, https://doi.org/10.1046/j.1360-0443.2001.961736.x.

9 **a process called "intertemporal bargaining":** Robert West and Jamie Brown, *Theory of Addiction*, 2nd ed. (Hoboken, NJ: Wiley-Blackwell, 2013), 59–63; George Ainslie, "Palpating the Elephant: Current Theories of Addiction in Light of Hyperbolic Delay Discounting," in Heather and Segal, *Addiction and Choice*, 227–44. The precise nature of this breakdown is debated. Choice models might put more or less emphasis on abnormal desires versus mistaken beliefs about the effects of drugs. See Richard Holton and Kent Berridge, "Compulsion and Choice in Addiction" in Heather and Segal, *Addiction and Choice*, 153–70.

9   **a voucher system:** Stephen T. Higgins et al., "Incentives Improve Outcome in Outpatient Behavioral Treatment of Cocaine Dependence," *Archives of General Psychiatry* 51, no. 7 (July 1994), 568–76, https://doi.org/10.1001/archpsyc.1994.03950070060011.

10 **strong evidence in its favor:** Michael Prendergast et al., "Contingency Management for Treatment of Substance Use Disorders: A Meta-Analysis," *Addiction* 101, no. 11 (November 2006): 1546–60, https://doi.org/10.1111/j.1360-0443.2006.01581.x; Jennifer Plebani Lussier et al., "A Meta-Analysis of Voucher-Based Reinforcement Therapy for Substance Use Disorders," *Addiction* 101, no. 2 (February 2006): 192–203, https://doi.org/10.1111/j.1360-0443.2006.01311.x.

10 **extraordinary five-year success rates:** A. Thomas McLellan et al., "Five Year Outcomes in a Cohort Study of Physicians Treated for Substance Use Disorders in the United States," *British Medical Journal* 337, no. 7679 (November 2008): 2038–44, https://doi.org/10.1136/bmj.a2038. It is important to note that the definition of "success rate" is open to debate, and could mean people completing the program, people testing negative for substance use, people licensed and working, or some other measure. The findings are further complicated by a fairly large proportion of initial enrollees who were lost to follow-up. Nevertheless, across several studies of physician health programs, it is clear they achieve very good results compared with treatment as usual.

12 **"a hissing cauldron of lust":** Augustine, *Confessions*, trans. R. S. Pine-Coffin (London: Penguin, 1961), 3.1.1.

12 **"surrendered myself entirely to lust":** Augustine, *Confessions*, 2.2.3.

12 **early example of addiction:** See, for example, Cynthia M. A. Geppert, "Aristotle, Augustine, and Addiction," *Psychiatric Times* 25, no. 7 (June 2008): 40, https://www.psychiatrictimes.com/view/aristotle-augustine-and-addiction; John M. Bowers, "Augustine as Addict: Sex and Texts in the *Confessions*," *Exemplaria* 2, no. 2 (1990): 403–48, https://doi.org/10.1179/exm.1990.2.2.403.

12 **"obviously one of us":** Janice M. Irvine, *Disorders of Desire: Sexuality and Gender in Modern American Sexology* (Philadelphia: Temple University Press, 2005), 166; Janice M. Irvine, "Regulated Passions: The Invention of Inhibited Sexual Desire and Sex Addiction," *Social Text*, no. 37 (Winter 1993): 203–26, https://doi.org/10.2307/466269.

12 **he was still tortured:** Augustine, *Confessions*, 10.30.41.

13 **"the spirit of Perverseness":** Edgar Allan Poe, "The Black Cat," in *Tales* (London: Wiley and Putnam, 1845), 37–46, https://books.google.com/books?id=nQ0EAAAAQAAJ.

13 **transformed all of human nature:** Christian Tornau, "Saint Augustine," in *The Stanford Encyclopedia of Philosophy*, ed. Edward N. Zalta (Palo Alto, CA: Metaphysics Research Lab, 2020), https://plato.stanford.edu/archives/sum2020/entries/augustine/.

13 **"I have no time for reading":** Augustine, *Confessions*, 6.11.18.

13 **sinful misdirection of the will:** See Bruce K. Alexander's excellent framing of this issue at more length: *The Globalization of Addiction* (New York: Oxford University Press, 2010), loc. 4242 of 15778, Kindle.

14 **retreat to quiet their thinking:** Karen Armstrong, *The Case for God* (New York: Knopf, 2009), 111.

14 **sought to practice *Gelassenheit*:** Joel F. Harrington, *Dangerous Mystic: Meister Eckhart's Path to the God Within* (New York: Penguin Press, 2018), 9.

14 **human suffering, *dukkha*:** Piyadassi Thera, trans., *Dhammacakkappavattana Sutta: Setting in Motion the Wheel of Truth*, SN 56.11, Access to Insight, http://www.accesstoinsight.org/tipitaka/sn/sn56/sn56.011.piya.html. "The five aggregates subject to grasping are suffering. The Noble Truth of the Origin (cause) of Suffering is this: It is this craving (thirst) which produces re-becoming (rebirth) accompanied by passionate greed, and finding fresh delight now here, and now there, namely craving for sense pleasure, craving for existence and craving for non-existence (self-annihilation)." See also Chonyi Taylor, *Enough! A Buddhist Approach to Finding Release from Addictive Patterns* (Ithaca, NY: Snow Lion, 2010); Darren Littlejohn, *The 12-Step Buddhist: Enhance Recovery from Any Addiction* (New York: Atria, 2009).

14 **"the intoxicating inclinations":** Vince Cullen, trans., *Roga Sutta*, AN 4.157 (unpublished translation, 2019), prepared for the International Buddhist Recovery Summit. A variant translation is available here: Bhikkhu Sujato, trans., *Roga Sutta*, AN 4.157, https://suttacentral.net/an4.157/en/sujato. Cullen is using "intoxicating inclinations" as a translation for *Āsava*, which is also used by the scholar Peter Harvey. See Peter Harvey, "In Search of the Real Buddha," *Buddhist News*, November 28, 2019, https://thebuddhist.news/headline-news/in-search-of-the-real-buddha/; Peter Harvey, *Introduction to Buddhism* (New York: Cambridge University Press, 2013).

14 **ordinary, though detrimental, psychological processes:** Brendan Dill and Richard Holton, "The Addict in Us All," *Frontiers in Psychiatry*, October 9, 2014, https://doi.org/10.3389/fpsyt.2014.00139.

14 **"psychological inflexibility":** Stephen C. Hayes, Kirk D. Strosahl, and Kelly G. Wilson, *Acceptance and Commitment Therapy: The Process and Practice of Mindful Change*, 2nd ed. (New York: Guilford Press, 2012), vii–x, 95–98. See also Caroline Davis and Gordon Claridge, "The Eating Disorders as Addiction: A Psychobiological Perspective," *Addictive Behaviors* 23, no. 4 (July 1, 1998): 463–75, https://doi.org/10.1016/S0306-4603(98)00009-4; Jason Luoma et al., "Substance Abuse and Psychological Flexibility: The Development of a New Measure," *Addiction Research & Theory* 19, no. 1 (February 1, 2011): 3–13, https://doi.org/10.3109/16066359.2010.524956; Manuel Alcaraz-Ibáñez, José M. Aguilar-Parra, and Joaquín F. Álvarez-Hernández, "Exercise Addiction: Preliminary Evidence on the Role of Psychological Inflexibility," *International Journal of Mental Health and Addiction* 16, no. 1 (February 1, 2018): 199–206, https://doi.org/10.1007/s11469-018-9875-y; Wei-Po Chou, Cheng-Fang Yen, and Tai-Ling Liu, "Predicting Effects of Psychological Inflexibility/Experiential Avoidance and Stress Coping Strategies for Internet Addiction, Significant Depression, and Suicidality in College Students: A Prospective Study," *International Journal of Environmental Research and Public Health* 15, no. 4 (April 2018): 788, https://doi.org/10.3390/ijerph15040788. This notion has resonances with findings from both contemplative and psychedelic research. See Judson Brewer, *The Craving Mind: From Cigarettes to Smartphones to Love—Why We Get Hooked and How We Can Break Bad Habits* (New Haven, CT: Yale University Press, 2017), 115; Michael Pollan, *How to Change Your Mind: What the New Science of Psychedelics Teaches Us about Consciousness, Dying, Addiction, Depression, and Transcendence* (New York: Penguin Press, 2018), 358–68.

15 **a kind of self-medication:** Against a superficial account of self-medication, see in particular West and Brown, *Theory of Addiction*, 49–51.

15 **mental disorders were categorical, fixed entities:** Peter Zachar and Kenneth S. Kendler, "Psychiatric Disorders: A Conceptual Taxonomy," *American Journal of Psychiatry* 164, no. 4 (April 2007): 57–65, https://doi.org/10.1176/ajp.2007.164.4.557; Nick Haslam, "Psychiatric Categories as Natural Kinds: Essentialist Thinking about Mental Disorder," *Social Research* 67, no. 4 (Winter 2000): 1031–58.

15 **a neatly graded spectrum:** Deborah Hasin, "Truth (Validity) and Use Despite Consequences: The DSM-5 Substance Use Disorder Unidimensional Syndrome," *Addiction* 109, no. 11 (November 2014): 1781–82, https://doi.org/10.1111/add.12686; Deborah Hasin, "DSM-5 SUD Diagnoses: Changes, Reactions, Remaining Open Questions," *Drug and Alcohol Dependence* 148, no. 3 (March 1, 2015): 226–29, https://doi.org/10.1016/j.drugalcdep.2014.12.006; Deborah Hasin et al., "DSM-5 Criteria for Substance Use Disorders: Recommendations and Rationale," *American Journal of Psychiatry* 170, no. 8 (August 1, 2013): 834, https://doi.org/10.1176/appi.ajp.2013.12060782.

15 **the neurodiversity movement:** Steve Silberman, *NeuroTribes: The Legacy of Autism and the Future of Neurodiversity* (New York: Avery, 2015); Christina Nicolaidis, "What Can Physicians Learn from the Neurodiversity Movement?," *AMA Journal of Ethics* 14, no. 6 (June 2012): 503–10, https://doi.org/10.1001/virtualmentor.2012.14.6.oped1-1206. More generally on the notion of spectrum concepts: Thomas Insel et al., "Research Domain Criteria (RDoC): Toward a New Classification Framework for Research on Mental Disorders," *American Journal of Psychiatry* 167, no. 7 (July 2010): 748–51, https://doi.org/10.1176/appi.ajp.2010.09091379; William E. Narrow and Emily A. Kuhl, "Dimensional Approaches to Psychiatric Diagnosis in DSM-5," *Journal of Mental Health Policy and Economics* 14, no. 4 (December 2011): 197–200, PMID: 22345361; Kristian E. Markon, Michael Chmielewski, and Christopher J. Miller, "The Reliability and Validity of Discrete and Continuous Measures of Psychopathology: A Quantitative Review," *Psychological Bulletin* 137, no. 5 (2011): 856–79, https://doi.apa.org/doi/10.1037/a0023678; Michael P. Hengartner and Sandrine N. Lehmann, "Why Psychiatric Research Must Abandon Traditional Diagnostic Classification and Adopt a Fully Dimensional Scope: Two Solutions to a Persistent Problem," *Frontiers in Psychiatry* 8 (June 2017), https://doi.org/10.3389/fpsyt.2017.00101.

15 **part of a complex system:** Reinout W. Wiers and Paul Verschure, "Curing the Broken Brain Model of Addiction: Neurorehabilitation from a Systems Perspective," *Addictive Behaviors* 112 (January 2021): 106602, https://doi.org/10.1016/j.addbeh.2020.106602.

16 **heroin "is momentary freedom":** William S. Burroughs, *Junky*, ed. Oliver Harris (New York: Penguin Classics, 2008), 128; Caroline Knapp, *Drinking: A Love Story* (New York: Dial Press, 1996), 104, quoted in Jason David Gray, "Philosophy, Phenomenology, and Neuroscience: The Groundwork for an Interdisciplinary Approach to a Comprehensive Understanding of Addiction" (PhD diss., University of California, Riverside, 2013), 88.

16 **"an existential anxiety":** Owen Flanagan, "What Is It Like to Be an Addict?," in *Addiction and Responsibility*, ed. Jeffrey Poland and George Graham (Cambridge, MA: MIT Press, 2011), 275.

16 **"My two wills":** Augustine, *Confessions*, 8.5.1.

NOTES

17 German physicians called *das Nichtaufhörenkönnen*: E. M. Jellinek, *The Disease Concept of Alcoholism* (New Haven, CT: Hillhouse Press, 1960), 41.

17 *"akrasia"* is the best way: Heather, "Addiction as a Form of *Akrasia*."

17 several other historical figures: Regarding the problems with retrospective diagnosis, see Axel Karenberg, "Retrospective Diagnosis: Use and Abuse in Medical Historiography," *Prague Medical Report* 110, no. 2 (2009): 140–45.

17 "gobbets of wine-reeking food": Marcus Tullius Cicero, *Selected Works*, trans. Michael Grant (New York: Penguin Classics, 1960), 129. Though it is worth noting that this quotation comes from Cicero, an avowed enemy of Mark Antony.

17 a chief factor in his downfall: Seneca, *Moral Letters to Lucilius*, 83.25, https://en.wikisource.org/wiki/Moral_letters_to_Lucilius/Letter_83.

17 Alexander III of Macedon: Quintus Curtius Rufus, *History of Alexander the Great of Macedon*, 5.7.1; Marcus Junianus Justinus, *Epitome of the Phillipic History of Pompeius Trogus*, trans. John Selby Watson (London, 1853), 9.8.15, http://www.forumromanum.org/literature/justin/english/index.html. Peter Green, Alexander's definitive recent biographer, scatters his text with liberal references to Alexander's "alcoholism": *Alexander of Macedon, 356–323 B.C.* (Berkeley: University of California Press, 1991), 443, 453. John O'Brien has argued that Alexander not only exhibited the classic symptoms of alcoholism, but also that it was the primary reason for his decline, his "critical problem": John O'Brien, *Alexander the Great: The Invisible Enemy* (New York: Routledge, 1992), 230.

18 patient with severe alcohol addiction: Ryan P. McCormack et al., "Commitment to Assessment and Treatment: Comprehensive Care for Patients Gravely Disabled by Alcohol Use Disorders," *Lancet* 382, no. 9896 (September 2013): 995–97, https://doi.org/10.1016/s0140-6736(12)62206-5.

18 "substance use disorder": Nick Heather, "On Defining Addiction," in Heather and Segal, *Addiction and Choice*, 3–28; Michael S. Moore, "Addiction, Responsibility, and Neuroscience," *University of Illinois Law Review* 202, no. 2: 375–470, https://illinoislawreview.org/wp-content/uploads/2020/04/Moore.pdf. Note also that the supposedly objective criteria cannot help but attach value judgments about what counts as "a lot" and "problems."

18 reliability comes at the expense: Note also that the SUD criteria aren't all that reliable. Deborah Hasin et al., "The DSM-5 Field Trials and Reliability of Alcohol Use Disorder," *Drug and Alcohol Dependence* 148 (March 2015): 226–29, https://doi.org/10.1016/j.drugalcdep.2014.12.006.

19 "willing" and "unwilling" addicts: Harry G. Frankfurt, "Freedom of the Will and the Concept of a Person," *Journal of Philosophy* 68, no. 1 (January 1971): 12, https://doi.org/10.2307/2024717.

19 an enormously significant determination: Herbert Fingarette, "Philosophical and Legal Aspects of the Disease Concept of Alcoholism," in *Research Advances in Alcohol and Drug Problems*, vol. 7, ed. Reginald G. Smart et al. (New York: Plenum Press, 1983), 4.

20 first to use the word "addict": Jose Murgatroyd Cree, "Protestant Evangelicals and Addiction in Early Modern English," *Renaissance Studies* 32, no. 3 (June 2018): 446–62, https://doi.org/10.1111/rest.12328; Jose Murgatroyd Cree, "The Invention of Addiction in Early Modern England" (PhD diss., University of Sheffield, 2018). See also Augustus Charles Bickley, "John Frith," in *Dictionary of National Biography*, ed. Leslie Stephen (London: Smith, Elder, 1889), https://en.wikisource.org/wiki/Frith,_John_(DNB00); Thomas Russell, "The Story, Life, and Martyrdom of John Frith, with the Godly and Learned Works and Writings of the Said Author, Hereafter Appearing," in *The Works of the English Reformers: William Tyndale and John Frith*, ed. Thomas Russell (London: Ebenezer Palmer, 1831), 2:77, https://archive.org/details/theworksoftheeng03tynduoft/page/n7/mode/2up.

20 debtor could be enslaved: Rebecca Lemon, *Addiction and Devotion in Early Modern England* (Philadelphia: University of Pennsylvania Press, 2018), ix.

20 referred to a strong devotion: Cree, "Protestant Evangelicals," 3.

20 "be not partially *addict*": John Frith, *Antithesis* [. . .], in Russell, *Works of the English Reformers*, 318 (emphasis added).

20 between free will and compulsion: Cree, "The Invention of Addiction," chap. 4. Specifically, the word came from Neo-Latin, where it may have already taken on the meaning used by Frith.

21 almost heroic devotion and commitment: Cree, "Protestant Evangelicals," 174, 448.

21 addict to sin: Cree, "Protestant Evangelicals," 455.

21 paradoxical sense of "willed compulsion": Lemon, *Addiction and Devotion*, 10.

21 the idea of self-discipline: Gabriel, "Gods and Monsters," 86–90; Christopher Cook, *Alcohol, Addiction, and Christian Ethics* (New York: Cambridge University Press, 2006); Mariana Valverde, *Diseases of the Will: Alcohol and the Dilemmas of Freedom* (New York: Cambridge University Press, 1998).

21 Marlowe's **1604 play** *Doctor Faustus*: Rebecca Lemon, "Scholarly Addiction: *Doctor Faustus* and the Drama of Devotion," *Renaissance Quarterly* 69, no. 3 (Fall 2016): 865–98, https://doi.org/10.1086/689036; Genevieve Guenther, "Why Devils Came When Faustus Called Them," *Modern Philology* 109, no. 1 (August 2011): 46–70, https://doi.org/10.1086/662147.

21 describes **Faust as "addicted"**: Henri Logeman, ed., *The English Faust-Book of 1592* (Ghent, 1900), 1, https://books.google.com/books?id=Q0RHAAAAcAAJ.

Chapter Two

23 **on the verge of mutiny**: Laurence Bergreen, *Columbus: The Four Voyages, 1492–1504* (New York: Penguin, 2012), 26–28.

23 **rolling up an unfamiliar plant**: Bergreen, *Columbus*, 19, 27; Count Corti, *A History of Smoking*, trans. Paul England (New York: Harcourt, Brace, 1932), 35–39. Columbus was given tobacco by the first group of Taíno people he met in the Bahamas, but he discarded the leaves.

24 **De Jerez was imprisoned**: Rudi Mathee, "Exotic Substances: The Introduction and Global Spread of Tobacco, Coffee, Cocoa, Tea, and Distilled Liquor, Sixteenth to Eighteenth Centuries," in *Drugs and Narcotics in History*, ed. Roy Porter and Mikuláš Teich (New York: Cambridge University Press, 1995), 33.

24 **slippery and sometimes outright harmful**: Zachary Siegel, "Is the U.S. Knee-Deep in 'Epidemics,' or Is That Just Wishful Thinking?," *New York Times*, August 14, 2018, https://www.nytimes.com/2018/08/14/magazine/epidemic-disaster-tragedy.html.

25 **the "psychoactive revolution"**: David T. Courtwright, *Forces of Habit: Drugs and the Making of the Modern World* (Cambridge, MA: Harvard University Press, 2001), 1–6.

25 **mass-produced "soft drugs"**: Jordan Goodman, "Excitantia: Or, How Enlightenment Europe Took to Soft Drugs," in *Consuming Habits: Global and Historical Perspectives on How Cultures Define Drugs*, 2nd ed., ed. Jordan Goodman, Paul E. Lovejoy, and Andrew Sherratt (New York: Routledge, 2007), 121. Sugar: Andrew Sherratt, introduction to *Consuming Habits*, 7.

25 **Indian society used opium**: Garcia da Orta, *Colloquies on the Simples & Drugs of India*, ed. Conde de Ficalho, trans. Clements Markham (Lisbon, 1895), https://archive.org/stream/colloquiesonsimp00orta/colloquiesonsimp00orta_djvu.txt. ("The men who eat it go about sleepily, and they say that they take it so as not to feel any trouble. . . . If it is not used there is danger of death ensuing . . . and there is a very strong desire for it among those who use it.") See also Benjamin Breen, *The Age of Intoxication: Origins of the Global Drug Trade* (Philadelphia: University of Pennsylvania Press, 2019), 58–59; Marcus Boon, *The Road of Excess: A History of Writers on Drugs* (Cambridge, MA: Harvard University Press, 2005), chap. 1.

26 **Jean Nicot**: It's from Nicot's name that we get the word "nicotine." Larry Harrison, "Tobacco Battered and the Pipes Shattered: A Note on the Fate of the First British Campaign against Tobacco Smoking," *British Journal of Addiction* 81, no. 4 (April 1986): 553–58, https://doi.org/10.1111/j.1360-0443.1986.tb00367.x.

26 **pipes were lit with coal**: Corti, *History of Smoking*, 69; Alfred H. Dunhill, "Smoking in England—Elizabethan," in *The Gentle Art of Smoking* (New York: Putnam, 1954), https://web.archive.org/web/20181109095246/http://archive.tobacco.org:80/History/Elizabethan_Smoking.html; Iain Gately, *Tobacco: A Cultural History of How an Exotic Plant Seduced Civilization* (New York: Grove Press, 2001), 45.

26 **threatened snuff users**: Patrizia Russo et al., "Tobacco Habit: Historical, Cultural, Neurobiological, and Genetic Features of People's Relationship with an Addictive Drug," *Perspectives in Biology and Medicine* 54, no. 4 (Autumn 2011): 557–77, https://doi.org/10.1353/pbm.2011.0047. Specifically, the pope was threatening excommunication for people who used snuff in churches: J. D. Rolleston, "On Snuff Taking," *British Journal of Inebriety* 34, no. 1 (July 1936): 1–16.

26 **Russian, Japanese, and Chinese rulers**: Carol Benedict, *Golden-Silk Smoke: A History of Tobacco in China, 1555–2010* (Berkeley: University of California Press, 2011), 24; Corti, *History of Smoking*, 141.

26 **"the severest torture"**: David Courtwright, *The Age of Addiction: How Bad Habits Became Big Business* (Cambridge, MA: Harvard University Press, 2019), 70. See also James Grehan, "Smoking and 'Early Modern' Sociability: The Great Tobacco Debate in the Ottoman Middle East (Seventeenth to Eighteenth Centuries)," *American Historical Review* 111, no. 5 (December 2006): 1352–77, https://doi.org/10.1086/ahr.111.5.1352.

26 *A Counterblaste to Tobacco*: King James I, *A Counterblaste to Tobacco* (London, 1604), 16, https://books.google.com/books?id=EasUAAAAYAAJ. See also David Harley, "The Beginnings of the Tobacco Controversy: Puritanism, James I, and the Royal Physicians," *Bulletin of the History of Medicine* 67, no. 1 (Spring 1993): 28–50, PMID: 8461637.

26 **"a Plague intolerable":** Joshua Sylvester, *Tobacco Battered and the Pipes Shattered (About Their Ears, That Id'ly Idolize So Base and Barbarous a Weed: Or, at Least-Wise Over-Love So Loathsome Vanity)* (London, 1676; Ann Arbor, MI: Text Creation Partnership, 2011), https://quod.lib.umich.edu/e/eebo /A87472.0001.001/1:6?rgn=div1;view=fulltext.

29 **Purdue executives testified:** *OxyContin: Its Use and Abuse, Hearing before the Subcommittee on Oversight and Investigations of the Committee on Energy and Commerce, House of Representatives*, 107th Cong. 54 (2001) (prepared statement of Michael Friedman, executive vice president, chief operating officer, Purdue Pharma L.P.). For other information on the current opioid overdose crisis, see in particular Patrick Radden Keefe, "The Family That Built an Empire of Pain," *New Yorker*, October 30, 2017, https://www .newyorker.com/magazine/2017/10/30/the-family-that-built-an-empire-of-pain; Barry Meier, *Pain Killer: An Empire of Deceit and the Origin of America's Opioid Epidemic* (New York: Random House, 2003); Sam Quinones, *Dreamland: The True Tale of America's Opiate Epidemic* (New York: Bloomsbury Press, 2015); Anne Case and Angus Deaton, *Deaths of Despair and the Future of Capitalism* (Princeton, NJ: Princeton University Press, 2020); Art Van Zee, "The Promotion and Marketing of OxyContin: Commercial Triumph, Public Health Tragedy," *American Journal of Public Health* 99, no. 2 (February 2009): 221–27, https://doi.org/10.2105/AJPH.2007.131714.

29 **$225 million in civil penalties:** Gerald Posner, "How to Hold Purdue Pharma Accountable for Its Role in the Opioid Epidemic," *Los Angeles Times*, May 17, 2020, https://www.latimes.com/opinion /story/2020-05-17/sacklers-opioid-epidemic-bankruptcy; Katie Benner, "Purdue Pharma Pleads Guilty to Role in Opioid Crisis as Part of Deal with Justice Dept.," *New York Times*, November 24, 2020, https://www.nytimes.com/2020/11/24/us/politics/purdue-pharma-opioids-guilty-settlement.html; "2020 America's Richest Families Net Worth—#30 Sackler Family," *Forbes*, December 16, 2020, https://www.forbes.com/profile/sackler/?sh=53c8914b5d63.

29 **"addiction supply industries":** Jim Orford, *Power, Powerlessness, and Addiction* (New York: Cambridge University Press, 2013), 131.

29 **Raise prices on heroin:** William Rhodes et al., *Illicit Drugs: Price Elasticity of Demand and Supply* (Washington, DC: National Criminal Justice Reference Service, 2002), 60–67, https://www.ojp.gov /pdffiles1/nij/grants/191856.pdf.

30 **one-quarter of cannabis buyers:** Jonathan P. Caulkins and Rosalie Liccardo Pacula, "Marijuana Markets: Inferences from Reports by the Household Population," *Journal of Drug Issues* 38, no. 1 (January 2006): 173–200, https://doi.org/10.1177/002204260603600108.

30 **high cost of importing tobacco:** Alfred Rive, "A Brief History of the Regulation and Taxation of Tobacco in England," *William and Mary Quarterly* 9, no. 1 (January 1929), https://doi.org/10.2307 /1920374; Mathee, "Exotic Substances," 33.

30 **Parliament had discarded prohibitionist taxes:** Harrison, "Tobacco Battered," 556.

30 **In late-seventeenth-century Russia:** Courtwright, *Forces of Habit*, 156; Corti, *History of Smoking*, 141.

30 **other leaders followed suit:** Corti, *History of Smoking*, 149.

31 **taxes on alcohol, tobacco, and tea:** Courtwright, *Forces of Habit*, 4–5.

31 **the need for tax revenue:** Courtwright, *Forces of Habit*, 156, 197.

31 **systems of subjugation and conquest:** Orford, *Power, Powerlessness, and Addiction*.

31 **the first enslaved Africans:** Peter C. Mancall, "Tales Tobacco Told in Sixteenth-Century Europe," *Environmental History* 9, no. 4 (2004): 648–78, https://doi.org/10.2307/3986264; Marcy Norton, *Sacred Gifts, Profane Pleasures: A History of Tobacco and Chocolate in the Atlantic World* (Ithaca, NY: Cornell University Press, 2008), 221–22.

31 **obstructed antislavery movements:** Harrison, "Tobacco Battered," 557.

31 **Caribbean sugar:** Sidney W. Mintz, *Sweetness and Power: The Place of Sugar in Modern History* (New York: Penguin, 1986); James Walvin, *Sugar, the World Corrupted: From Slavery to Obesity* (New York: Pegasus, 2018).

31 **promoting the use of cocaine:** Joseph F. Spillane, *Cocaine: From Medical Marvel to Modern Menace in the United States, 1884–1920* (Baltimore: Johns Hopkins University Press, 2000), 32. See also David F. Musto, "Opium, Cocaine and Marijuana in American History," *Scientific American*, July 1991, https:// doi.org/10.1038/scientificamerican0791-40. Regarding Merck: H. Richard Friman, "Germany and the Transformations of Cocaine, 1860–1920," in *Cocaine: Global Histories*, ed. Paul Gootenberg (New York: Routledge, 2002), 85.

31 **"industrial epidemics":** René I. Jahiel and Thomas F. Babor, "Industrial Epidemics, Public Health Advocacy and the Alcohol Industry: Lessons from Other Fields," *Addiction* 102, no. 9 (September 2007): 1335–39, https://doi.org/10.1111/j.1360-0443.2007.01900.x.

32 **smoking was safe:** Richard Kluger, *Ashes to Ashes: America's Hundred-Year Cigarette War, the Public Health, and the Unabashed Triumph of Philip Morris* (New York: Vintage, 1997), chaps. 4–9.

32 **"Doubt is our product":** Unknown, memo to R. A. Pittman, August 21, 1969, Brown & Williamson Records, Truth Tobacco Industry Records, University of California, San Francisco, https://www .industrydocuments.ucsf.edu/tobacco/docs/#id=xqkd0134; David Michaels, *Doubt Is Their Product* (New York: Oxford University Press, 2008).

32 **manufacture doubt about climate change:** Graham Readfearn, "Doubt over Climate Science Is a Product with an Industry behind It," *Guardian*, March 5, 2015, https://www.theguardian.com /environment/planet-oz/2015/mar/05/doubt-over-climate-science-is-a-product-with-an-industry -behind-it; David Michaels, *The Triumph of Doubt: Dark Money and the Science of Deception* (New York: Oxford University Press, 2020).

33 **"the love of single causes":** Frederick Turner and Ernst Pöppel, "The Neural Lyre: Poetic Meter, the Brain, and Time," *Poetry* 142, no. 5 (August 1983): 277–309, https://www.jstor.org/stable/20599567.

33 **heavy toll on Native cultures:** Peter C. Mancall, *Deadly Medicine: Indians and Alcohol in Early America* (Ithaca, NY: Cornell University Press, 1997), chaps. 4–5; Samson Occom, *A Sermon, Preached at the Execution of Moses Paul, an Indian* [. . .] (New Haven, 1772; Ann Arbor, MI: Text Creation Partnership, 2011), https://quod.lib.umich.edu/e/evans/N09814.0001.001/1:4?rgn=div1;view=fulltext.

34 **Wheelock was blown away:** Joanna Brooks and Robert Warrior, eds., *The Collected Writings of Samson Occom, Mohegan* (New York: Oxford University Press, 2006), 13–15; Bernd Peyer, *The Tutor'd Mind: Indian Missionary-Writers in Antebellum America* (Amherst: University of Massachusetts Press, 1997), 65.

34 **deliberate instrument of oppression:** Occom, *A Sermon*.

34 **restrictions on the liquor trade:** Mancall, *Deadly Medicine*, 44, 103–7, 114, 124; James Axtell, *The European and the Indian: Essays in the Ethnohistory of Colonial North America* (New York: Oxford University Press, 1981), 49, 65; Don L. Coyhis and William L. White, *Alcohol Problems in Native America: The Untold Story of Resistance and Recovery—the Truth about the Lie* (Colorado Springs, CO: Coyhis, 2006), chap. 3.

35 **better control their appetites:** "Journal of Indian Affairs," February 25, 1767, in *The Papers of Sir William Johnson*, vol. 12, ed. Milton W. Hamilton and Albert B. Corey (Albany: University of the State of New York, 1957), 273, https://archive.org/details/papersofsirwill12john.

35 **"devilish men":** Occom, *A Sermon*.

35 **most popular sermon:** Bernd Peyer, "Samson Occom: Mohegan Missionary and Writer of the 18th Century," *American Indian Quarterly* 6, no. 3–4 (Winter 1982): 208–17, https://doi.org/10.2307 /1183629.

35 **raised at least £11,000:** Peyer, *Tutor'd Mind*, 74–79; "Five Ways to Compute the Relative Value of a UK Pound Amount, 1270 to Present," Measuring Worth Foundation (website), accessed February 27, 2021, https://www.measuringworth.com/calculators/ukcompare/.

35 **just indenture the boy:** Brooks and Warrior, *Collected Writings of Samson Occom*, 78.

36 **grew into Dartmouth College:** Peyer, *Tutor'd Mind*, 74–79. To its credit, Dartmouth appears now to have a much more robust Native American program: "The Native Legacy at Dartmouth College," Dartmouth Native American Program, Dartmouth College (website), accessed February 2, 2021, https://students.dartmouth.edu/nap/about/history.

36 **the Brothertown movement:** Brooks and Warrior, *Collected Writings of Samson Occom*, 28.

36 **"firewater myths":** Joy Leland, *Firewater Myths: North American Indian Drinking and Alcohol Addiction* (New Brunswick, NJ: Rutgers Center of Alcohol Studies, 1976).

36 **myths have been roundly disproven:** Coyhis and White, *Alcohol Problems*, preface, chaps. 2–3.

36 **The Opium Wars:** Frank Dikötter, Lars Laamann, and Xun Zhou, *Narcotic Culture: A History of Drugs in China* (Chicago: University of Chicago Press, 2004), 1; Bruce K. Alexander, *The Globalization of Addiction* (New York: Oxford University Press, 2010), 131; Carl Trocki, *Opium, Empire and the Global Political Economy* (New York: Routledge, 1999), chap. 5. On the evolution of the British anti-opium movement and its motivations, which biased nineteenth-century portrayals of the problem, see Virginia Berridge, *Opium and the People*, rev. ed. (New York: Free Association Books, 1999), 175–80.

37 **seemingly unending series of plagues:** Courtwright, *Age of Addiction*, 70.

37 **"dislocation theory of addiction":** Alexander, *Globalization of Addiction*, 1–84.

39 **wrong key on their computer:** Case and Deaton, *Deaths of Despair*, 1–16.

39 **More people were living alone:** Esteban Ortiz-Ospina, "The Rise of Living Alone: How One-Person Households Are Becoming Increasingly Common around the World," Our World in Data, December 10, 2019, https://ourworldindata.org/living-alone.

39 **highest income inequality:** Katherine Schaeffer, "Six Facts about Economic Inequality in the U.S.," Pew Research Center, February 7, 2020, https://www.pewresearch.org/fact-tank/2020/02/07/6-facts-about-economic-inequality-in-the-u-s/.

39 **more than 150,000 deaths of despair:** Case and Deaton, *Deaths of Despair*, 94; Department of Veterans Affairs, *America's Wars* (Washington, DC: Office of Public Affairs, 2020), https://www.va.gov/opa/publications/factsheets/fs_americas_wars.pdf.

39 **the "Lost Generation":** John W. Crowley, "'Alcoholism' and the Modern Temper," in *The Serpent in the Cup: Temperance in American Literature* (Amherst: University of Massachusetts Press, 1997), 165.

39 **Sartre smoked two packs:** Roger Kimball, "Sartre Resartus," *New Criterion*, May 1987, https://newcriterion.com/issues/1987/5/sartre-resartus.

40 **the Beat generation:** Ted Morgan, *Literary Outlaw: The Life and Times of William S. Burroughs* (New York: W. W. Norton, 1988), loc. 2932 and 3194 of 14351, Kindle.

40 **Persistent health inequities:** Nabarun Dasgupta, Leo Beletsky, and Daniel Ciccarone, "Opioid Crisis: No Easy Fix to Its Social and Economic Determinants," *American Journal of Public Health* 108, no. 2 (February 2018): 182–86, https://doi.org/10.2105/AJPH.2017.304187.

40 **exclusive focus on white problems:** Julie Netherland and Helena B. Hansen, "The War on Drugs That Wasn't: Wasted Whiteness, 'Dirty Doctors,' and Race in Media Coverage of Prescription Opioid Misuse," *Culture, Medicine, and Psychiatry* 40, no. 4 (December 2016): 664–86, https://doi.org/10.1007/s11013-016-9496-5.

41 **"their deadly *beson*":** Neolin, quoted in Mancall, *Deadly Medicine*, 116.

41 **a man named Papunhank:** Richard W. Pointer, "An Almost Friend: Papunhank, Quakers, and the Search for Security amid Pennsylvania's Wars, 1754–65," *Pennsylvania Magazine of History and Biography* 138, no. 3 (2014): 237–68; Coyhis and White, *Alcohol Problems*, 78–79.

41 **Seneca man named Handsome Lake:** William L. White, "Pre-A.A. Alcohol Mutual Aid Societies," *Alcoholism Treatment Quarterly* 19, no. 1 (2001): 1–21; Coyhis and White, *Alcohol Problems*, 93–101; Christopher M. Finan, *Drunks: An American History* (Boston: Beacon Press, 2017), 5–23.

42 **Native American recovery tradition, Wellbriety:** *The Red Road to Wellbriety: In the Native American Way* (Colorado Springs, CO: White Bison, 2002). Thanks to Jon Soske for this connection.

42 **the largest city in Europe:** Matthew White, "Health, Hygiene and the Rise of 'Mother Gin' in the 18th Century," British Library, October 14, 2009, https://www.bl.uk/georgian-britain/articles/health-hygiene-and-the-rise-of-mother-gin-in-the-18th-century.

42 **fearful new threat:** Spontaneous combustion: Jessica Warner, "Old and in the Way: Widows, Witches, and Spontaneous Combustion in the Age of Reason," *Contemporary Drug Problems* 23, no. 2 (June 1996): 197–220, https://doi.org/10.1177/009145099602300204; Emily Anne Adams, "'Ladies' Delight?': Women in London's 18th Century Gin Craze, *Crimson Historical Review* 2, no. 1 (Fall 2019), https://crimsonhistorical.ua.edu/wp-content/uploads/2019/12/LadiesDelight.pdf. Grace Pitt's case is described also in Thomas Trotter's essay, discussed in the next chapter. Thomas Trotter, *An Essay, Medical, Philosophical, and Chemical* [. . .] (London, 1804), 87–89, https://www.google.com/books/edition/An_Essay_Medical_Philosophical_and_Chemi/b2NHAAAAYAAJ. In *Bleak House,* Dickens uses her case as an example of why he believes in spontaneous combustion. On the Gin Craze in general, see Warner's excellent book *Craze: Gin and Debauchery in an Age of Reason* (New York: Four Walls Eight Windows, 2002), 74–81.

43 **twice as strong:** Mark Forsyth, "The 18th-Century Craze for Gin," *History Extra*, December 2017, https://www.historyextra.com/period/georgian/gin-craze-panic-18th-century-london-when-came-england-alcohol-drinking-history/.

43 **doubled from 1700 to 1720:** Warner, *Craze*, 3.

43 **industry funded pamphleteers:** Daniel Defoe, *A Brief Case of the Distillers* [. . .] (London, 1726; Ann Arbor, MI: Text Creation Partnership, 2011), https://quod.lib.umich.edu/e/ecco/004834050.0001.000?view=toc. See also Warner, *Craze*, ix–xii.

43 **"poorer Sort of People":** John Gonson, *Five Charges to Several Grand Juries*, 3rd ed. (London, 1740), 103, https://www.google.com/books/edition/Five_Charges_to_several_Grand_Juries_Thi/vYhz5NMQtE0C.

44 **a massive shift:** Alexander, *Globalization of Addiction*, chap. 6.

44 **120,000 outlets selling gin:** Warner, *Craze*, 35–47.

44 **a bad mother:** *Proceedings of the Old Bailey*, February 27, 1734, 10, https://www.oldbaileyonline.org/images.jsp?doc=173402270010.

45 **"Wretches stretched upon the Pavement":** Henry Lowther, Viscount Lonsdale, 1743, quoted in Warner, *Craze*, 13.

45 **largely composed of landowners:** Ernest L. Abel, "The Gin Epidemic: Much Ado about What?," *Alcohol and Alcoholism* 36, no. 5 (September 2001): 401–5, https://doi.org/10.1093/alcalc/36.5.401. After the "Tippling Act" of 1751, which issued stricter controls on retail, consumption declined.

45 **A 1736 act of Parliament:** An Act for Laying a Duty upon the Retailers of Spiritous Liquors, and for Licensing the Retailers Thereof, 1736, 9 Geo. 2, c. 23.

46 **an act of political protest:** Warner, *Craze*, 132; James Nicholls, *The Politics of Alcohol* (Manchester, UK: Manchester University Press, 2009), 51.

46 **a contagion sweeping the city:** Daniel Defoe, *Augusta Triumphans: Or, the Way to Make London the Most Flourishing City in the Universe* (London, 1728), http://www.gutenberg.org/files/32405/32405-h /32405-h.htm.

46 **drinking as a medical problem:** Roy Porter, "The Drinking Man's Disease: The 'Pre-History' of Alcoholism in Georgian Britain," *British Journal of Addiction* 80, no. 4 (December 1985): 385–96, https:// doi.org/10.1111/j.1360-0443.1985.tb03010.x.

46 **a reductionist account:** Stephen Hales, *A Friendly Admonition to the Drinkers of Gin, Brandy and Other Distilled Spiritous Liquors* [. . .] (London, 1734), 6, Eighteenth Century Collections Online.

47 ***Daintiemouthde Droonkardes:*** George Gascoigne, *A Delicate Diet, for Daintiemouthde Droonkardes* [. . .] (London, 1576; Ann Arbor, MI: Text Creation Partnership, 2011), https://quod.lib.umich.edu/e /eebo/A01517.0001.001?view=toc.

47 **"Loathsom Sin of Drunkenness":** "House of Commons Journal Volume 1: 03 March 1607," in *Journal of the House of Commons*, vol. 1, 1547–1629 (London, 1802), 346–47, https://www.british-history .ac.uk/commons-jrnl/vol1/pp346-347.

47 **"addicted to this vice":** John Downame, *Foure Treatises Tending to Disswade All Christians from Foure no Lesse Hainous Then Common Sinnes* [. . .] (London, 1609; Ann Arbor, MI: Text Creation Partnership, 2011), https://quod.lib.umich.edu/e/eebo2/A20760.0001.001?view=toc.

47 **also a condition:** Nicholls, *The Politics of Alcohol*, 64.

47 **"diligent and fervent prayer":** Hales, *Friendly Admonition*, 26.

47 **just deserts of sinful behavior:** Porter, "Drinking Man's Disease," 390.

Chapter Three

48 **birth of his first child:** On Rush in general, see the excellent biography by Stephen Fried, *Rush: Revolution, Madness, and Benjamin Rush, the Visionary Doctor Who Became a Founding Father* (New York: Crown, 2018), 207.

48 **Alcohol problems were rife:** Peter Andreas, *Killer High: A History of War in Six Drugs* (New York: Oxford University Press, 2020), 27.

49 **he returned to Philadelphia:** Fried, *Rush*, 232–38.

49 **"Elegant not great":** *Diary and Autobiography of John Adams*, vol. 2 (Cambridge, MA: Belknap Press of Harvard University Press, 1962), http://www.masshist.org/publications/adams-papers/view?%20id =ADMS-01-02-02-0005-0003-0013.

49 **"quantity of rye destroyed":** Benjamin Rush Travel Diary, 1784 April 2–7, brpst023001:22, Benjamin and Julia Stockton Rush Papers, Duke University, https://repository.duke.edu/dc/rushbenjaminandjulia /brpst023001.

50 **enormously profitable distilleries:** Mark Edward Lender and James Kirby Martin, *Drinking in America: A History* (New York: Simon & Schuster, 1987), 30; Joseph Michael Gabriel, "Gods and Monsters: Drugs, Addiction, and the Origin of Narcotic Control in the Nineteenth-Century Urban North" (PhD diss., Rutgers University, 2006), 112–13.

50 **Quakers prohibited their members:** Michael Goode, "Dangerous Spirits: How the Indian Critique of Alcohol Shaped Eighteenth-Century Quaker Revivalism," *Early American Studies: An Interdisciplinary Journal* 14, no. 2 (Spring 2016): 256–83, https://doi.org/10.1353/eam.2016.0007.

50 **"as their GENEVA":** Benjamin Franklin, "To the Printer of the *Gazette*," *Pennsylvania Gazette*, July 22–August 2, 1736, Newspapers.com, https://www.newspapers.com/image/39391139/.

50 **caused by alcohol:** Fried, *Rush*, 264–65.

50 **special focus on willpower:** Christopher Cook, *Alcohol, Addiction, and Christian Ethics* (New York: Cambridge University Press, 2006), 117; Ernest Kurtz, *Not God: A History of Alcoholics Anonymous* (Center City, MN: Hazelden Educational Materials, 1979), 166; Harry Gene Levine, "The Discovery of Addiction: Changing Conceptions of Habitual Drunkenness in America," *Journal of Substance Abuse Treatment* 2, no. 1 (Winter 1985): 43–57; Gabriel, "Gods and Monsters," 119; Linda A. Mercadante, *Victims & Sinners: Spiritual Roots of Addiction and Recovery* (Louisville, KY: Westminster John Knox Press, 1996), 116, 143.

51 **"disease does not exist":** Charles E. Rosenberg, Janet Goldman, and Stephen Peitzman, "Framing Disease," *Hospital Practice* 27, no. 7 (July 1992): 179–221, https://doi.org/10.1080/21548331.1992.11705460. See also Charles E. Rosenberg, "Disease in History: Frames and Framers," *Milbank Quarterly* 67, no. S1 (1989): 1–15, https://doi.org/10.2307/3350182.

51 **calling something a disease:** On "jurisdictional" definition of disease, see Michael S. Moore, "Addiction, Responsibility, and Neuroscience," *University of Illinois Law Review* 202, no. 2: 384, https://illinoislawreview.org/wp-content/uploads/2020/04/Moore.pdf. Pickard argues that something need not be a disease in order for the medical profession to care for it: Hanna Pickard, "What We're Not Talking about When We Talk about Addiction," *Hastings Center Report* 50, no. 4 (July/August 2020): 37–46, https://doi.org/10.1002/hast.1172.

52 **located in reductionist biology:** Nick Haslam, "Psychiatric Categories as Natural Kinds: Essentialist Thinking about Mental Disorder," *Social Research* 67, no. 4 (Winter 2000): 1032.

52 **prayer and religion:** Benjamin Rush, *An Inquiry into the Effects of Ardent Spirits* [. . .], 8th ed. (Boston, 1823), 31, https://books.google.com/books?id=-6UoAAAAYAAJ.

52 **"a disease of the mind":** Thomas Trotter, *An Essay, Medical, Philosophical, and Chemical* [. . .] (London, 1804), 1–5, 172, https://www.google.com/books/edition/An_Essay_Medical_Philosophical_and_Chemi/b2NHAAAAYAAJ.

52 **claimed to be the first:** Roy Porter, "Introduction," in *An Essay Medical, Philosophical, and Chemical on Drunkenness and Its Effects on the Human Body*, by Thomas Trotter, ed. Roy Porter (London, 1804; New York: Routledge, 1988), xiv. Trotter didn't have anything like Rush's reach, but he still made an impact, with his essay published in several editions and translated into German and Swedish.

53 **"Drops beget Drams":** George Cheyne, *An Essay of Health and Long Life* (London, 1724; Ann Arbor, MI: Text Creation Partnership, 2011), 52–53, https://quod.lib.umich.edu/e/ecco/004834818.0001.000?rgn=main;view=fulltext. See also Roy Porter, "The Drinking Man's Disease: The 'Pre-History' of Alcoholism in Georgian Britain," *British Journal of Addiction*, 80, no. 4 (December 1985):" 392; Christopher M. Finan, *Drunks: An American History* (Boston: Beacon Press, 2017), 57.

53 **"milk and vegetables":** James Nicholls, *The Politics of Alcohol* (Manchester, UK: Manchester University Press, 2009), 60; George Cheyne, *The English Malady: Or, a Treatise of Nervous Diseases of All Kinds* [. . .] (London, 1733), 325–26, https://archive.org/details/englishmaladyort00cheyuoft/page/324/mode/2up.

53 **"bound in slavery to these infernal spirits":** Anthony Benezet, *The Mighty Destroyer Displayed* [. . .] (Philadelphia, 1774; Ann Arbor, MI: Text Creation Partnership, 2011), 8, https://quod.lib.umich.edu/e/evans/N32312.0001.001/1:2?rgn=div1;view=fulltext. Benezet's prescription for abstinence is why his pamphlet is often cited as the first piece of American temperance literature, though Occom's came two years earlier.

53 **an "odious disease":** Rush, *An Inquiry into the Effects of Ardent Spirits*, 8.

53 **put medicine at the center:** Rush regularly revised and expanded his popular inquiry, and each time, he increased the focus on habitual drunkenness as a disease of the mind. On Rush's thought, the historian Matthew Osborn has nicely described the evolution of his views on drunkenness, which changed across Rush's life. Matthew Warner Osborn, *Rum Maniacs: Alcoholic Insanity in the Early American Republic* (Chicago: University of Chicago Press, 2014), 23–24; Gabriel, "Gods and Monsters," 117.

57 **so much blood was spilled:** Robert L. North, "Benjamin Rush, MD: Assassin or Beloved Healer?," *Baylor University Medical Center Proceedings* 13, no. 1 (January 2000): 45–49, https://dx.doi.org/10.1080%2F08998280.2000.11927641; "Politics of Yellow Fever in Alexander Hamilton's America," U.S. National Library of Medicine, updated November 16, 2018, https://www.nlm.nih.gov/exhibition/politicsofyellowfever/index.html; Kenneth R. Foster, Mary F. Jenkins, and Anna Coxe Toogood, "The Philadelphia Yellow Fever Epidemic of 1793," *Scientific American*, February 1998, 88–93; Jacquelyn C. Miller, "The Wages of Blackness: African American Workers and the Meanings of Race during Philadelphia's 1793 Yellow Fever Epidemic," *Pennsylvania Magazine of History and Biography* 129, no. 2 (April 2005): 163–94, https://www.jstor.org/stable/20093783.

58 **cures for just about anything:** William L. White, *Slaying the Dragon: The History of Addiction Treatment and Recovery in America*, 2nd ed. (Chicago: Lighthouse Institute, 2014), 88.

58 **"bi-chloride of gold":** Finan, *Drunks*, 102.

58 **"liberate[d] the will":** Leslie E. Keeley, *Opium: Its Use, Abuse, and Cure; or, from Bondage to Freedom* (Chicago, 1897), 82, https://books.google.com/books?id=LAhq6YjNIq0C.

58 **more than 500,000 people:** Timothy A. Hickman, *The Secret Leprosy of Modern Days: Narcotic Addiction and Cultural Crisis in the United States, 1870–1920* (Amherst: University of Massachusetts Press, 2007), 51–57; White, *Slaying the Dragon*, 68–86; H. Wayne Morgan, *Drugs in America: A Social History, 1800–1980* (Syracuse, NY: Syracuse University Press), 75–82.

58 **"Drunkenness is a disease":** White, *Slaying the Dragon*, 69.

58 **advertising cure rates:** Eliyahu Kamisher, "Dueling Lawsuits between Malibu Rehab Centers Expose the Shady Side of the Recovery Industry," *Los Angeles Magazine*, February 12, 2020, https://www .lamag.com/citythinkblog/dueling-lawsuits-between-malibu-rehab-centers-expose-the-shady -side-of-the-recovery-industry/.

59 **disease of "morphinism":** Keeley, *Opium*, 46; Timothy A. Hickman, "Keeping Secrets: Leslie E. Keeley, the Gold Cure, and the 19th-Century Neuroscience of Addiction," *Addiction* 113, no. 9 (June 2018): 1739–49, https://doi.org/10.1111/add.1422.

59 **"Addiction Is a Brain Disease":** Alan I. Leshner, "Addiction Is a Brain Disease, and It Matters," *Science* 278, no. 5335 (October 1997): 45–47, https://doi.org/10.1126/science.278.5335.45.

60 **more than two thousand times:** "Leshner: 'Addiction Is a Brain Disease, and It Matters,'" Google Scholar, accessed February 6, 2021, https://scholar.google.com/scholar?cites=16995262381563870016. For comparison, Leshner's editorial beats out a *Science* editorial published that year by Stanley Prusiner, who won the Nobel Prize that year: "Prion Diseases and the BSE Crisis," *Science* 278, no. 5336 (October 1997): 245–51, https://doi.org/10.1126/science.278.5336.245.

60 **congressional funding for addiction research:** Sally Satel and Scott O. Lilienfeld, "Addiction and the Brain-Disease Fallacy," *Frontiers in Psychiatry* 4 (2014): 141, https://doi.org/10.3389/fpsyt.2013.00141.

60 **a blistering critique:** Derek Heim, "Addiction: Not Just Brain Malfunction," *Nature* 507, no. 40 (March 2014), https://doi.org/10.1038/507040e.

61 **"a *primary*, chronic disease":** American Society of Addiction Medicine, "Public Policy Statement: Definition of Addiction," April 12, 2011, https://www.asam.org/docs/default-source/public-policy -statements/1definition_of_addiction_long_4-11.pdf (emphasis added). Further discussion: David E. Smith, "The Process Addictions and the New ASAM Definition of Addiction," *Journal of Psychoactive Drugs* 44, no. 1 (January 2012): 1–4, https://doi.org/10.1080/02791072.2012.662105.

61 **"a disorder in the imagination":** John Locke, "Madness," in *The Life of John Locke: With Extracts from His Correspondence, Journals and Common-Place Books*, ed. Lord Peter King (London, 1829), 328, https://books.google.com/books?id=AuFSCJWCcwEC&pg=PA328; Osborn, *Rum Maniacs*, chap. 1. To attribute this tabula rasa belief to Locke himself would be an oversimplification. Arguably, Locke himself took a more balanced view. See Han-Kyul Kim, "Locke and the Mind-Body Problem: An Interpretation of His Agnosticism," *Philosophy* 83, no. 326 (2008): 439–58, https://doi.org/10.1017 /S003181910800082X.

61 **Thomas Trotter insisted:** Trotter, *An Essay, Medical, Philosophical, and Chemical*, 1–5, 172.

61 **Philippe Pinel, a contemporaneous pioneer:** Edward A. Shorter, *A History of Psychiatry: From the Era of the Asylum to the Age of Asylum* (New York: John Wiley & Sons, 1997), 10–16.

62 **"bodies before books":** Roy Porter, *The Greatest Benefit to All Mankind: A Medical History of Humanity* (1997; repr. New York: W. W. Norton, 1998), 305.

62 **the disease of "*Trunksucht*":** William F. Bynum, "Chronic Alcoholism in the First Half of the 19th Century," *Bulletin of the History of Medicine* 42, no. 2 (March 1968): 160–85, https://www.jstor.org /stable/44450720.

62 **Napoleon's 1812 invasion:** Friedrich-Wilhelm Kielhorn, "The History of Alcoholism: Brühl-Cramer's Concepts and Observations," *Addiction* 91, no. 1 (January 1996): 121–28, https://doi.org/10.1046/j.1360 -0443.1996.91112114.x.

62 **vodka supplies like firebombs:** Andreas, *Killer High*, 39.

62 **fundamentally a biological problem:** Kielhorn, "History of Alcoholism," 123–25. Of note, Brühl-Cramer also forcefully argued that biological causation meant dipsomania should be treated compassionately as a disease rather than a moral problem.

62 **Jean-Étienne-Dominique Esquirol:** Porter, *Greatest Benefit*, 502; Bynum, "Chronic Alcoholism," 164, 185.

63 **mental treatments indirectly healed the body:** Eric T. Carlson and Jeffrey L. Wollock, "Benjamin Rush and His Insane Son," *Bulletin of the New York Academy of Medicine* 51, no. 11 (1975): 1326.

63 **only substitutes one level:** Following Daniel Dennett, the psychiatrist Sally Satel and the late psychologist Scott Lilienfeld, two conceptually rigorous critics of the brain disease model, call the idea of addiction as a primary brain disease a form of "greedy reductionism": Sally Satel and Scott O. Lilienfeld, "If Addiction Is Not Best Conceptualized a Brain Disease, Then What Kind of Disease Is It?," *Neuroethics* 10, no. 1 (April 2017): 19–24, https://doi.org/10.1007/s12152-016-9287-2. More generally, see Gregory A. Miller, "Mistreating Psychology in the Decades of the Brain," *Perspectives on Psychological Science* 5, no. 6 (December 2010): 716–43, https://doi.org/10.1177/1745691610388774.

63 **Neuroscience can help to clarify:** Kent C. Berridge, "Is Addiction a Brain Disease?," *Neuroethics* 10, no. 1 (April 2017): 1–5, https://doi.org/10.1007/s12152-016-9286-3; Moore, "Addiction, Responsibility, and Neuroscience."

63 **long and worrying drift:** Lorraine T. Midanik, "Biomedicalization and Alcohol Studies: Implications for Policy," *Journal of Public Health Policy* 25, no. 2 (April 2004): 211–28, https://doi.org/10.1057/palgrave.jphp.3190021; Lorraine T. Midanik, *Biomedicalization of Alcohol Studies: Ideological Shifts and Institutional Challenges* (Piscataway, NJ: Transaction, 2006).

64 **biological explanations increase aversion:** Amy Loughman and Nick Haslam, "Neuroscientific Explanations and the Stigma of Mental Disorder: A Meta-Analytic Study," *Cognitive Research: Principles and Implications* 3, no. 45 (November 2018), https://doi.org/10.1186/s41235-018-0136-1; Erlend P. Kvaale, Nick Haslam, and William H. Gottdiener, "The 'Side-Effects' of Medicalization: A Meta-Analytic Review of How Biogenetic Explanations Affect Stigma," *Clinical Psychology Review* 33, no. 6 (August 2013): 782–94, https://doi.org/10.1016/j.cpr.2013.06.002. Reducing blame: Brett J. Deacon and Grayson L. Baird, "The Chemical Imbalance Explanation of Depression: Reducing Blame at What Cost?," *Journal of Social & Clinical Psychology* 28, no. 4 (April 2009): 415–35, https://doi.org/10.1521/jscp.2009.28.4.415.

64 **"free will":** Nora Volkow, "Addiction Is a Disease of Free Will," *Nora's Blog*, National Institute on Drug Abuse, June 12, 2015, https://archives.drugabuse.gov/about-nida/noras-blog/2015/06/addiction-disease-free-will.

64 **Brühl-Cramer stopped short:** Carl von Brühl-Kramer, *Über die Trunksucht* [. . .] (Berlin, 1819), 21–22, quoted in Bynum, "Chronic Alcoholism," 170.

64 **Rush refused to say:** Benjamin Rush, *Medical Inquiries and Observations upon the Diseases of the Mind*, 5th ed. (Philadelphia, 1835), 358, https://books.google.com/books?id=l-oRAAAAYAAJ&pg=PA358.

64 **John Adams lost his son:** Finan, *Drunks*, 1–2.

65 **"anatomy of the human mind":** Amos A. Evans, letter to Benjamin Rush, June 16, 1809, quoted in Carlson and Wollock, "Benjamin Rush," 1324; Fried, *Rush*, 444.

65 **wrote ruefully to Adams:** Benjamin Rush, letter to John Adams, April 26, 1810, Founders Online, National Archive, https://founders.archives.gov/documents/Adams/99-02-02-5523.

66 **"cell in the Pennsylvania Hospital":** Benjamin Rush, letter to Thomas Jefferson, January 2, 1811, Founders Online, National Archives, https://founders.archives.gov/documents/Jefferson/03-03-02-0203.

66 **"passing before that cannon":** Rush, *Medical Inquiries*, 261–68, https://books.google.com/books?id=l-oRAAAAYAAJ&pg=PA264; Fried, *Rush*, 465–77.

66 **many doctors doubted:** Eric T. Carlson and Meribeth M. Simpson, "Benjamin Rush's Medical Use of the Moral Faculty," *Bulletin of the History of Medicine* 39, no. 1 (January 1965): 22–33, https://www.jstor.org/stable/44447102; Osborn, *Rum Maniacs*, 33–41.

66 **termed *Alcoholismus Chronicus*:** Jean-Charles Sournia, *A History of Alcoholism*, trans. Nicholas Hindley and Gareth Stanton (Cambridge, MA: Basil Blackwell, 1990), 44–50.

67 **"empire of Habit":** Benjamin Rush, letter to John Adams, September 16, 1808, in *Letters of Benjamin Rush*, vol. 2, *1793–1813*, ed. Lyman Henry Butterfield (Princeton, NJ: Princeton University Press, 2019), 977–79.

67 **called "Rush's walk":** Fried, *Rush*, 478; Carlson and Wollock, "Benjamin Rush," 1312.

Chapter Four

74 **a scholar named Zhang Bin:** Edwin Van Bibber-Orr, "Alcoholism and Song Literati," in *Behaving Badly in Early and Medieval China*, ed. N. Harry Rothschild and Leslie V. Wallace (Honolulu: University of Hawai'i Press, 2017), 135.

75 **like an alien spirit:** Robin Room, "The Cultural Framing of Addiction," *Janus Head* 6, no. 2 (2003): 226.

75 **an indestructible junkie worm:** Jaime S. Jorquez, "Heroin Use in the Barrio: Solving the Problem of Relapse or Keeping the Tecato Gusano Asleep," *American Journal of Drug and Alcohol Abuse* 10, no. 1 (1984): 63–75, https://doi.org/10.3109/00952998409002656.

75 **a "midbrain mutiny":** Owen Flanagan, "Addiction Doesn't Exist, but It Is Bad for You," *Neuroethics* 10 (2017): 93, https://doi.org/10.1007/s12152-016-9298-z.

75 **Beecher was a zealous believer:** John Kobler, *Ardent Spirits: The Rise and Fall of Prohibition* (New York: Putnam, 1973), 53.

75 **Second Great Awakening:** Frances FitzGerald, *The Evangelicals: The Struggle to Shape America* (New York: Simon & Schuster, 2017), 2–16.

76 **"it shouldn't be so":** *Autobiography, Correspondence, Etc., of Lyman Beecher, D.D.,* vol. 1, ed. Charles Beecher (New York: Harper & Brothers, 1866), 92–124, 176–78, https://play.google.com/books/reader?id =gxEai3oXdKAC&hl=en&pg=GBS.PA92; Jessica Warner, *All or Nothing: A Short History of Abstinence in America* (Toronto: Emblem, 2010), chap. 2.

77 **reached its all-time high:** W. J. Rorabaugh, *The Alcoholic Republic: An American Tradition* (New York: Oxford University Press, 1979), 9, chart 1.2; Warner, *All or Nothing,* 31; Mark Edward Lender and James Kirby Martin, *Drinking in America: A History* (New York: Simon & Schuster, 1987), 35–46; "Total Alcohol Consumption per Capita (Liters of Pure Alcohol, Projected Estimates, 15+ Years of Age)," World Health Organization, Global Health Observatory Data Repository, World Bank Data-Bank (website), accessed February 28, 2021, https://data.worldbank.org/indicator/SH.ALC.PCAP.LI.

77 **"general addiction to hard drinking":** Rorabaugh, *Alcoholic Republic,* chaps. 2 and 6.

77 **fanatical movement for total abstinence:** Christopher Cook, *Alcohol, Addiction, and Christian Ethics* (New York: Cambridge University Press, 2006), 77.

78 **creation of God:** 1 Cor. 5:11, 6:10; Gal. 5:19–21; 1 Tim. 4:4.

78 **excessive use was a sin:** Gregory A. Austin, *Alcohol in Western Society from Antiquity to 1800* (Santa Barbara, CA: ABC-Clio Information Services, 1985), 44, 47–48.

78 **the "good creature of God":** Rorabaugh, *Alcoholic Republic,* 30.

78 **"Moral Inability":** Jonathan Edwards, *A Careful and Strict Enquiry into the Modern Prevailing Notions of That Freedom of the Will* [. . .] (Glasgow, 1790), 37, https://www.google.com/books/edition/A_Careful _and_Strict_Inquiry_Into_the_Mo/xikqAAAAYAAJ.

78 **working all night by candlelight:** Ian R. Tyrrell, *Sobering Up: From Temperance to Prohibition in Antebellum America, 1800–1860* (Westport, CT: Greenwood Press, 1979), 42, 58; Warner, *All or Nothing,* 40; Lyman Beecher, "Address on the Abuse of Spirituous Liquors," *The Panoplist, and Missionary Magazine United,* September 1812, 188–90, https://www.google.com/books/edition/The_Panoplist_and _Missionary_Magazine_Un/RbAPAAAAIAA.

78 **an address on temperance:** Lender and Martin, *Drinking in America,* 66–67.

78 **preachers per person:** Louis Menand, *The Metaphysical Club* (New York: Farrar, Straus and Giroux, 2001), 80.

79 **eagerly quoting Rush:** Joseph Michael Gabriel, "Gods and Monsters: Drugs, Addiction, and the Origin of Narcotic Control in the Nineteenth-Century Urban North" (PhD diss., Rutgers University, 2006), 114.

79 ***Six Sermons:*** Lyman Beecher, *Six Sermons* [. . .] (Boston, 1827), https://www.google.com/books/edition /Six_Sermons_on_the_Nature_Occasions_Sign/CmpgIP2W5lIC; Lyman Beecher, *Autobiography,* vol. 2 (New York, 1865), 78. While several secondary sources claim he gave the sermons in 1825, the historical record is muddled. Jack S. Blocker, *American Temperance Movements: Cycles of Reform* (Boston: Twayne, 1989), 22–23.

79 **uniquely dangerous, unlike beer:** Rorabaugh, *The Alcoholic Republic,* 101–2.

80 **"cries are hushed in death":** Beecher, *Six Sermons,* 105.

80 **poisoning, diseasing, or invading entity:** Elaine Frantz Parsons, *Manhood Lost: Fallen Drunkards and Redeeming Women in the Nineteenth-Century United States* (Baltimore: Johns Hopkins University Press, 2003), loc. 1510–14 of 3566, Kindle.

80 **"insatiable desire," a "moral ruin":** Beecher, *Six Sermons,* 8, 26.

80 **"marked with blood":** John Marsh, *Putnam and the Wolf* [. . .] (Hartford, CT, 1830), 10–11, https:// books.google.com/books?id=DvYoAAAAYAAJ&pg=PA10. "Satan is in Eden. And if no check is put to the ravages of the demon, our benevolent institutions must die, our sanctuaries be forsaken, our beautiful fields be wastes."

81 **"pharmacological determinism":** Craig Reinarman and Harry G. Levine, "Crack in Context: Politics and Media in the Making of a Drug Scare," *Contemporary Drug Problems* 16, no. 4 (Winter 1989): 535–77. See also Bruce K. Alexander and Linda S. Wong, "The Myth of Drug-Induced Addiction," BruceKAlexander.com, last updated June 2010, https://www.brucekalexander.com/articles-speeches /demon-drug-myths/164-myth-drug-induced.

81 **demons manufacturing casks:** George Barrell Cheever, *The Dream, or The True History of Deacon Giles' Distillery* [. . .] (New York, 1848), 18, https://www.google.com/books/edition/The_Dream_Or |_The_True_History_of_Deacon/CTMMAQAAMAAJ.

81 **more than two million people:** Lender and Martin, *Drinking in America,* 71; Kobler, *Ardent Spirits,* 56; Blocker, *American Temperance Movements,* 22–23; Campbell Gibson and Kay Jung, "Historical Census Statistics on Population Totals by Race, 1790 to 1990, and by Hispanic Origin, 1970 to 1990, for Large Cities and Other Urban Places in the United States," U.S. Census Bureau, Population Division

Working Paper no. 76, https://www.census.gov/content/dam/Census/library/working-papers/2005/demo/POP-twps0076.pdf.

81 the "teetotal" movement urged abstinence: Blocker, *American Temperance Movements*, 22–23.

82 dropped by almost half: Rorabaugh, *The Alcoholic Republic*, 223–36.

83 died four days after that: His cause of death is a topic of controversy, but it is highly suspicious for complications of alcohol problems. Edgar Allan Poe, "The Black Cat," in *Tales* (London: Wiley and Putnam, 1845), 38–39; Matthew Warner Osborn, *Rum Maniacs: Alcoholic Insanity in the Early American Republic* (Chicago: University of Chicago Press, 2014), 169–204; David S. Reynolds, "Black Cats and Delirium Tremens: Temperance and the American Renaissance," in *The Serpent in the Cup: Temperance in American Literature* (Amherst: University of Massachusetts Press, 1997), 22–59; J. Gerald Kennedy, "Edgar Allan Poe, 1809–1849: A Brief Biography," in *A Historical Guide to Edgar Allan Poe*, ed. J. Gerald Kennedy (New York: Oxford University Press, 2001), 19–59; Jeffrey Andrew Weinstock, "Introduction: The American Gothic," in *The Cambridge Companion to American Gothic*, ed. Jeffrey Andrew Weinstock (New York: Cambridge University Press, 2017), 4.

83 this "drunkard narrative": Parsons, *Manhood Lost*, loc. 173 of 3566; John Crowley, ed., *Drunkard's Progress: Narratives of Addiction, Despair, and Recovery* (Baltimore: Johns Hopkins University Press, 1999).

84 Whitman later denounced the book: William G. Lulloff, "Franklin Evans; or the Inebriate," in *Walt Whitman: An Encyclopedia*, ed. J. R. LeMaster and Donald D. Kummings (New York: Garland, 1998), reproduced with permission at https://whitmanarchive.org/criticism/current/encyclopedia/entry_81.html.

84 Herman Melville won praise: Herman Melville, *White-Jacket; or, The World in a Man-of-War* (Boston, 1850), 166, https://www.google.com/books/edition/White_jacket_Or_The_World_in_a_Man_of_wa/fzI2AQAAMAAJ.

84 *Ten Nights in a Bar-Room*: T. S. Arthur, "The Experience Meeting," in Crowley, *Drunkard's Progress*, 29; Janet Chrzan, *Alcohol: Social Drinking in Cultural Context* (New York: Routledge, 2013), 75–76.

84 the horrors of delirium tremens: Osborn, "The Pursuit of Happiness," in *Rum Maniacs*, 147–84.

84 12 percent of American novels: James D. Hart, *The Popular Book: A History of America's Literary Taste* (New York: Oxford University Press, 1950), 108.

84 bemoaning the "hackneyed" stories: *Knickerbocker, or New York Monthly Magazine*, May 1837, 512, cited in Elizabeth Ann Salem, "Gendered Bodies and Nervous Minds: Creating Addiction in America, 1770–1910" (PhD diss., Case Western Reserve University, 2016), 89.

85 inherently and irresistibly dangerous: Alexander and Wong, "Myth of Drug-Induced Addiction"; Harry Gene Levine, "The Alcohol Problem in America: From Temperance to Alcoholism," *British Journal of Addiction* 79, no. 1 (March 1984): 109–19, https://doi.org/10.1111/j.1360-0443.1984.tb00252.x.

85 why did this keep happening: William Cope Moyers, *Broken: My Story of Addiction and Redemption* (New York: Penguin, 2006), 1–4, 300.

85 son's brain had been "hijacked": Moyers, *Broken*, 80; "Portrait of Addiction," BillMoyers.com, March 29, 1998, https://billmoyers.com/content/moyers-on-addiction-close-to-home/; Christopher S. Wren, "Celebrity's Son: Big Connections and Addictions; Ordeal of Moyers Family Underlies a TV Documentary," *New York Times*, March 20, 1998, B1, https://www.nytimes.com/1998/03/20/nyregion/celebrity-s-son-big-connections-addictions-ordeal-moyers-family-underlies-tv.html.

86 "usurp" the "pleasure circuit": *Moyers on Addiction: Close to Home*: episode 1, "Portrait of Addiction," produced by Amy Schatz and Bill D. Moyers; episode 2, "The Hijacked Brain," produced by Gail Pellett and Bill Moyers; both aired March 29, 1998, on PBS, https://billmoyers.com/content/moyers-on-addiction-close-to-home/.

86 the "pleasure center": Kent C. Berridge and Morten L. Kringelbach, "Pleasure Systems in the Brain," *Neuron* 86, no. 3 (May 2015): 646–64, https://dx.doi.org/10.1016%2Fj.neuron.2015.02.018. See also Adam Alter's account of these studies, for which he did some primary research with Olds's students: *Irresistible: The Rise of Addictive Technology and the Business of Keeping Us Hooked* (New York: Penguin, 2017), 56, 328.

86 button up to 1,500 times: R. G. Heath, "Pleasure and Brain Activity in Man: Deep and Surface Electroencephalograms during Orgasm," *Journal of Nervous and Mental Disease* 154, no. 1 (January 1972): 3–18, https://doi.org/10.1097/00005053-197201000-00002.

86 wasn't well recognized: "Conversation with Conan Kornetsky," interview, *Addiction* 98, no. 7 (July 2003): 875–82, https://doi.org/10.1046/j.1360-0443.2003.00423.x.

87 but researchers doubted: Charles A. Marsden, "Dopamine: The Rewarding Years," *British Journal of Pharmacology* 147, no. 51 (February 2009): S136–44, https://doi.org/10.1038/sj.bjp.0706473.

87 **a provocative hypothesis:** Robert A. Yokel and Roy A. Wise, "Increased Lever Pressing for Amphetamine after Pimozide in Rats: Implications for a Dopamine Theory of Reward," *Science* 187, no. 4187 (February 1975): 547–49, https://doi.org/10.1126/science.1114313; Roy A. Wise, "The Dopamine Synapse and the Notion of 'Pleasure Centers' in the Brain," *Trends in Neuroscience* 3, no. 4 (April 1980): 91–95, https://doi.org/10.1016/0166-2236(80)90035-1; Kent C. Berridge and Terry E. Robinson, "What Is the Role of Dopamine in Reward: Hedonic Impact, Reward Learning, or Incentive Salience?," *Brain Research Reviews* 28, no. 3 (December 1998): 309–69, https://doi.org/10.1016/S0165-0173(98)00019-8.

87 **crack cocaine sparked:** Craig Reinarman and Harry G. Levine, eds., *Crack in America: Demon Drugs and Social Justice* (Berkeley: University of California Press, 1997), chaps. 1–2.

87 **purchased crack on camera:** Reinarman and Levine, *Crack in America*, 20; Jacob V. Lamar Jr., "Rolling Out the Big Guns," *Time*, September 22, 1986, http://content.time.com/time/subscriber/article /0,33009,962371,00.html.

88 **violent competition for market share:** David Farber, *Crack: Rock Cocaine, Street Capitalism, and the Decade of Greed* (New York: Cambridge University Press, 2019); Roland G. Fryer et al., "Measuring Crack Cocaine and Its Impact," *Economic Inquiry* 51, no. 3 (July 2013): 1651–81, https://doi.org/10.1111 /j.1465-7295.2012.00506.x; Eric C. Schneider, *Smack: Heroin and the American City* (Philadelphia: University of Pennsylvania Press, 2013), 193–94.

88 **most crack users were white:** National Institute on Drug Abuse, *National Household Survey on Drug Abuse: Main Findings, 1988*, DHHS Publication No. 90-1681 (Rockville, MD: Department of Health and Human Services, 1990), 50. See also Marsha Lillie-Blanton, James C. Anthony, and Charles R. Schuster, "Probing the Meaning of Racial/Ethnic Group Comparisons in Crack Cocaine Smoking," *JAMA* 269, no. 8 (January 1993): 993–97, https://doi.org/10.1001/jama.1993.03500080041029.

88 **series of high-profile articles:** Peter Kerr, "Crack Addiction Spreads among the Middle Class," *New York Times*, June 8, 1986, https://www.nytimes.com/1986/06/08/nyregion/crack-addiction-spreads -among-the-middle-class.html; Tessa Melvin, "Hearing Called to Explore Use of 'Crack' by Teen-Agers," *New York Times*, April 27, 1986, https://www.nytimes.com/1986/04/27/nyregion/hearing -called-to-explore-use-of-crack-by-teen-agers.html; Peter Kerr, "Extra-Potent Cocaine: Use Rising Sharply among Teen-Agers," *New York Times*, March 20, 1986, https://www.nytimes.com/1986/03/20 /nyregion/extra-potent-cocaine-use-rising-sharply-among-teen-agers.html. In a 2018 editorial, *The New York Times* apologized for its coverage of crack and its demonization of Black women with reports drawing on shoddy science about "crack babies": "Slandering the Unborn," editorial, *New York Times*, December 28, 2018, https://www.nytimes.com/interactive/2018/12/28/opinion/crack-babies -racism.html.

88 **"almost instantaneous addiction":** Arnold Washton, quoted in "Kids and Cocaine: An Epidemic Strikes Middle America," *Newsweek*, March 17, 1986, 58–65.

88 **"intense and unrelenting drug hunger":** Mark S. Gold, *800-Cocaine* (New York: Bantam, 1984), 78.

89 **"prefer that she try heroin":** Gina Kolata, "Drug Researchers Try to Treat a Nearly Unbreakable Habit," *New York Times*, June 25, 1988, https://www.nytimes.com/1988/06/25/nyregion/drug -researchers-try-to-treat-a-nearly-unbreakable-habit.html.

89 **dopamine only grew:** As early as 1988, the popular press was starting to describe in more detail how this elusive pleasure center was the brain area called the nucleus accumbens, the "hotspot" of drug activity and a brain area closely associated with dopamine. "Addiction Clue: Just Say Dopamine," *Science News*, July 30, 1988, https://www.sciencenews.org/archive/addiction-clue-just-say-dopamine.

89 **addictive drugs release dopamine:** G. Di Chiara and A. Imperato, "Drugs Abused by Humans Preferentially Increase Synaptic Dopamine Concentrations in the Mesolimbic System of Freely Moving Rats," *Proceedings of the National Academy of Sciences* 85, no. 14 (July 1988): 5274–78, https://doi.org /10.1073/pnas.85.14.5274; David J. Nutt et al., "The Dopamine Theory of Addiction: 40 Years of Highs and Lows," *Nature Reviews Neuroscience* 16, no. 5 (May 2015): 305–12, https://doi.org/10.1038/nrn3939.

89 **"hijacking a natural reward system":** J. Madeleine Nash, "Addicted: Why Do People Get Hooked?," *Time*, May 5, 1997, http://content.time.com/time/magazine/article/0,9171,986282,00.html; and for more on Volkow, see David Courtwright, *The Age of Addiction: How Bad Habits Became Big Business* (Cambridge, MA: Harvard University Press, 2019), 165.

89 **"hijacking" metaphor is omnipresent:** "Biology of Addiction: Drugs and Alcohol Can Hijack Your Brain," *NIH News in Health*, October 2015, https://newsinhealth.nih.gov/2015/10/biology-addiction; Howard J. Shaffer, "What Is Addiction?," *Harvard Health Blog*, June 19, 2017, https://www.health .harvard.edu/blog/what-is-addiction-2-2017061914490; Cynthia M. Kuhn and Wilkie A. Wilson, "How Addiction Hijacks Our Reward System," *Cerebrum* (blog), Dana Foundation, April 1, 2005, https:// www.dana.org/article/how-addiction-hijacks-our-reward-system/; "Addiction: The Hijacker, Episode

1," Addiction Policy Forum, posted July 17, 2018, YouTube video, 3:17, https://www.youtube.com /watch?v=MbOAKmzKmJo.

89 **"reboot the brain":** Chris Stokel-Walker, "Is 'Dopamine Fasting' Silicon Valley's New Productivity Fad?," *BBC*, November 19, 2019, https://www.bbc.com/worklife/article/20191115-what-is-dopamine-fasting.

90 **Wise retracted his hypothesis:** Ingrid Wickelgren, "Getting the Brain's Attention," *Science* 278, no. 5335 (October 1997): 35–37, https://doi.org/10.1126/science.278.5335.35; Berridge and Kringelbach, "Pleasure Systems in the Brain," 656–57. Specifically, the experiments showed that disrupting dopamine pathways didn't actually interfere with the experience of pleasure. Wise was quoted as saying, "I no longer believe that the amount of pleasure felt is proportional to the amount of dopamine floating around in the brain."

90 **cannabis and opioids do not:** Nutt et al., "Dopamine Theory," 307. Nutt also discusses several studies strongly challenging the notion that dopamine release is central to the rewarding effects of opioids, though it bears noting that there is one recent study showing significant dopamine release in the ventral striatum after morphine administration. Primavera A. Spagnolo et al., "Striatal Dopamine Release in Response to Morphine: A [11C]Raclopride Positron Emission Tomography Study in Healthy Men," *Biological Psychiatry* 86, no. 5 (September 2019): 356–64, https://doi.org/10.1016/j.biopsych.2019.03.965.

90 **have such a special power:** Kenneth W. Tupper, "Psychoactive Substances and the English Language: 'Drugs,' Discourses, and Public Policy," *Contemporary Drug Problems* 39, no. 3 (September 2012): 462–92, https://doi.org/10.1177/009145091203900306.

90 **do not develop significant problems:** Discussed at length in Carl L. Hart, *Drug Use for Grown-Ups: Chasing Liberty in the Land of Fear* (New York: Penguin Press, 2021), 11.

90 **Beecher spun medical stories:** Beecher, *Six Sermons*, 12–14.

91 **alcohol is a poison:** Thomas R. Pegram, *Battling Demon Rum: The Struggle for a Dry America, 1800–1933* (Chicago: Ivan R. Dee Press, 1998), loc. 774–76 of 2089, Kindle; David Hanson, "Scientific Temperance Instruction: Temperance Teachings," Alcohol Problems and Solutions (website), accessed February 11, 2021, https://www.alcoholproblemsandsolutions.org/scientific-temperance-instruction -temperance-teachings/; Parsons, *Manhood Lost*, loc. 154 of 3566.

91 **a time of escalating fears:** Osama bin Laden, interview by Peter Arnett, "Osama bin Laden Declares Jihad in 1997 in CNN Interview," CNN, posted May 2, 2011, YouTube video, 1:23, https://www .youtube.com/watch?v=orawG7vt68o; Susan Michelle Gerling, "Louisiana's New 'Kill the Carjacker' Statute: Self-Defense or Instant Injustice?," *Journal of Urban and Contemporary Law* 55, no. 1 (January 1999): 109–34.

92 **a growth in inequality:** Anne Case and Angus Deaton, *Deaths of Despair and the Future of Capitalism* (Princeton, NJ: Princeton University Press, 2020), 1–16.

92 **"free will becomes hijacked":** Beth Macy, *Dopesick: Dealers, Doctors, and the Drug Company That Addicted America* (New York: Little, Brown, 2018), 113.

92 **primordial fish-human:** Nash, "Addicted."

92 **"intemperate will soon be dead":** Justin Edwards, letter to William Allen Hallock, in William Allen Hallock, *Light and Love: A Sketch of the Life and Labors of the Rev. Justin Edwards* (New York, 1855), 195, https://books.google.com/books?id=ObpEAAAAIAAJ.

93 **"all a parcel of hypocrites":** American Temperance Union, "Sixth Annual Report," in *Permanent Temperance Documents*, vol. 2 (New York, 1853), 332, https://www.google.com/books/edition/Permanent _Temperance_Documents_Annual_re/DNsXAAAAYAAJ.

93 **describing their own problems:** Milton A. Maxwell, "The Washingtonian Movement," *Quarterly Journal of Studies on Alcohol* 11, no. 3 (1950): 410–51, https://doi.org/10.15288/qjsa.1950.11.410; Christopher M. Finan, *Drunks: An American History* (Boston: Beacon Press, 2017), chap. 2; A Member of the Society, *Foundation, Progress and Principles of the Washington Temperance Society* [. . .] (Baltimore, 1842), https:// www.google.com/books/edition/The_Foundation_Progress_and_Principles_o/iS1CAQAAMAAJ; David Harrisson Jr., *A Voice from the Washingtonian Home* [. . .] (Boston, 1860), https://babel.hathitrust .org/cgi/pt?id=pst.000052997631&view=1up&seq=9; T. S. Arthur, *Six Nights with the Washingtonians: A Series of Temperance Tales* (Philadelphia, 1843), https://babel.hathitrust.org/cgi/pt?id=hvd.32044051143683 &view=1up&seq=9; John Marsh, *Hannah Hawkins, the Reformed Drunkard's Daughter* (New York, 1844), https://play.google.com/books/reader?id=vA0qAAAAYAAJ.

93 **The Washingtonians' egalitarian leanings:** Finan, *Drunks*, 37–39.

93 **"Martha Washingtonian" meetings:** Gabriel, "Gods and Monsters," 132.

93 **women in the temperance movement:** Michelle L. McClellan, *Lady Lushes: Gender, Alcoholism, and Medicine in Modern America* (New Brunswick, NJ: Rutgers University Press, 2017), 41–42.

94 they reported millions: Blocker, *American Temperance Movements*, 41; Tyrrell, *Sobering Up*, 166.

94 "a new era": Arthur, *Six Nights*, 43.

94 young Abraham Lincoln: Abraham Lincoln, "Temperance Address Delivered before the Springfield Washington Temperance Society, on the 22nd February, 1842," in *Collected Works of Abraham Lincoln*, vol. 1, ed. Roy P. Balser (New Brunswick, NJ: Rutgers University Press, 1953; Ann Arbor, MI: Text Creation Partnership, 2011), 271–79.

94 "exerted a moral power": John B. Gough, *An Autobiography* [. . .], in Crowley, *Drunkard's Progress*, 158.

94 "Try it—Try it": William George Hawkins, *Life of John H. W. Hawkins* (Boston, 1862), 90–92, https:// babel.hathitrust.org/cgi/pt?id=uc2.ark:/13960/t7fq9t07q&view=1up&seq=9.

94 "Drunken devils are cast out": Lincoln, "Temperance Address," in *Collected Works*, 271–76.

95 They banned prayers: Crowley, introduction to *Drunkard's Progress*, 6.

95 they held sober concerts: Tyrrell, *Sobering Up*, 176.

95 "grand blow out at night": [Walt Whitman], "Temperance among the Firemen!," *New York Aurora*, March 30, 1842, in *Walt Whitman, the Journalism*, vol. 1, *1834–1846*, ed. Herbert Bergman, Douglas A. Noverr, and Edward J. Recchia (New York: Peter Lang, 1998), https://whitmanarchive.org/published /periodical/journalism/tei/per.00420.xml; Reynolds, "Black Cats," 48.

95 the "master passion" of drink: Gough, *An Autobiography*, 136–40.

96 "narration of horrible 'experiences'": Reynolds, "Black Cats," 26.

96 John Gough had multiple relapses: Crowley, *Drunkard's Progress*, 15.

96 "fetters the immortal mind": "Evils of Intemperance," *Sailors' Magazine*, October 1842, 301, https:// www.google.com/books/edition/The_Pilot_or_Sailors_magazine_Continued/6DoEAAAAQAAJ.

96 The Washingtonians collapsed: William L. White, *Slaying the Dragon: The History of Addiction Treatment and Recovery in America*, 2nd ed. (Chicago: Lighthouse Institute, 2014), 19.

97 What could we expect: Reynolds, "Black Cats," 31; Finan, *Drunks*, 51; Parsons, *Manhood Lost*, loc. 660–61 of 3566.

97 other mutual-help organizations: Finan, *Drunks*, 49; Maxwell, "Washingtonian Movement," 439–40.

Chapter Five

98 opium was a commonplace: Louise Foxcroft, *The Making of Addiction: The "Use and Abuse" of Opium in Nineteenth Century Britain* (Burlington, VT: Ashgate, 2007), 10–26. It's possible De Quincey suffered from trigeminal neuralgia, an excruciating, chronic disorder of one of the major facial nerves. Thomas De Quincey, *Confessions of an English Opium-Eater* (London, 1821), 73, 115, https://archive .org/details/confessionsanen04quingoog.

99 overshadowed by the psychic: De Quincey, *Opium-Eater*, 74.

99 "teeming with power and beauty": Thomas De Quincey, "Samuel Taylor Coleridge, by the English Opium-Eater," in *The Works of Thomas De Quincey, Part II*, vol. 10, ed. Grevel Lindop and Barry Symonds (New York: Routledge, 2016), 287.

99 he could see the intricate harmonies: De Quincey, *Opium-Eater*, 85.

99 soon reached astronomical levels: De Quincey, *Opium-Eater*, 104, 140; Virginia Berridge, *Opium and the People*, rev. ed. (New York: Free Association Books, 1999), 51; 24 Fed. Reg. 5348 (July 1, 1959); Food and Drug Administration, *Highlights of Prescribing Information: Morphine Sulfate Tablets, CII* (Washington, DC: Food and Drug Administration, 2012), https://www.accessdata.fda.gov/drugsatfda_docs/label /2012/022207s004lbl.pdf; "Opioid Oral Morphine Milligram Equivalent (MME) Conversion Factors," Centers for Medicare & Medicaid Services, February 2018, https://www.cms.gov/Medicare/Prescription -Drug-Coverage/PrescriptionDrugCovContra/Downloads/Oral-MME-CFs-vFeb-2018.pdf.

99 "one general discourtesy of silence": Thomas De Quincy, letter to William Blackwood, 1820, quoted in Colin Dickey, "The Addicted Life of Thomas De Quincey," *Lapham's Quarterly*, March 19, 2013, https://www.laphamsquarterly.org/roundtable/addicted-life-thomas-de-quincey.

100 a true landmark: Marcus Boon, *The Road of Excess: A History of Writers on Drugs* (Cambridge, MA: Harvard University Press, 2005), 13.

100 "Pains of Opium": De Quincey, *Opium-Eater*, 80, 104, 118.

100 "Lies! Lies! Lies!": De Quincey, *Opium-Eater*, 76.

101 "god within": John O'Brien, *Alexander the Great: The Invisible Enemy* (New York: Routledge, 1992), 1–15. It is from that word that "entheogen" was derived in the mid-twentieth century by proponents of LSD and psilocybin.

101 celebrate imagination, subjectivity, and feeling: Martin Booth, *Opium: A History* (New York: Thomas Dunne, 1996), 35; Foxcroft, *Making of Addiction*, 17; Joseph Michael Gabriel, "Gods and Monsters:

Drugs, Addiction, and the Origin of Narcotic Control in the Nineteenth-Century Urban North" (PhD diss., Rutgers University, 2006), 176, 190–99.

102 **shake off the limitations:** Susan Zieger, *Inventing the Addict* (Amherst, MA: University of Massachusetts Press, 2008), 36.

102 **list of British Romantic figures:** Booth, *Opium*, 46.

102 **not blind to the dangers:** Wilkie Collins, *The Moonstone* (Oxford, 1868), 184, https://www.google .com/books/edition/The_moonstone/FmsOAAAAQAAJ.

102 **"sunless sea":** Samuel Taylor Coleridge, *Kubla Khan*, st. 1, line 5; Boon, *Road of Excess*, 21.

102 **a "dread agent":** De Quincey, *Opium-Eater*, 73, 105–10, 137.

102 **a "double game":** Mike Jay, "The Pope of Opium," *London Review of Books*, May 13, 2010, https:// www.lrb.co.uk/the-paper/v32/n09/mike-jay/drink-it-don-t-eat-it-or-smoke-it.

103 **"no man is likely":** Thomas De Quincey, quoted in H. A. Page, *Thomas De Quincey: His Life and Writings, with Unpublished Correspondence*, vol. 2 (London, 1879), 273.

103 **"always neglected to read":** William Blair, "An Opium-Eater in America," *Knickerbocker, or New-York Monthly Magazine*, July 1842, 49, https://www.google.com/books/edition/The_Knickerbocker /L60RAAAAYAAJ.

103 **manly or sophisticated achievement:** Jack London, *John Barleycorn* (New York: Century, 1913), 49, https://www.google.com/books/edition/_/cEnmTtCi9cYC; Charles Jackson, *The Lost Weekend* (1944; New York: Vintage, 2013), 16. See also Owen Flanagan, "Identity and Addiction: What Alcoholic Memoirs Teach," in *The Oxford Handbook of Philosophy and Psychiatry* (New York: Oxford University Press, 2013), 865–88.

103 **an early introduction to cannabis:** Peter Andreas, *Killer High: A History of War in Six Drugs* (New York: Oxford University Press, 2020), chap. 2; David T. Courtwright, *Forces of Habit: Drugs and the Making of the Modern World* (Cambridge, MA: Harvard University Press, 2001), chap. 2; William A. Emboden Jr., "Ritual Use of *Cannabis sativa* L.: A Historical-Ethnographic Survey," in *Flesh of the Gods*, ed. Peter T. Furst (Prospect Heights, IL: Waveland Press, 1990), 214–36.

104 **his own experiences with hashish:** Boon, *Road of Excess*, 45.

104 **writers called the Decadents:** Boon, *Road of Excess*, 51–53.

104 **artistic groups incorporating drug use:** Meyer Berger, "Tea for a Viper," *New Yorker*, March 5, 1938.

104 **"not just an odd dosing regimen":** Owen Flanagan, "Addiction Doesn't Exist, but It Is Bad for You," *Neuroethics* 10 (2017): 98, https://doi.org/10.1007/s12152-016-9298-z.

104 **heroin's popularity among jazz musicians:** Red Rodney, quoted in Jill Jonnes, *Hep-Cats, Narcs, and Pipe Dreams: A History of America's Romance with Illegal Drugs* (Baltimore: Johns Hopkins University Press, 1999).

105 **Even William Burroughs warned:** William S. Burroughs, interview, in David T. Courtwright, Herman Joseph, and Don Des Jarlais, *Addicts Who Survived: An Oral History of Narcotic Use in America before 1965* (Knoxville: University of Tennessee Press, 2012), 276.

105 **One of his biographers:** Richard Holmes, "De Quincey: So Original, So Truly Weird," *New York Review of Books*, November 24, 2016, https://www.nybooks.com/articles/2016/11/24/de-quincey-so -original-so-truly-weird/.

105 **masked a devastating reality:** Booth, *Opium*, 39.

108 **"books, ill health, and musing":** Fitz Hugh Ludlow, *The Hasheesh Eater: Being Passages from the Life of a Pythagorean* (New York, 1857), 62, https://archive.org/details/66640730R.nlm.nih.gov/page/n65 /mode/2up. For more on Ludlow's life, see Dave Gross, "A Brief Biography of Fitz Hugh Ludlow," Lycaeum (website), archived September 18, 2015, https://web.archive.org/web/20150918165744/http:// www.lycaeum.org/nepenthes/Ludlow/THE/Biography/biography.html; Timothy A. Hickman, *The Secret Leprosy of Modern Days: Narcotic Addiction and Cultural Crisis in the United States, 1870–1920* (Amherst: University of Massachusetts Press, 2007), 25–32.

108 **"every strange drug and chemical":** Ludlow, *Hasheesh Eater*, 16.

108 **"a blush of exquisite languor":** Fitz Hugh Ludlow, "The Apocalypse of Hasheesh," *Putnam's Monthly*, December 1856, https://web.archive.org/web/20140503090034/http:/www.lycaeum.org/nepenthes/Ludlow /Texts/apocalyp.html.

108 **"storm-wrapped peaks of sublimity":** Ludlow, *Hasheesh Eater*, ix–x.

109 **"horrible mental bondage":** Fitz Hugh Ludlow, "What Shall They Do to Be Saved?," *Harper's New Monthly Magazine*, August 1867, 377–87; Gross, "Brief Biography."

109 **"any other chronic disease":** Fitz Hugh Ludlow, letter to the editor, *Harper's New Monthly Magazine*, August 1870, 458, https://www.google.com/books/edition/Harper_s_New_Monthly_Magazine /xkhGAAAAcAAJ.

110 "this species of intemperance": "Confessions of an English Opium-Eater," *North American Review*, January 1824, 92, https://www.google.com/books/edition/The_North_American_Review /haJKAAAAcAAJ.

110 most significant was morphine: H. Wayne Morgan, *Drugs in America: A Social History, 1800–1980* (Syracuse, NY: Syracuse University Press), 11–27. Opium contains several naturally occurring psychoactive opioids, the most abundant of which is morphine, first isolated in the 1800s but not mass-produced until 1827, by Heinrich Emanuel Merck, who turned his family's apothecary shop into what eventually became the enormous pharmaceutical dynasty.

110 mainstream doctors distinguished themselves: Paul Starr, *The Social Transformation of American Medicine: The Rise of a Sovereign Profession and the Making of a Vast Industry* (New York: Basic Books, 1982), 47, 65, 96–108; Berridge, *Opium and the People*, 64.

110 Developed in Britain: Hickman, *Secret Leprosy*, 38.

110 The hypodermic needle was professional: Berridge, *Opium and the People*, 135–42.

111 company introduced OxyContin: Anne Case and Angus Deaton, *Deaths of Despair and the Future of Capitalism* (Princeton, NJ: Princeton University Press, 2020), 117.

111 opioid addiction increased sixfold: David T. Courtwright, *Dark Paradise: A History of Opiate Addiction in America* (Cambridge, MA: Harvard University Press, 2001), 9. It is always debatable whether we can diagnose people in the past with "addiction," but Courtwright had a rigorous methodology, which he describes in his chapter 1. See also Courtwright, *Forces of Habit*, 36–37.

111 "temporary relief from their sufferings": Horace B. Day, *The Opium Habit* [. . .] (New York, 1868), 7, https://quod.lib.umich.edu/m/moa/AEU2766.0001.001.

112 called "the army disease": Jonathan S. Jones, "Then and Now: How Civil War-Era Doctors Responded to Their Own Opiate Epidemic," *Civil War Monitor*, November 3, 2017, https://www.civilwarmonitor .com/blog/then-and-now-how-civil-war-era-doctors-responded-to-their-own-opiate-epidemic; David T. Courtwright, "Opiate Addiction as a Consequence of the Civil War," *Civil War History* 24, no. 2 (June 1978), 101–11, https://doi.org/10.1353/cwh.1978.0039.

112 the epidemic was already developing: Mark A. Quinones, "Drug Abuse during the Civil War (1861–1865)," *International Journal of the Addictions* 10, no. 6 (1975), https://doi.org/10.3109/10826087509028357.

112 *Scientific American* also warned: Gabriel, "Gods and Monsters," 210.

112 "frightful endemic demoralization": Oliver Wendell Holmes Sr., *Currents and Counter-Currents in Medical Science* [. . .] (Boston, 1860), 35, https://www.google.com/books/edition/Currents_and_Counter _currents_in_Medical/XaYrAQAAMAAJ.

112 the "pernicious habit": Day, *The Opium Habit*, 5, 7.

112 injected morphine was entirely safe: Morgan, *Drugs in America*, 22–27.

112 honeymoon period of uncritical use: William White has his own framework of dormancy, hibernation, and cyclical reemergence: William L. White and Randall Webber, "Substance Use Trends: History and Principles," *Counselor* 4, no. 3 (2003): 18–20.

113 large and desperate market: Joseph F. Spillane, *Cocaine: From Medical Marvel to Modern Menace in the United States, 1884–1920* (Baltimore: Johns Hopkins University Press, 2000), 8–22, 84–86; Courtwright, *Forces of Habit*, 47.

113 two more pounds?: W. H. Bentley, "*Erythoxylon coca*," *Chicago Medical Times* 12, no. 10 (January 1881): 504–5, https://books.google.com/books?id=4ZavVd0VBfQC&pg=PA504; W. H. Bentley, "*Erythoxylon coca*," *Therapeutic Gazette* 1, no. 12 (December 1880): 350–51, https://books.google.com /books?id=RHVMAQAAMAAJ&pg=PA350.

113 specialized treatment centers for addiction: William L. White, *Slaying the Dragon: The History of Addiction Treatment and Recovery in America*, 2nd ed. (Chicago: Lighthouse Institute, 2014), 31–33.

114 the Cure of Inebriates: Sarah W. Tracy, *Alcoholism in America: From Reconstruction to Prohibition* (Baltimore: Johns Hopkins University Press, 2005), 28–40; White, *Slaying the Dragon*, 31; John W. Crowley and William L. White, *Drunkard's Refuge: The Lessons of the New York State Inebriate Asylum* (Amherst: University of Massachusetts Press, 2004); Arnold Jaffe, *Addiction Reform in the Progressive Age: Scientific and Social Responses to Drug Dependence in the United States, 1870–1930* (Lexington: University of Kentucky Press, 1976); Mariana Valverde, *Diseases of the Will: Alcohol and the Dilemmas of Freedom* (New York: Cambridge University Press, 1998); Christopher M. Finan, *Drunks: An American History* (Boston: Beacon Press, 2017), 80–83.

114 its own eighteen-page chapter: Roberts Bartholow, *The Treatment of Diseases by the Hypodermatic Method* (Philadelphia, 1879), 6, 90–107, https://books.google.com/books?id=oyvePAtztLsC.

114 morphine use as a disease: Berridge, *Opium and the People*, 142.

114 **New York State Inebriate Asylum:** Crowley and White, *Drunkard's Refuge*, 29–39; Finan, *Drunks*, 72–77; Jaffe, *Addiction Reform*, 27.

115 **emphasized non-medical means:** Jim Baumohl, "Inebriate Institutions in North America, 1840–1920," *British Journal of Addiction* 85, no. 9 (September 1990): 1187–204, https://doi.org/10.1111/j.1360 -0443.1990.tb03444.x; Jim Baumohl and Robin Room, "Inebriety, Doctors, and the State: Alcoholism Treatment Institutions before 1940," in *Recent Developments in Alcoholism*, vol. 5, ed. Marc Galanter (New York: Springer, 1987), 135–74; Finan, *Drunks*, 50–70.

115 **a grassroots evangelical Christian approach:** Katherine A. Chavigny, "'An Army of Reformed Drunkards and Clergymen': The Medicalization of Habitual Drunkenness, 1857–1910," *Journal of the History of Medicine and Allied Sciences* 69, no. 3 (July 2014): 383–425, https://doi.org/10.1093/jhmas /jrs082.

115 **considerable overlap between these efforts:** White, *Slaying the Dragon*, 62–67. For more on how the phenomenon of drug addiction became a topic of medical and popular discourses, see Zieger, *Inventing the Addict*, 51–60.

117 **"addiction" implies substances:** Carl Erik Fisher, "Food, Sex, Gambling, the Internet: When Is It Addiction?," *Scientific American Mind*, January 2016, https://www.scientificamerican.com/article /food-sex-gambling-the-internet-when-is-it-addiction/; David J. Ley, *The Myth of Sex Addiction* (Lanham, MD: Rowman & Littlefield, 2014).

117 **"miss them when we stop":** Allen Frances, "Behavioral Addictions: A Dangerous and Slippery Slope," *HuffPost*, May 16, 2016, https://www.huffpost.com/entry/behavioral-addictions-a-d_b_9959140; Joël Billieux et al., "Are We Overpathologizing Everyday Life? A Tenable Blueprint for Behavioral Addiction Research," *Journal of Behavioral Addictions* 4, no. 3 (September 2015): 119–23, https://dx.doi.org /10.1556%2F2006.4.2015.009.

117 **cast a wide net:** Tracy, *Alcoholism in America*, 39–40.

117 **addicting properties of other foods:** Adrian Meule, "Back by Popular Demand: A Narrative Review on the History of Food Addiction Research," *Yale Journal of Biology and Medicine* 88, no. 3 (September 2013): 295–302, https://www.ncbi.nlm.nih.gov/pubmed/26339213.

118 **in reference to chocolate:** Barbara Weiner and William White, "The Journal of Inebriety (1876–1914): History, Topical Analysis, and Photographic Images," *Addiction* 102, no. 1 (January 2007): 15–23, https://doi.org/10.1111/j.1360-0443.2006.01680.x.

118 **"disease in the will":** Benjamin Rush, *Medical Inquiries and Observations upon the Diseases of the Mind*, 5th ed. (Philadelphia, 1835), 268; Eric T. Carlson and Meribeth M. Simpson, "Benjamin Rush's Medical Use of the Moral Faculty," *Bulletin of the History of Medicine* 39, no. 1 (January 1965): 22–33.

118 **gambling as a medical problem:** Peter Ferentzy and Nigel E. Turner, *The History of Problem Gambling: Temperance, Substance Abuse, Medicine, and Metaphors* (New York: Springer, 2013), 17.

118 **Sexual behaviors, too:** Andreas De Block and Pieter R. Adriaens, "Pathologizing Sexual Deviance: A History," *Journal of Sex Research* 50, no. 3–4 (March 2013): 276–98, https://doi.org/10.1080 /00224499.2012.738259.

118 **marred by acrimonious infighting:** White, *Slaying the Dragon*, 41–42.

118 **a considerable opium problem:** Berridge, *Opium and the People*, 54; Booth, *Opium*, 42–45; Foxcroft, *Making of Addiction*, 32.

118 **"ACCURSED Habit ignorantly":** Samuel Taylor Coleridge, letter to Joseph Cottle, April 26, 1814, in Day, *Opium Habit*, 150–51; Berridge, *Opium and the People*, 52.

119 **"slavery to opium":** William Rosser Cobbe, *Doctor Judas: A Portrayal of the Opium Habit* (Chicago, 1895), 13, 17, 40; for general discussion of iatrogenic addiction during this time, see Courtwright, *Dark Paradise*, 50–52.

119 **blamed inattentive medical providers:** David Herzberg, *White Market Drugs: Big Pharma and the Hidden History of Addiction in America* (Chicago: University of Chicago Press, 2020), 25.

119 **Industrialization was rocketing forward:** Frances FitzGerald, *The Evangelicals: The Struggle to Shape America* (New York: Simon & Schuster, 2017), 58–59; Hickman, *Secret Leprosy*, 34.

119 **"American disease" of "neurasthenia":** American Association for the Study and Cure of Inebriety, *Proceedings, 1870–1875* (New York: Arno Press, 1981), 52, https://books.google.com/books?id =yXDs45f2S5sC. On Beard's thought, see also Hickman, *Secret Leprosy*, 42; Baumohl, "Inebriate Institutions," 1194.

120 **the root cause of inebriety:** American Association for the Study and Cure of Inebriety, *Proceedings*, 64.

120 **addiction of O'Neill's mother:** Jonnes, *Hep-Cats*, 18. See also Courtwright, *Dark Paradise*, 36.

120 **William Halsted became addicted:** Howard Markel, *An Anatomy of Addiction: Sigmund Freud, William Halsted, and the Miracle Drug, Cocaine* (New York: Vintage, 2011), 4–6.

120 **90 percent of such "habitués":** Barry Milligan, "Morphine-Addicted Doctors, the English Opium-Eater, and Embattled Medical Authority," *Victorian Literature and Culture* 33, no. 2 (September 2005): 541–53, https://doi.org/10.1017/S1060150305050977.

120 **professionals' seduction and fall:** Morgan, *Drugs in America*, 42.

120 **dangerous industrial products:** Herzberg, *White Market Drugs*, 17.

121 **actually undermining those values:** Morgan, *Drugs in America*; Helen Keane, *What's Wrong with Addiction?* (Melbourne: Melbourne University Press, 2002); Gabriel, "Gods and Monsters"; Harry G. Levine, "The Discovery of Addiction: Changing Conceptions of Habitual Drunkenness in America," *Journal of Substance Abuse Treatment* 2, no. 1 (January 1985): 43–57, https://doi.org/10.1016/0740-5472(85)90022-4; Eve Kosofsky Sedgwick, "Epidemics of the Will," in *Tendencies* (Durham, NC: Duke University Press, 1993), 130–42.

121 **only thirty were left standing:** T. D. Crothers, *The Disease of Inebriety* [. . .] (New York, 1893), 24, http://www.williamwhitepapers.com/pr/1893%20The%20Disease%20of%20Inebriety.pdf.

121 **converted to general insane asylums:** Baumohl, "Inebriate Institutions," 1189; White, *Slaying the Dragon*, 40.

121 **anti-vice activism:** David T. Courtwright, "A Short History of Drug Policy or Why We Make War on Some Drugs but Not on Others," *History Faculty Publications*, no. 23 (October 2012), https://digitalcommons.unf.edu/ahis_facpub/23/.

121 ***Drunkenness a Vice, Not a Disease:*** *The Combined Addiction Disease Chronologies of William White, MA, Ernest Kurtz, PhD, and Caroline Acker, PhD* (unpublished study, 2001), 12, http://www.williamwhitepapers.com/pr/2001Addiction%20as%20Disease%20Chronology.pdf.

Chapter Six

122 **pounds of confiscated opium:** John H. Halpern, *Opium: How an Ancient Flower Shaped and Poisoned Our World* (New York: Hachette, 2019), 130–35. For other accounts of the Opium Wars, see Frank Dikötter, Lars Laamann, and Xun Zhou, *Narcotic Culture: A History of Drugs in China* (Chicago: University of Chicago Press, 2004), 42–46; David T. Courtwright, *Forces of Habit: Drugs and the Making of the Modern World* (Cambridge, MA: Harvard University Press, 2001), 32–36.

123 **impoverished and politically destabilized:** Dikötter, Laaman, and Xun, *Narcotic Culture*, 46; Liping Zhu, *A Chinaman's Chance: The Chinese on the Rocky Mountain Mining Frontier* (Niwot: University of Colorado, 1997), 19.

123 **Chinese people collected in "Chinatowns":** Gordon H. Chang and Shelley Fisher Fishkin, eds., *The Chinese and the Iron Road: Building the Transcontinental Railroad* (Palo Alto, CA: Stanford University Press, 2019); Manu Karuka, *Empire's Tracks: Indigenous Nations, Chinese Workers, and the Transcontinental Railroad* (Oakland: University of California Press, 2019); Zhu, *Chinaman's Chance*, 24–25.

123 **Smoking opium helped laborers:** Courtwright, *Forces of Habit*, 135–36; David T. Courtwright, Herman Joseph, and Don Des Jarlais, *Addicts Who Survived: An Oral History of Narcotic Use in America before 1965* (Knoxville: University of Tennessee Press, 2012), 207.

123 **anti-immigrant sentiment grew:** David T. Courtwright, *Dark Paradise: A History of Opiate Addiction in America* (Cambridge, MA: Harvard University Press, 2001), 66; Joseph Michael Gabriel, "Gods and Monsters: Drugs, Addiction, and the Origin of Narcotic Control in the Nineteenth-Century Urban North" (PhD diss., Rutgers University, 2006), 380–85; John Helmer and Thomas Vietorisz, *Drug Use, the Labor Market and Class Conflict* (Washington, DC: Drug Abuse Council, 1974), 10–13, https://files.eric.ed.gov/fulltext/ED108098.pdf.

124 **Stigma is often cited:** German Lopez, "The Single Biggest Reason America Is Failing in Its Response to the Opioid Epidemic," *Vox*, December 18, 2017, https://www.vox.com/science-and-health/2017/12/18/16635910/opioid-epidemic-lessons. It is also common in certain advocacy circles to cite the NSDUH, table 7.67B (combining several categories into one), to say that stigma is the largest reason people with SUD do not seek treatment, but this is contestable. For extensive discussion on this point, see Jason Schwartz, "Reasons for Not Receiving Substance Use Treatment," *Recovery Review* (blog), September 14, 2020, https://recoveryreview.blog/2020/09/14/reasons-for-not-receiving-substance-use-treatment/; Substance Abuse and Mental Health Services Administration, *Key Substance Use and Mental Health Indicators in the United States: Results from the 2019 National Survey on Drug Use and Health* (Washington, DC: Department of Health and Human Services, 2020), table 7.67B, https://www.samhsa.gov/data/report/2019-nsduh-annual-national-report.

124 **a Chinese social club:** Virginia Berridge, *Opium and the People*, rev. ed. (New York: Free Association Books, 1999), 200–2.

125 **returned with stories:** For one such account, see J. J. Acheson, "A Night in an Opium Den," *Centennial Magazine*, April 1890, 668, https://www.google.com/books/edition/The_Centennial_Magazine /H7ICAAAAIAAJ. For Chinatowns being a focus of anti-Chinese fears, see H. Wayne Morgan, *Drugs in America: A Social History, 1800–1980* (Syracuse, NY: Syracuse University Press), 7, 33–35; Courtwright, *Forces of Habit*, 32–33, 135–36, 177; Timothy A. Hickman, *The Secret Leprosy of Modern Days: Narcotic Addiction and Cultural Crisis in the United States, 1870–1920* (Amherst: University of Massachusetts Press, 2007), 29, 61; Doris Marie Provine, *Unequal Under Law: Race in the War on Drugs* (Chicago: University of Chicago Press, 2007), loc. 964 of 2874.

125 **corrupting force of Chinese opium:** Berridge, *Opium and the People*, 196–97; Virginia Berridge, *Demons: Our Changing Attitudes to Alcohol, Tobacco, and Drugs* (New York: Oxford University Press, 2013), 82. Other contemporaneous examples of opium and middle-class corruption include several of the Sherlock Holmes stories and Oscar Wilde's *The Picture of Dorian Gray*.

125 **reformers set about suppressing vices:** Arnold Jaffe, *Addiction Reform in the Progressive Age: Scientific and Social Responses to Drug Dependence in the United States, 1870–1930* (Lexington: University of Kentucky Press, 1976), 46–79.

126 **the "worthy" and "unworthy":** Sarah W. Tracy, *Alcoholism in America: From Reconstruction to Prohibition* (Baltimore: Johns Hopkins University Press, 2005), 20, 68; Michael B. Katz, *The Undeserving Poor: America's Enduring Confrontation with Poverty* (New York: Oxford University, 2013); Alice O'Connor, *Poverty Knowledge: Social Science, Social Policy and the Poor in Twentieth-Century U.S. History* (Princeton, NJ: Princeton University Press, 2001).

127 **contagious form of substance use:** Morgan, *Drugs in America*, 7–8.

127 **Journalists denounced opium smoking:** William Rosser Cobbe, *Doctor Judas: A Portrayal of the Opium Habit* (Chicago, 1895), 125, 133.

127 **merely different ways of using:** David Herzberg, *White Market Drugs: Big Pharma and the Hidden History of Addiction in America* (Chicago: University of Chicago Press, 2020), 17.

128 **opium smoking as a purposeless vice:** William White, "Addiction as a Disease: Birth of a Concept," *Counselor* 1, no. 1 (2000): 46–51, 73, http://www.williamwhitepapers.com/pr/2000HistoryoftheDisease ConceptSeries.pdf; Hickman, *Secret Leprosy*.

128 **opium for smoking was banned:** Herzberg, *White Market Drugs*, 20–21, 32–34.

128 **among New Orleans dockworkers:** Morgan, *Drugs in America*, 92–93.

128 **a relatively benign drug:** Joseph F. Spillane, *Cocaine: From Medical Marvel to Modern Menace in the United States, 1884–1920* (Baltimore: Johns Hopkins University Press, 2000), 18–19, 32, 43–44.

128 **made Black people physically strong:** *Importation and Use of Opium: Hearings Before the Committee on Ways and Means of the House of Representatives on H.R. 25240, H.R. 25241, H.R. 25242, and H.R. 28971*, 61st Cong. 72 (1911) (statement of Dr. Christopher Koch, vice president of the State Pharmaceutical Examining Board of Pennsylvania).

128 **"the cocaine[n——]":** Edward Huntington Williams, "The Drug-Habit Menace in the South," *Medical Record* 85, no. 6 (February 1914): 247–49, https://www.google.com/books/edition/Medical_Record /e20cAQAAMAAJ.

129 **".38 special":** David F. Musto, *The American Disease: Origins of Narcotic Control*, 3rd ed. (New York: Oxford University Press, 1999), 7.

129 **widely manufactured and promoted:** Gabriel, "Gods and Monsters," 438–46; Spillane, *Cocaine*, 32–34, 91–94; Hickman, *Secret Leprosy*, 72.

129 **the southern convict population grew:** Gabriel, "Gods and Monsters," 480. See also Spillane, *Cocaine*, 119–21; Musto, *American Disease*, 5–8; Courtwright, *Dark Paradise*, 96–98; David Courtwright, "The Hidden Epidemic: Opiate Addiction and Cocaine in the South, 1860–1920," *Journal of Southern History* 49, no. 1 (February 1983): 69–71, http://www.ncbi.nlm.nih.gov/pubmed /11614816.

129 **into a "wild frenzy":** "Negro Cocaine Evil," *New York Times*, March 20, 1905, https://timesmachine .nytimes.com/timesmachine/1905/03/20/223718772.pdf.

129 **the most serious drug problem:** S. Doc No. 61-377, at 48 (1910), https://books.google.com/books?id =L_NGAQAAIAAJ; Richard DeGrandpre, *The Cult of Pharmacology* (Durham, NC: Duke University Press, 2006), 132.

129 **Heroin was first widely produced:** David Musto, "Introduction: The Origins of Heroin," in *One Hundred Years of Heroin*, ed. David Musto, Pamela Korsmeyer, and Thomas W. Maulucci Jr. (Westport, CT: Greenwood, 2002), xiii–xv. Heroin was the first widely used semisynthetic opioid. It is formed by attaching two acetyl groups to the morphine molecule to make it more potent and faster-acting, hence its other name, diacetylmorphine.

130 **portrait of heroin addiction:** David Courtwright, "The Roads to H: The Emergence of the American Heroin Complex, 1898–1956," in Musto, Korsmeyer, and Maulucci, *One Hundred Years of Heroin*, 7–8.

130 **non-medical channels like street peddlers:** Herzberg, *White Market Drugs*, 17–18; David Herzberg, "Entitled to Addiction? Pharmaceuticals, Race, and America's First Drug War," *Bulletin of the History of Medicine* 91, no. 3 (Fall 2017): 586–623, https://doi.org/10.1353/bhm.2017.0061.

130 **racist stigma was attached:** Berridge, *Demons*, 71.

130 **the victims of bad drugs:** Beth Macy, interview with Chris Hayes, "On the Frontlines of Opioid Addiction with Beth Macy," *NBC News*, February 11, 2020, https://www.nbcnews.com/think/opinion/frontlines-opioid-addiction-beth-macy-podcast-transcript-ncna1132471; Matthew D. Lassiter, "Impossible Criminals: The Suburban Imperatives of America's War on Drugs," *Journal of American History* 102, no. 1 (June 2015): 126–40, https://doi.org/10.1093/jahist/jav243.

130 **sensationalistic stories of middle-class users:** Harry Hubbell Kane, *Opium-Smoking in America and China: A Study* [. . .] (New York, 1882), 68, https://books.google.com/books?id=sDsZAAAAYAAJ.

133 **first woman convicted for "delivering":** Loren Siegel, "The Pregnancy Police," in Craig Reinarman and Harry G. Levine, eds., *Crack in America: Demon Drugs and Social Justice* (Berkeley: University of California Press, 1997), 249–60; "Mother Sentenced for Giving Babies Cocaine," *UPI*, August 25, 1989, https://www.upi.com/Archives/1989/08/25/Mother-sentenced-for-giving-babies-cocaine/5274620020800/. Johnson's sentence was later overturned: Tamar Lewin, "Mother Cleared of Passing Drug to Babies," *New York Times*, July 24, 1992, https://www.nytimes.com/1992/07/24/news/mother-cleared-of-passing-drug-to-babies.html. She is now an advocate for pregnant women: "NAPW Activist Update: A New President, a New Day—New York," National Advocates for Pregnant Women (website), January 22, 2021, http://www.nationaladvocatesforpregnantwomen.org/napw-activist-update-a-new-president-a-new-day/.

134 **"cocaine babies whose biological inferiority":** Charles Krauthammer, "Children of Cocaine," *Washington Post*, July 30, 1989, https://www.washingtonpost.com/archive/opinions/1989/07/30/children-of-cocaine/41a8b4db-dee2-4906-a686-a8a5720bf52a/. For one important research finding and a discussion of 1990s failures to replicate the original "crack baby" reports, see Gale A. Richardson, Mary L. Conroy, Nancy L. Day, "Prenatal Cocaine Exposure: Effects on the Development of School-Age Children," *Neurotoxicology and Teratology* 18, no. 6 (November–December 1996): 627–34, https://doi.org/10.1016/S0892-0362(96)00121-3.

134 **droves of "mentally useless children":** Berridge, *Demons*, 64.

134 **"must be an habitual drunkard":** Francis Galton, "Of the Causes Which Operate to Create Scientific Men," *Fortnightly Review*, March 1, 1873, 351, https://www.google.com/books/edition/The_Fortnightly_Review/MB4_AQAAMAAJ. For more on degeneration, see William L. White, *Slaying the Dragon: The History of Addiction Treatment and Recovery in America*, 2nd ed. (Chicago: Lighthouse Institute, 2014), 120. The idea was outdated by that time, because it was more Lamarckian than Darwinian.

134 **insanity down the generations:** Andrew Scull, *Madness in Civilization: A Cultural History of Insanity, from the Bible to Freud, from the Madhouse to Modern Medicine* (Princeton, NJ: Princeton University Press, 2015), 243; Marcus Boon, *The Road of Excess: A History of Writers on Drugs* (Cambridge, MA: Harvard University Press, 2005), 50.

135 **predestined to his criminal behavior:** Susan Zieger, *Inventing the Addict* (Amherst, MA: University of Massachusetts Press, 2008), 207–8.

135 **described as "ape-like":** Stephen D. Arata, "The Sedulous Ape: Atavism, Professionalism, and Stevenson's *Jekyll and Hyde*," *Criticism* 37, no. 2 (Spring 1995): 233–59, https://www.jstor.org/stable/23116549.

135 **vices caused degeneration:** Berridge, *Opium and the People*, 157.

135 **"throw up some wall":** Alonzo Calkins, *Opium and the Opium-Appetite* [. . .] (Philadelphia, 1876), 20, https://collections.nlm.nih.gov/bookviewer?PID=nlm:nlmuid-66640160R-bk.

135 **people could be incarcerated indefinitely:** Jim Baumohl and Robin Room, "Inebriety, Doctors, and the State: Alcoholism Treatment Institutions before 1940," in *Recent Developments in Alcoholism*, vol. 5, ed. Marc Galanter (New York: Springer, 1987), 144–60.

136 **people with addiction were sterilized:** White, *Slaying the Dragon*, 121.

136 **"greatest evil in Filipino society":** Frederick Ward Kates, "Charles Henry Brent: Ambassador of Christ," *Trinity College School Record*, October 1946, 4–6.

136 **1909 opium meeting:** United Nations Office on Drugs and Crime, Shanghai Opium Commission (January 1, 1959), https://www.unodc.org/unodc/en/data-and-analysis/bulletin/bulletin_1959-01-01_1_page006.html.

137 **"direct, idealistic, uncompromising, and unpopular":** J. M. Scott, *The White Poppy: The History of Opium* (New York: Funk & Wagnalls, 1969), quoted in William White, "The Early Criminalization

of Narcotics Addiction," *Selected Papers of William L. White*, 2014, http://www.williamwhitepapers .com/pr/dlm_uploads/The-Early-Criminalization-of-Narcotic-Addiction.pdf.

137 **domestic anti-drug laws:** Courtwright, *Dark Paradise*, 28. This was an urgent issue: reformers felt that the United States had to craft its own powerful prohibitory laws if it wanted to seize the leadership of international anti-narcotic efforts.

137 **"unfortunate women and their hangers-on":** S. Doc No. 61-377, at 47 (1910).

137 **"most pernicious drug known to humanity":** Edward Marshall, "Uncle Sam Is the Worst Drug Fiend in the World," *New York Times*, March 12, 1911, https://timesmachine.nytimes.com/timesmachine /1911/03/12/104858335.pdf.

138 **move to criminalize drug possession:** David T. Courtwright, Herman Joseph, and Don Des Jarlais, *Addicts Who Survived: An Oral History of Narcotic Use in America before 1965* (Knoxville: University of Tennessee Press, 2012), 7–10; Musto, *American Disease*, 6, 54–69.

138 **smuggling Chinese laborers:** Scott D. Seligman, *Three Tough Chinamen* (Hong Kong: Earnshaw Books, 2012). At the immigration case, he offered a bag containing $6,000 of jewelry as bail, but that was declined: "On Charge of Smuggling," *Bemidji Daily Pioneer*, May 4, 1911, https://chroniclingamerica .loc.gov/lccn/sn86063381/1911-05-04/ed-1/seq-1/.

138 **prescribe huge quantities of morphine:** Jin Fuey Moy v. United States, 254 U.S. 189 (1920).

138 **allowed doctors to prescribe normally:** Edward M. Brecher and the Editors of *Consumer Reports* Magazine, *The Consumers Union Report on Licit and Illicit Drugs* (New York: Consumers Union, 1972), chap. 8, http://www.druglibrary.net/schaffer/Library/studies/cu/cu8.html.

138 **prescriptions for people with addiction:** Herzberg, *White Market Drugs*, 37.

139 **a crime merely to possess:** United States v. Jin Fuey Moy, 241 U.S. 394 (1916). See also O. Hayden Griffin, "The Role of the United States Supreme Court in Shaping Federal Drug Policy," *American Journal of Criminal Justice* 39, no. 3 (September 2014): 660–79, http://doi.org/10.1007/s12103-013-9224-4.

139 **"foreign invasion of undeveloped races":** Elizabeth Tilton diaries, June 26, 1928, Reel 993, Papers of Elizabeth Tilton, 1914–1949, Schlesinger Library, Radcliffe Institute, Cambridge, MA, quoted in Lisa McGirr, *The War on Alcohol: Prohibition and the Rise of the American State* (New York: W. W. Norton, 2015), chap. 6. See also Susan L. Speaker, "Demons for the Twentieth Century," in *Altering American Consciousness*, ed. Sarah W. Tracy and Caroline Jean Acker (Amherst, MA: University of Massachusetts Press, 2004), 203–24.

139 **stereotypes of drunken Irishmen:** Richard Stivers, *A Hair of the Dog: Irish Drinking and American Stereotype* (University Park: Pennsylvania State University Press, 1976).

139 **helped to revive the Klan:** Lisa McGirr, "How Prohibition Fueled the Klan," *New York Times*, January 16, 2019, https://www.nytimes.com/2019/01/16/opinion/prohibition-immigration-klan.html.

139 **As the fatal disease spread:** John M. Barry, *The Great Influenza: The Story of the Deadliest Pandemic in History* (New York: Random House, 2005). See also John M. Barry, "1918 Revisited: Lessons and Suggestions for Further Inquiry," in *The Threat of Pandemic Influenza: Are We Ready?*, ed. S. L. Nobler et al. (Washington, DC: National Academies Press, 2005), https://www.ncbi.nlm.nih.gov/books /NBK22148/#_a2000c209ddd00079_.

140 **starting to look feasible:** Musto, *American Disease*, 134. On the rise of Prohibition as the genesis of the contemporary penal state, see McGirr, *War on Alcohol*.

140 **a new Prohibition Unit:** Herzberg, *White Market Drugs*, 40.

140 **a series of drug treaties:** Berridge, *Demons*, 130–34.

140 **"attempted cure of the habit":** Webb et al. v. United States, 249 U.S. 96 (1919).

140 **serving two years in prison:** Seligman, *Three Tough Chinamen*, 201.

141 **cost of Prohibition:** David J. Hanson, "Was Prohibition Really a Success? You Be the Judge," Alcohol Problems and Solutions, accessed February 27, 2021, https://www.alcoholproblemsandsolutions.org /was-prohibition-really-a-success-you-be-the-judge/.

141 **Reverend Brent had his doubts:** David Courtwright, *The Age of Addiction: How Bad Habits Became Big Business* (Cambridge, MA: Harvard University Press, 2019), 107–19.

141 **numerous poppy fields sprung up:** Harry C. A. Damm, dispatch to Department of State, May 7, 1926, in *Drugs in the Western Hemisphere: An Odyssey of Cultures in Conflict*, ed. William O. Walker (Wilmington, DE: Scholarly Resources, 1996), 59–60, https://books.google.com/books/about/Drugs_in _the_Western_Hemisphere.html?id=Rkk50NzEdmEC.

141 **potent forms of administration:** Jill Jonnes, *Hep-Cats, Narcs, and Pipe Dreams: A History of America's Romance with Illegal Drugs* (Baltimore: Johns Hopkins University Press, 1999), 49.

141 **the "iron law of prohibition":** Richard Cowan, "How the Narcs Created Crack: A War against Ourselves," *National Review*, December 5, 1986, 26.

141 **more deadly fentanyl:** Leo Beletsky and Corey S. Davis, "Today's Fentanyl Crisis: Prohibition's Iron Law Revisited," *International Journal of Drug Policy* 46 (2017): 1–5, https://doi.org/10.1016/j.drugpo.2017.05.050.

141 **right and wrong kinds of drugs:** Herzberg, *White Market Drugs*, 40–44.

142 **"maintenance treatment" might be allowed:** David T. Courtwright, "A Century of American Narcotic Policy," in *Treating Drug Problems*, vol. 2, ed. D. R. Gerstein and H. J. Harwood (Washington, DC: National Academies Press, 1992), 1–62, https://www.ncbi.nlm.nih.gov/books/NBK234755/.

142 **roughly one dozen "narcotic clinics":** Musto, *American Disease*, 143.

142 **A significant public backlash ensued:** Morgan, *Drugs in America*, 107–11.

142 **they were regularly harassed:** Courtwright, *Dark Paradise*, 123, 251.

142 **went after the clinics:** Courtwright, "Century of American Narcotic Policy," 10.

142 **gray market of morphine thrived:** Herzberg, "Entitled to Addiction?," 593–98.

142 **25,000 physicians were reported:** Henry Smith Williams, *Drug Addicts Are Human Beings: The Story of Our Billion-Dollar Racket* (Washington, DC: Shaw, 1938), 88, https://archive.org/details/DrugAddictsAreHumanBeingsTheStoryOfOurBillion-dollarDrugRacketHow_485.

143 **"maintenance" treatment with high doses:** United States v. Berhman, 258 U.S. 280 (1922).

143 **relieve the symptoms of addiction:** Linder v. United States, 268 U.S. 5 (1925), at 6.

143 **a "disease" or a "vice":** Musto, *American Disease*, 137; Tracy, *Alcoholism in America*, 25.

143 **divided on whether indefinite maintenance:** Herzberg, *White Market Drugs,* 37–38.

144 **"The shallow pretense":** "Proceedings of the New Orleans Session: Minutes of the Seventy-First Annual Session of the American Medical Association, Held at New Orleans, April 26–30, 1920," *JAMA* 74, no. 19 (May 1920): 1317–28, http://doi.org/10.1001/jama.1920.02620190023014; Alfred C. Prentice, "The Problem of the Narcotic Drug Addict," *JAMA* 76, no. 23 (June 1921): 1553, http://doi.org/10.1001/jama.1921.02630230013002; Caroline Jean Acker, "From All Purpose Anodyne to Marker of Deviance: Physicians' Attitudes towards Opiates in the US from 1890 to 1940," in *Drugs and Narcotics in History*, ed. Roy Porter and Mikuláš Teich (New York: Cambridge University Press, 1995), 124.

144 **"chaos of contradictory opinion":** Charles E. Terry and Mildred Pellens, *The Opium Problem* (New York: Committee on Drug Addictions, 1928), 928, https://catalog.hathitrust.org/Record/001133723. See also Caroline Acker, *Creating the American Junkie: Addiction Research in the Classic Era of Narcotic Control* (Baltimore: Johns Hopkins University Press, 2002), 54.

144 **"carriers" of a disease:** Winifred Black and Fremont Older, *Dope: The Story of the Living Dead* (New York: J. J. Little & Ives, 1928), 48.

144 **uncannily echoes the rhetoric:** Doctor Springwater, *The Cold-Water-Man; or, a Pocket Companion for the Temperate* (Albany, 1832), 22, https://www.google.com/books/edition/The_Cold_water_man/BNAXAAAAYAAJ.

144 **better word would be "oppression":** Helena Hansen, "Racism and the Opioid Crisis (a Clinical Perspective)" (presentation, National Academy of Medicine's Opioid Collaborative Virtual Town Hall on Health Equity, Tuesday, July 21, 2020).

145 **subhuman, contagious, and possessed:** Speaker, "Demons for the Twentieth Century," 203–24.

145 **scavenging failed construction sites:** Beth Macy, *Dopesick: Dealers, Doctors, and the Drug Company That Addicted America* (New York: Little, Brown, 2018), 25; Wilbert L. Cooper, "Scrape or Die," *Vice*, December 26, 2013, https://www.vice.com/en/article/ppmdbg/scrap-or-die-0000117-v20n10; Courtwright, *Dark Paradise*, 110.

Chapter Seven

150 **What, exactly, was wrong with her?:** Sally Brown and David R. Brown, *A Biography of Mrs. Marty Mann: The First Lady of Alcoholics Anonymous* (Center City, MN: Hazelden, 2011), 80–90.

150 **she would return drunk:** Brown and Brown, *Mrs. Marty Mann*, 100–5.

151 **scrappy, informal fellowship:** William H. Schaberg, *Writing the Big Book* (Las Vegas: Central Recovery Press, 2019), 127, Kindle. Official AA lore holds that the Big Book was a collaborative project written collectively by the group, but more recent scholarship has shown that its core teachings come almost exclusively from Bill Wilson himself.

151 **brewed dandelion wine:** Matthew J. Raphael, *Bill W. and Mr. Wilson: The Legend and Life of A.A.'s Cofounder* (Amherst: University of Massachusetts Press, 2000), 57.

151 **from a scalp wound:** Alcoholics Anonymous, *"Pass It On": The Story of Bill Wilson and How the A.A. Message Reached the World* (New York: Alcoholics Anonymous World Services, 1984), 100–11.

151 **paranoid and suicidal:** Alcoholics Anonymous, *"Pass It On,"* 106.

152 **simply prescribed more willpower:** Ernest Kurtz, *Not God: A History of Alcoholics Anonymous* (Center City, MN: Hazelden Educational Materials, 1979), 14.

152 **Charles B. Towns Hospital:** Kurtz, *Not God*, 14–15; William L. White, *Slaying the Dragon: The History of Addiction Treatment and Recovery in America*, 2nd ed. (Chicago: Lighthouse Institute, 2014), 117.

152 **diphtheria antitoxin serum:** "Emil von Berhing Facts," The Nobel Prize (website), last updated 2021, https://www.nobelprize.org/prizes/medicine/1901/behring/facts/. Anti-syphilis medication: K. J. Williams, "The Introduction of 'Chemotherapy' Using Arsphenamine—the First Magic Bullet," *Journal of the Royal Society of Medicine* 102, no. 8 (August 2009): 343–48, https://doi.org/10.1258/jrsm.2009.09k036.

152 **supposed antitoxin serum:** Cited in White, *Slaying the Dragon*, 126; David T. Courtwright, *Dark Paradise: A History of Opiate Addiction in America* (Cambridge, MA: Harvard University Press, 2001), 128–29.

152 **This didn't stop entrepreneurial hucksters:** Nancy D. Campbell, *Discovering Addiction: The Science and Politics of Substance Abuse Research* (Ann Arbor: University of Michigan Press, 2007), 18.

152 **patient-run societies:** Christopher M. Finan, *Drunks: An American History* (Boston: Beacon Press, 2017), 110–13; White, *Slaying the Dragon*, 68–87.

153 **exercises to strengthen the will:** White, *Slaying the Dragon*, 116.

153 **"I won't go in. I won't":** Robert Thomsen, *Bill W.: The Absorbing and Deeply Moving Life Story of Bill Wilson, Co-Founder of Alcoholics Anonymous* (Carter City, MN: Hazelden, 1975), chap. 6, Kindle.

153 **"a little cracked":** *Alcoholics Anonymous*, 4th ed. (New York: Alcoholics Anonymous World Services, 2001), 9, https://www.aa.org/pages/en_US/alcoholics-anonymous.

154 **"let him show himself!":** Alcoholics Anonymous, *"Pass It On,"* 120–21.

154 **powerful psychoactive substances:** Kurtz, *Not God*, 15–16; White, *Slaying the Dragon*, 117.

154 **"The only radical remedy I know":** William James, *The Varieties of Religious Experience* (New York: Modern Library, 1929), 263, https://books.google.com/books?id=Qi4XAAAAIAAJ.

154 **"by its results exclusively":** James, *Varieties of Religious Experience*, 22.

154 **"harmoniously adjusting ourselves thereto":** James, *Varieties of Religious Experience*, 53.

155 **a surgeon named Bob Smith:** White, *Slaying the Dragon*, 172–73.

155 **"threefold nature" of alcoholism:** Kurtz, *Not God*, 199.

155 **ongoing work to change:** Kurtz, *Not God*, 179. See also White, *Slaying the Dragon*, 193–94.

155 **prevailing stereotypes of female alcoholics:** Michelle L. McClellan, *Lady Lushes: Gender, Alcoholism, and Medicine in Modern America* (New Brunswick, NJ: Rutgers University Press, 2017), 1–26.

156 **Bob in Akron was particularly notorious:** Schaberg, *Writing the Big Book*, chap. 18.

156 **"Under every skirt there's a slip":** McClellan, *Lady Lushes*, 80.

156 **"woman-on-the-make":** White, *Slaying the Dragon*, 208.

156 **men outnumber women in AA:** "2014 A.A. Membership Survey Reveals Current Trends," *About AA: A Newsletter for Professionals*, Fall 2015, https://www.aa.org/newsletters/en_US/f-13_fall15.pdf.

156 **"Thirteen Statements of Acceptance":** White, *Slaying the Dragon*, 478–79. See also Finan, *Drunks*, 254–55.

156 **she hid upstairs:** McClellan, *Lady Lushes*, 76.

156 **"I could finish their sentences!":** Brown and Brown, *Mrs. Marty Mann*, 112.

156 **community in the group's success:** John F. Kelly, Keith Humphreys, and Marica Ferri, "Alcoholics Anonymous and Other 12-Step Programs for Alcohol Use Disorder," *Cochrane Database of Systematic Reviews*, no. 3 (2020), CD012880, https://doi.org/10.1002/14651858.CD012880.pub2.

157 **"I wasn't alone any more":** *Alcoholics Anonymous*, 206.

157 **It was a joke:** Brown and Brown, *Mrs. Marty Mann*, 128.

159 **Denial is a profound obstacle:** Substance Abuse and Mental Health Services Administration, *Key Substance Use and Mental Health Indicators in the United States: Results from the 2019 National Survey on Drug Use and Health* (Washington, DC: Department of Health and Human Services, 2020), 54; Hanna Pickard, "Denial in Addiction," *Mind & Language* 31, no. 3 (June 2016): 277–99, https://doi.org/10.1111/mila.12106.

157 **two measly pages:** Shannon C. Miller et al., *The ASAM Principles of Addiction Medicine*, 6th ed. (Philadelphia: Wolters Kluwer, 2019). The *APA Textbook of Substance Abuse Treatment* (5th ed.) has a little more, with "denial" appearing on about 26 of 960 pages according to that index, but it still doesn't get its own section or heading, appearing only in casual mentions scattered throughout the book. Marc Galanter, Herbert D. Kleber, and Kathleen T. Brady, *The American Psychiatric Publishing Textbook of Substance Abuse Treatment*, 5th ed. (Arlington, VA: American Psychiatric Publishing, 2015).

157 **self-deception is actually beneficial:** Robert Trivers, *Deceit and Self-Deception: Fooling Yourself the Better to Fool Others* (New York: Penguin, 2011).

160 **her partner, Priscilla Peck:** Brown and Brown, *Mrs. Marty Mann*, 138–51.

160 **article by Jack Alexander:** Jack Alexander, "Alcoholics Anonymous," *Saturday Evening Post*, March 1, 1941, https://aa-show-low-az.tripod.com/webonmediacontents/AA_Jack_Alexander.html; Kurtz, *Not God*, 100–1, 113.

161 **spacious office near Grand Central Station:** Kurtz, *Not God*, 112.

161 **barely even mentioned meetings in the Big Book:** *Alcoholics Anonymous*, 160. The book mentions that "casual get-togethers and once-weekly meetings" were starting to emerge. See Keith Humphreys, "An International Tour of Addiction-Related Mutual-Help Organizations," in *Circles of Recovery* (New York: Cambridge University Press, 2004), 33–93, for further discussion.

161 **Her plan was to reach:** Bruce Holley Johnson, "The Alcoholism Movement in America: A Study in Cultural Innovation" (PhD diss., University of Illinois at Urbana–Champaign, 1973), 266–68. See also White, *Slaying the Dragon*, 242–44.

161 **public health advocacy movements:** Keith Humphreys, "Definitions, Scope, and Origin of the Health-Related Self-Help Group Movement," in *Circles of Recovery*, 1–32; also Virginia Berridge, *Demons: Our Changing Attitudes to Alcohol, Tobacco, and Drugs* (New York: Oxford University Press, 2013), 165.

161 **National Tuberculosis Association:** Brown and Brown, *Mrs. Marty Mann*, 34–35, 166. On public health in general: Paul Starr, *The Social Transformation of American Medicine: The Rise of a Sovereign Profession and the Making of a Vast Industry* (New York: Basic Books, 1982), 191; Sigard Adolphus Knopf, *A History of the National Tuberculosis Association: The Anti-Tuberculosis Movement in the United States* (New York: National Tuberculosis Association, 1922), https://books.google.com/books?id=ldw9MrxLjUIC.

162 **important publication framing alcoholism:** Johnson, "Alcoholism Movement," 103.

162 **"regarded as a sick person":** Research Council on Problems of Alcohol, Scientific Committee Minutes, January 10, 1940, Lane Medical Archives, quoted in Ron Roizen, "The American Discovery of Alcoholism, 1933–1939" (PhD diss., University of California, Berkeley, 1991), chap. 8. See also Johnson, "Alcoholism Movement," 249.

162 **"responsibility of the healing professions":** Dwight Anderson, "Alcohol and Public Opinion," *Quarterly Journal of Studies on Alcohol* 3, no. 3 (September 1942): 376–92.

162 **currency-speculation-and-smuggling scheme:** Judith H. Ward et al., "Re-Introducing Bunky at 125: E. M. Jellinek's Life and Contributions to Alcohol Studies," *Journal of Studies on Alcohol and Drugs* 77, no. 3 (May 2016): 375–83, https://doi.org/10.15288/jsad.2016.77.375. See also Ron Roizen, "E. M. Jellinek and All That!" (H. Thomas Austern Lecture, ABMRF/The Foundation for Alcohol Research Annual Meeting, San Francisco, October 20–26, 2000), http://www.roizen.com/ron/jellinek-pres.htm; and Judith H. Ward, "E. M. Jellinek: The Hungarian Connection" (presented at 36th Annual Substance Abuse Librarians and Information Specialists Conference, New Brunswick, NJ, May 1, 2014), https://www.researchgate.net/publication/281906726_E_M_Jellinek_The_Hungarian_connection.

163 **"tall, smart looking blonde":** "Medicine: Help for Drunkards," *Time*, October 23, 1944, http://content.time.com/time/subscriber/article/0,33009,932497,00.html; Marty Mann, October 2, 1944 press conference at New York Biltmore Hotel, quoted in Joe Miller, *US of AA: How the Twelve Steps Hijacked the Science of Alcoholism* (Chicago: Chicago Review Press, 2019), 44.

163 **"alcoholism is a disease":** Johnson, "Alcoholism Movement," 272.

163 **two hundred public talks:** Brown and Brown, *Mrs. Marty Mann*, 172; Johnson, "Alcoholism Movement," 273.

163 **"alcoholism information centers":** White, *Slaying the Dragon*, 232–58.

164 **just shy of 100,000 members:** Johnson, "Alcoholism Movement," 287, quoting membership figures from the *World Directory,* published annually by the General Service Office of Alcoholics Anonymous, Inc.

164 **deliberately decentralized organizational structure:** White, *Slaying the Dragon* 180–204; Kurtz, *Not God*, 112–16.

164 **psychiatrist named Ruth Fox:** Johnson, "Alcoholism Movement," 262–64, regarding friendship. See also White, *Slaying the Dragon*, 245.

164 **"alcoholism as a medical problem":** "Reports of Officers," *JAMA* 162, no. 8 (October 1956): 750, https://doi.org/10.1001/jama.1956.02970250048013.

164 **American Hospital Association:** American Hospital Association, "Statement on Admission to the General Hospital of Patients with Alcohol and Other Drug Problems (Approved by the American Hospital Association September 29–October 2, 1957)," in *Hearings Before the Subcommittee on Public Health and Welfare of the Committee on Interstate and Foreign Commerce House of Representatives on H.R. 18874, H.R. 2707, H.R. 17788 and S. 3835*, 91st Cong. 77 (1970), at 437–38, https://www.google.com/books/edition/Hearings_Reports_and_Prints_of_the_House/Xug1AAAAIAAJ.

165 **at least thirty-four Hollywood films:** Robin Room, "Alcoholism and Alcoholics Anonymous in U.S. Films, 1945–1962: The Party Ends for the 'Wet Generations,'" *Journal of Studies on Alcohol and Drugs* 50, no. 4 (July 1989): 368–83, https://doi.org/10.15288/jsa.1989.50.368.

165 **disease concept of alcoholism:** Charles Jackson, *The Lost Weekend* (New York: Vintage, 2013), 224. See extensive discussion of Charles Jackson in Leslie Jamison's wonderful book *The Recovering: Intoxication and Its Aftermath* (New York: Hachette, 2018).

165 **directly consulted on several films:** Kurtz, *Not God*, 120; Brown and Brown, *Mrs. Marty Mann,* 177.

165 **AA members contributed powerfully:** Johnson, "Alcoholism Movement," 286.

165 **the tortured syntax:** Kurtz, *Not God*, 121; White, *Slaying the Dragon*, 203–7.

165 **a "sick person":** Stanton Peele, *Diseasing of America: How We Allowed Recovery Zealots and the Treatment Industry to Convince Us We Are Out of Control* (New York: Lexington Books, 1995), 45; White, *Slaying the Dragon*, 246–48.

166 **"a disease which will yield":** H.R. Rep. No. 89-395, at 7 (1966) (Message from the President of the United States).

166 **signed the bill into law:** Comprehensive Alcohol Abuse and Alcoholism Prevention, Treatment, and Rehabilitation Act of 1970, Pub. L. No. 91-616, 84 Stat. 1848, https://www.govinfo.gov/content/pkg/STATUTE-84/pdf/STATUTE-84-Pg1848.pdf. See also Nancy Olson, "Problems in the House," in *With a Lot of Help from Our Friends: The Politics of Alcoholism* (Lincoln, NE: Writers Club Press, 2003), 84–93; White, *Slaying the Dragon*, 378.

166 **end to "America's 150-year war":** Marty Mann, "America's 150-Year War: Alcohol vs. Alcoholism," *Alcohol Health and Research World* 1, no. 1 (Spring 1973): 5–7, https://babel.hathitrust.org/cgi/pt?id=uc1.c069821021&view=1up&seq=13.

167 **photographed stoking the flames:** Roizen, "American Discovery of Alcoholism," chap. 6, http://www.roizen.com/ron/dissch6.htm; J. A. Waddell and H. B. Haag, *Alcohol in Moderation and Excess: A Study of the Effects of the Use of Alcohol on the Human System*, 3rd ed. (Richmond, VA: William Byrd Press, 1940), https://babel.hathitrust.org/cgi/pt?id=coo.31924003194986&view=1up&seq=7.

167 **make *alcoholism* its single focus:** Roizen, "American Discovery of Alcoholism," chap. 8.

167 **Burnham argues that industrialism:** John C. Burnham, *Bad Habits: Drinking, Smoking, Taking Drugs, Gambling, Sexual Misbehavior, and Swearing in American History* (New York: New York University Press, 1993).

169 **"not in the bottle":** Thomas F. McCarthy, president of Licensed Beverage Industries, Inc., 1947, quoted in Burnham, *Bad Habits*, 83.

169 **"potentially valuable allies":** Randolph W. Childs, *Making Repeal Work* (Philadelphia: Pennsylvania Alcoholic Beverage Study, Inc., 1947), 256, quoted in Burnham, *Bad Habits*, 82.

169 **most of the harmful effects:** Thomas F. Babor et al., *Alcohol: No Ordinary Commodity*, 2nd ed. (New York: Oxford University Press, 2010), summarizing numerous sources. See also Gerhard Gmel et al., "Revising the Preventative Paradox: The Swiss Case," *Addiction* 96, no. 2 (February 2001): 273–84, https://doi.org/10.1046/j.1360-0443.2001.96227311.x; Ingeborg Rossow and Anders Romelsjö, "The Extent of the 'Prevention Paradox' in Alcohol Problems as a Function of Population Drinking Patterns," *Addiction* 101, no. 1 (January 2006): 84–90, https://doi.org/10.1111/j.1360-0443.2005.01294.x.

169 **account for the most revenue:** Aveek Bhattacharya et al., "How Dependent Is the Alcohol Industry on Heavy Drinking in England?," *Addiction* 113, no. 12 (December 2018): 2225–32, https://doi.org/10.1111/add.14386; Sarah Boseley, "Problem Drinkers Account for Most of Alcohol Industry's Sales, Figures Reveal," *Guardian*, January 22, 2016, https://www.theguardian.com/society/2016/jan/22/problem-drinkers-alcohol-industry-most-sales-figures-reveal; *The Public Health Burden of Alcohol and the Effectiveness and Cost-Effectiveness of Alcohol Control Policies* (London: Public Health England, 2016), https://assets.publishing.service.gov.uk/government/uploads/system/uploads/attachment_data/file/733108/alcohol_public_health_burden_evidence_review_update_2018.pdf. See also Babor et al., *Alcohol: No Ordinary Commodity*.

170 **"hard core drunk drivers":** Thomas F. Babor, "Alcohol Research and the Alcoholic Beverage Industry: Issues, Concerns and Conflicts of Interest," *Addiction* 104, no. S1 (February 2009): 34–47, https://doi.org/10.1111/j.1360-0443.2008.02433.x.

170 **focused on individual responsibility:** Craig Reinarman, "The Social Construction of an Alcohol Problem," *Theory and Society* 17, no. 1 (January 1, 1988): 91–120, https://doi.org/10.1007/BF00163727. See also Burnham, *Bad Habits*, 81.

170 **more than $1.5 trillion:** David H. Jernigan, "The Global Alcohol Industry: An Overview," *Addiction* 104, no. S1 (February 2009): 6–12, https://doi.org/10.1111/j.1360-0443.2008.02430.x; Allied Market Research, *Alcoholic Beverages Market [. . .] Global Opportunity Analysis and Industry Forecast, 2018–2025*

(Portland, OR: Allied Market Research, 2018), https://www.alliedmarketresearch.com/alcoholic
-beverages-market.

170 **"industrial epidemics":** René I. Jahiel and Thomas F. Babor, "Industrial Epidemics, Public Health
Advocacy and the Alcohol Industry: Lessons from Other Fields," *Addiction* 102, no. 9 (September
2007): 1335–39, https://doi.org/10.1111/j.1360-0443.2007.01900.x. Regarding efforts to open Southeast
Asia and Africa to alcohol, and similar efforts by global food marketers, see also David Courtwright,
The Age of Addiction: How Bad Habits Became Big Business (Cambridge, MA: Harvard University
Press, 2019), 150, 190.

170 **a team of Norwegian researchers:** Øystein Bakke and Dag Endal, "Vested Interests in Addiction
Research and Policy Alcohol Policies Out of Context: Drinks Industry Supplanting Government Role
in Alcohol Policies in Sub-Saharan Africa," *Addiction* 105, no. 1 (January 2010): 22–28, https://doi.org
/10.1111/j.1360-0443.2009.02695.x.

171 **promoted soft strategies:** Bakke and Endal, "Vested Interests in Addiction Research," 26.

171 **"torches of freedom":** Sarah Milov, *The Cigarette: A Political History* (Cambridge, MA: Harvard Uni-
versity Press, 2019); David T. Courtwright, *Forces of Habit: Drugs and the Making of the Modern World*
(Cambridge, MA: Harvard University Press, 2001), 114–22; Iris Mostegel, "The Original Influencer,"
History Today, February 6, 2019, https://www.historytoday.com/miscellanies/original-influencer. For
additional images, see Wendy Christensen, "Torches of Freedom: Women and Smoking Propaganda,"
Sociological Images (blog), February 27, 2012, https://thesocietypages.org/socimages/2012/02/27/torches
-of-freedom-women-and-smoking-propaganda/.

171 **rift between alcohol and tobacco and other drugs:** David T. Courtwright, "Mr. ATOD's Wild Ride:
What Do Alcohol, Tobacco, and Other Drugs Have in Common?," *Social History of Alcohol and Drugs*
20, no. 1 (Fall 2005): 105–24, https://doi.org/10.1086/SHAD20010105.

173 **Betty, reluctantly, told her family:** Betty Ford and Chris Chase, *Betty: A Glad Awakening* (New York:
Doubleday, 1987), 53–60. See also White, *Slaying the Dragon*, 396–97. It bears noting that to many
feminist critics, the Betty Ford story is not inspiring, but a twisted tale of a domesticated woman who
had failed to live up to what others saw as her wifely duties, then was coerced into a paternalistic
treatment system when she did not comply.

173 **Elizabeth Taylor went public:** John Duka, "Elizabeth Taylor: Journal of a Recovery," *New York Times*,
February 4, 1985, https://www.nytimes.com/1985/02/04/style/elizabeth-taylor-journal-of-a-recovery.html.

174 **TV shows and movies:** White, *Slaying the Dragon*, 395.

174 **almost one million in 1990:** Trysh Travis, *Language of the Heart* (Chapel Hill: University of North
Carolina, 2009), 274.

174 **"healing ourselves and our planet":** Vince R. Miller, "The Twelve Steps: Meeting the Challenge of
Our Success," *Recovering*, January 1991, 1–9, quoted in Robin Room, "Healing Ourselves and Our
Planet: The Emergence and Nature of a Generalized Twelve-Step Consciousness," *Contemporary
Drug Problems* 19 (Winter 1992): 717–40.

174 **punishing speaking schedule:** Brown and Brown, *Mrs. Marty Mann*, 217.

174 **approximately 80 percent:** Stanton Peele, *The Meaning of Addiction* (San Francisco: Jossey-Bass, 1985), 28.

174 **"I was a sick person":** Her story is in the Big Book, titled "Women Suffer Too," *Alcoholics Anonymous*, 205.

175 **"threefold nature" of alcoholism:** Kurtz, *Not God*, 199.

175 **"between the sacred and the secular":** Raphael, *Bill W. and Mr. Wilson*, 60.

175 **"AAs have never called alcoholism a disease":** Bill Wilson, lecture to the National Clergy Conference
on Alcoholism, 1960, http://www.a-1associates.com/aa/LETS_ASK_BILL/wilsonstalktotheclergy
.htm.

175 **Mann insisted that alcoholism:** Marty Mann, *New Primer on Alcoholism: How People Drink, How to
Recognize Alcoholics, and What to Do about Them* (New York: Holt, Rinehart and Winston, 1958). See
in particular chap. 2.

176 **boundary between diabetic and healthy:** See, for example, Nicholas J. Wareham and Stephen O'Rahilly,
"The Changing Classification and Diagnosis of Diabetes: New Classification Is Based on Pathogenesis,
Not Insulin Dependence," *British Medical Journal* 317, no. 7155 (August 1998): 359–60, https://dx.doi.org
/10.1136%2Fbmj.317.7155.359; Steven H. Woolf and Stephen F. Rothemich, "New Diabetes Guidelines:
A Closer Look at the Evidence," *American Family Physician* 58, no. 6 (October 1998): 1287–89, PMID:
9803186; Barbara Brooks-Worrell and Jerry P. Palmer, "Is Diabetes Mellitus a Continuous Spectrum?,"
Clinical Chemistry 57, no. 2 (February 2011): 158–61, https://doi.org/10.1373/clinchem.2010.148270.

177 **"dyed-in-the-wool AA":** Marty Mann, letter to Julian Armstrong, September 8, 1945, quoted in Johnson, "Alcoholism Movement," 289.

177 **"ignorance, fear, superstition, and stigma":** Mann, *New Primer*, 128–29.

177 **how often diseases are heavily moralized:** Robin Room and Wayne D. Hall, "Frameworks for Understanding Drug Use and Societal Responses," in *Drug Use in Australian Society*, 2nd ed., ed. A. Ritter, T. King, and M. Hamilton (Sydney: Oxford University Press, 2017).

177 **harder for people to recognize:** J. Morris et al., "Continuum Beliefs Are Associated with Higher Problem Recognition than Binary Beliefs among Harmful Drinkers without Addiction Experience," *Addictive Behaviors* 105 (June 2020): 106292, https://doi.org/10.1016/j.addbeh.2020.106292.

177 **most potent predictor of relapse:** William R. Miller et al., "What Predicts Relapse? Prospective Testing of Antecedent Models," *Addiction* 91, no. S1 (August 1996): S155–72, PMID: 8997790.

177 **"A Disease Like Any Other":** Bernice A. Pescosolido et al., "'A Disease Like Any Other'? A Decade of Change in Public Reactions to Schizophrenia, Depression, and Alcohol Dependence," *American Journal of Psychiatry* 167, no. 11 (November 2010): 1321–30, https://dx.doi.org/10.1176%2Fappi.ajp.2010.09121743. See also Emma E. McGinty and Colleen L. Barry, "Stigma Reduction to Combat the Addiction Crisis—Developing an Evidence Base," *New England Journal of Medicine* 382, no. 14 (April 2020): 1291–92, https://doi.org/10.1056/NEJMp2000227.

178 **declared them a "failure":** Keith Humphreys, email message to author, July 28, 2020. Relatively recently, the addiction nonprofit Shatterproof has started a new anti-stigma initiative that appears to be much more granular and much less organized around the notion of "disease": "Shatterproof Releases National Addiction Stigma Strategy as the COVID-19 Pandemic Continues to Worsen the Addiction Public Health Crisis," Shatterproof, accessed February 27, 2021, https://www.shatterproof.org/press/shatterproof-releases-national-addiction-stigma-strategy-covid-19-pandemic-continues-worsen.

178 **learn to drink like gentlemen:** William Seabrook, *Asylum* (New York: Dover, 2015). The writer Willie Seabrook is a key example of this phenomenon. "Willie Seabrook, Author, Is Suicide," *St. Petersburg Times*, September 21, 1945.

Chapter Eight

179 **federal agents were closing in quickly:** William S. Burroughs, *Junky*, ed. Oliver Harris (New York: Penguin Classics, 2008), 30–33; Ted Morgan, *Literary Outlaw: The Life and Times of William S. Burroughs* (New York: W. W. Norton, 1988), 61, 251.

179 **anti-drug, prohibitionist fervor:** David T. Courtwright, "A Century of American Narcotic Policy," in *Treating Drug Problems*, vol. 2, ed. D. R. Gerstein and H. J. Harwood (Washington, DC: National Academies Press, 1992), 4–7.

179 **uncle Horace:** Oliver Harris, "Editor's Introduction," in Burroughs, *Junky*, xxii. Also on Horace, see William S. Burroughs Jr., *Cursed from Birth*, ed. David Ohle (Brooklyn: Soft Skull Press, 2006), 31–32.

180 **United States Narcotic Farm:** Morgan, *Literary Outlaw*, 158; Burroughs, *Junky*, 62–64.

180 **twelve acres by itself:** Nancy D. Campbell, James P. Olsen, and Luke Walden, *The Narcotic Farm: The Rise and Fall of America's First Prison for Drug Addicts* (Lexington: University of Kentucky Press, 2021), 35–50.

180 **started buying up paregoric:** Burroughs, *Junky*, 69.

181 **That antitoxin theory:** David T. Courtwright, *Dark Paradise: A History of Opiate Addiction in America* (Cambridge, MA: Harvard University Press, 2001), 132–33. See also David F. Musto, *The American Disease: Origins of Narcotic Control*, 3rd ed. (New York: Oxford University Press, 1999), 336; William L. White, *Slaying the Dragon: The History of Addiction Treatment and Recovery in America*, 2nd ed. (Chicago: Lighthouse Institute, 2014), 126.

181 **born into poverty:** "Dr. Lawrence Kolb, 6645 32nd Street, N.W., Washington, DC, April 24, 1963," Reminiscences of Lawrence Kolb, Oral History Archives at Columbia, Rare Book & Manuscript Library, Columbia University, New York, 7.

182 **charged him with investigating addiction:** Courtwright, *Dark Paradise*, 130–31.

182 **Kolb was astounded to learn:** "Dr. Lawrence Kolb," 23–25.

182 **a "twisted personality":** Lawrence Kolb, "Types and Characteristics of Drug Addicts," *Mental Hygiene* 9, no. 2 (April 1925): 300–13, https://collections.nlm.nih.gov/ocr/nlm:nlmuid-2934112RX136-leaf; Caroline Acker, *Creating the American Junkie: Addiction Research in the Classic Era of Narcotic Control* (Baltimore: Johns Hopkins University Press, 2002), 141.

182 **predispose people to addiction:** William R. Miller, Alyssa A. Forcehimes, and Allen Zweben, *Treating Addiction: A Guide for Professionals*, 2nd ed. (New York: Guilford Press, 2019), 19. See also Maia Szalavitz, *Unbroken Brain* (New York: Macmillan, 2016), chap. 5.

183 **screening immigrants on Ellis Island:** Acker, *Creating the American Junkie*, 135.

183 **measuring intelligence was not enough:** Konrad Banicki, "The Character-Personality Distinction: An Historical, Conceptual, and Functional Investigation," *Theory & Psychology* 27, no. 1 (January 2017), https://doi.org/10.1177%2F0959354316684689.

183 **theories of addiction as a personality problem:** Courtwright, *Dark Paradise*, 129.

183 **"patients" rather than "prisoners":** Campbell, Olsen, and Walden, *Narcotic Farm*, 15, 52.

183 **"too good to be true":** Former Inmate No. 34, "Dope Addicts, 'America's Untouchables,' Described by Former Inmate of United States Narcotic Farm Here; Treatment Given at Government Institution Is Praised," *Lexington (KY) Herald*, December 1, 1935, 1, 18, https://www.newspapers.com/image /681291015.

183 **"multi-million dollar flophouse":** Nancy D. Campbell, *Discovering Addiction: The Science and Politics of Substance Abuse Research* (Ann Arbor: University of Michigan Press, 2007), 61, 65–68, 129.

184 **"the Nazi regime":** H. J. Anslinger and William Tompkins, *The Traffic in Narcotics* (New York: Funk & Wagnalls, 1953), 279, https://www.druglibrary.org/schaffer/people/anslinger/traffic/traffic.htm.

184 **Mexican Revolution to the U.S.:** John Burnett, "The Bath Riots: Indignity along the Mexican Border," NPR, January 28, 2006, https://www.npr.org/templates/story/story.php?storyId=5176177.

184 **tighter controls on the drug:** H. Wayne Morgan, *Drugs in America: A Social History, 1800–1980* (Syracuse, NY: Syracuse University Press, 1982), 138; see also Richard J. Bonnie and Charles H. Whitebread, *The Marijuana Conviction: A History of Marijuana Prohibition in the United States* (Charlottesville: University Press of Virginia, 1974), 42; Doris Marie Provine, *Unequal Under Law: Race in the War on Drugs* (Chicago: University of Chicago Press, 2007), loc. 1153–54 of 2874. It bears noting, as the historian Isaac Campos has documented at length, that anti-marijuana sentiment was not created in the U.S. but in a way imported from Mexico, where there was already a long tradition of vilifying marijuana users. Isaac Campos, *Home Grown: Marijuana and the Origins of Mexico's War on Drugs* (Chapel Hill: University of North Carolina Press, 2012).

184 **Anslinger realized the potential:** Bonnie and Whitebread, *The Marijuana Conviction*, 42, 100–17; Edward M. Brecher, "Marijuana Is Outlawed," in Brecher and the Editors of *Consumer Reports, The Consumers Union Report on Licit and Illicit Drugs* (New York: Consumers Union, 1972), chap. 56.

185 **script ideas about dangerous drugs:** Marcus Boon, *The Road of Excess: A History of Writers on Drugs* (Cambridge, MA: Harvard University Press, 2005), 157.

185 **1936's *Tell Your Children*:** Louis J. Gasnier, dir., *Reefer Madness*, 1936, https://archive.org/details /reefer_madness1938.

185 **"develop a delirious rage":** *Taxation of Marihuana: Hearings before the Committee on Ways and Means House of Representatives on H.R. 6385*, 75th Cong. 952 (1937) (additional statement of H. J. Anslinger, commissioner of narcotics), at 29, https://books.google.com/books?id=2EjVAAAAMAAJ.

185 **"created by infectious contact":** H. J. Anslinger and William Tompkins, *The Traffic in Narcotics* (New York: Funk & Wagnalls, 1953), 223. "In the third and largest group are found the psychopaths. These make up the bulk of the addict population . . ."

185 **addiction was the unstoppable combination:** Anslinger and Tompkins, *Traffic in Narcotics*, 170. Consider: The "young addict . . . should be plucked out of the community and quarantined, forced to undergo a cure. He will not do it voluntarily."

185 **"Whenever you find severe penalties":** Harry Anslinger and Kenneth W. Chapman, "Narcotic Addiction," *Modern Medicine* 25 (1957), 182, quoted in Courtwright, "Century of American Narcotic Policy," 14.

185 **"The best cure for addiction?":** Anslinger and Tompkins, *Traffic in Narcotics*, 241.

185 **"moral and physical scourge":** Richmond Hobson, "The Struggle of Mankind against Its Deadliest Foe," *Narcotic Education* 1, no. 4 (April 1928): 51–54. For Kolb's activities, see Musto, *American Disease*, 190, 372; Lawrence Kolb, "Drug Addiction as a Public Health Problem," *Scientific Monthly* 48, no. 5 (1939): 391–400; Courtwright, *Dark Paradise*, 132.

186 **surpassed 2,300 in 1950:** John C. Ball and Emily S. Cottrell, "Admissions of Narcotic Drug Addicts to Public Health Service Hospitals, 1935–63," *Public Health Reports* 80, no. 6 (June 1965): 471–75.

186 **Black admissions to Narco rose:** Courtwright, "Century of American Narcotic Policy," 17.

186 **chief of the Mental Hygiene Division:** Robert Felix, "Lawrence Kolb 1881–1972," *American Journal of Psychiatry* 130, no. 6 (June 1973): 718–19, https://doi.org/10.1176/ajp.130.6.718.

186 **"there was no program":** Eddie Flowers, interview with J. P. Olsen and Luke Walden, Alexandria, VA, 2004, quoted in Campbell, *Discovering Addiction*, 129, describing the late 1950s.

187 **influenced by Romantics like Coleridge:** Burroughs, *Junky*, 2; Morgan, *Literary Outlaw*, 61–62. Regarding the countercultural reclaiming of the word "junkie": Bruce K. Alexander, *The Globalization of Addiction* (New York: Oxford University Press, 2010), chap. 8.

187 **"permanent cellular alteration":** Burroughs, *Junky,* 163. It's also interesting to note how Burroughs mixed up allergic, metabolic, endocrinological, and other theories about withdrawal. See, for example, *Junky,* 167: "withdrawal sickness is an allergy"; *Junky,* 165: "When I say 'habit forming drug' I mean a drug that alters the endocrine balance of the body in such a way that the body requires that drug in order to function." This theme continues in his future work. See "Letter from a Master Addict to Dangerous Drugs," *Addiction* 53, no. 2 (January 1957): 119–32, https://doi.org/10.1111/j.1360-0443.1957 .tb05093.x: "The use of morphine leads to a metabolic dependence on morphine. Morphine becomes a biologic need just as water and the user may die if he is suddenly deprived of it."

187 **"no tolerance with C":** Burroughs, *Junky,* 122.

187 **"produce true addiction":** A. L. Tatum and M. H. Seevers, "Theories of Drug Addiction," *Physiological Reviews* 11 (1931): 107–21.

187 **stimulants were not truly addictive:** Kolb, "Drug Addiction as a Public Health Problem," 391–400. While Kolb was dismissive of stimulant addiction in general, his views on the addictiveness of cocaine are somewhat muddled. He did describe cocaine as a "stimulating addicting drug" but later in the piece said that the "cocaine addict . . . almost invariably changes over to opium" and that all addictions have a natural tendency to gravitate toward opium. Discussed further, including drug manufacturers' response, in Nicolas Rasmussen, *On Speed: From Benzedrine to Adderall* (New York: New York University Press, 2008), 49.

188 **a tiny laboratory:** Campbell, *Discovering Addiction,* 59–64.

188 **scientific cure for addiction:** Campbell, Olsen, and Walden, *Narcotic Farm,* 20.

188 **eradicate dangerous opioids entirely:** Acker, *Creating the American Junkie,* 62–69.

188 **mechanical workings of the brain:** Roy Porter, *The Greatest Benefit to All Mankind: A Medical History of Humanity* (1998; repr., New York: W. W. Norton, 1997), 570–72; Ben Ehrlich, *The Brain That Discovered Itself* (New York: Farrar, Straus and Giroux, forthcoming); Ben Ehrlich, *The Dreams of Santiago Ramón y Cajal* (New York: Oxford University Press, 2016).

188 **"the brains of these addicts":** Campbell, Olsen, and Walden, *Narcotic Farm,* 164. For more on EEG at Narco, see William R. Martin and Harris Isbell, eds., *Drug Addiction and the U.S. Public Health Service: Proceedings of the Symposium Commemorating the 40th Anniversary of the Addiction Research Center at Lexington, Ky* (Rockville, MD: National Institute on Drug Abuse, 1978), https://archive.org/stream /drugaddictionusp00mart/drugaddictionusp00mart_djvu.txt.

188 **"psychology lost its soul":** Robert Sessions Woodworth, *Psychology: A Study of Mental Life* (New York: Henry Holt, 1921), 2, https://www.google.com/books/edition/Psychology/oy7ARHvJ3eIC.

189 **behaviorism, an outright rejection:** Alexander, in *Globalization of Addiction,* loc. 4839 of 15778, writes in detail about behaviorism and its effects on conceptualizing addiction. See also George Graham, "Behaviorism," in *The Stanford Encyclopedia of Philosophy,* ed. Edward N. Zalta, last modified February 26, 2020 (Palo Alto, CA: Metaphysics Research Lab, 2020), https://plato.stanford.edu/archives /spr2019/entries/behaviorism.

189 **Behaviorism was immensely popular:** In the 1980s, Roy Wise, the architect of the dopamine theory of addiction, approvingly cited Skinner's argument that "psychic inner causes" were not the proper domain of psychology. Roy A. Wise, "The Neurobiology of Craving: Implications for the Understanding and Treatment of Addiction," *Journal of Abnormal Psychology* 97, no. 2 (1988): 118.

189 **"sine qua non of addiction":** Courtwright, "The Transformation of the Opiate Addict," in *Dark Paradise,* 110–44. Caroline Acker, "The Junkie as Psychopath," in *Creating the American Junkie,* 125–55.

189 **"very dependable kind of illness":** Clifton K. Himmelsbach, interview by Wyndham D. Miles, May 4, 1972, Oral History Interviews, Accession 613, History of Medicine Division, National Library of Medicine, quoted in Campbell, *Discovering Addiction,* 55.

189 **series of experiments:** Campbell, Olsen, and Walden, *Narcotic Farm,* 20, 180–81; Caroline Jean Acker, "Addiction and the Laboratory: The Work of the National Research Council's Committee on Drug Addiction," *Isis* 86, no. 2 (June 1995): 1–29, https://doi.org/10.1086/357152; Abraham Wikler, *Opiate Addiction: Psychological and Neurophysiological Aspects in Relation to Clinical Problems* (Springfield, IL: Charles C. Thomas, 1953), 17, https://babel.hathitrust.org/cgi/pt?id=mdp.39015042964331&view =1up&seq=7.

190 **"opioid withdrawal syndrome":** Campbell, *Discovering Addiction,* 70.

190 **increase the risk of overdose death:** John Strang et al., "Loss of Tolerance and Overdose Mortality after Inpatient Opiate Detoxification: Follow Up Study," *BMJ* 326, no. 7396 (May 2003): 959–60, https://doi.org/10.1136/bmj.326.7396.959. See also John Strang, "Death Matters: Understanding Heroin/Opiate Overdose Risk and Testing Potential to Prevent Deaths," *Addiction* 110, no. S2 (July 2015): 27–35, https://doi.org/10.1111/add.12904; James D. Wines et al., "Overdose after Detoxification: A

Prospective Study," *Drug and Alcohol Dependence* 89, no. 2 (July 2007): 161–69, https://doi.org/10.1016/j.drugalcdep.2006.12.019.

190 **boundary between "physical" and "psychological":** Nicolas Rasmussen, "Maurice Seevers, the Stimulants and the Political Economy of Addiction in American Biomedicine," *BioSocieties* 5, no. 1 (March 1, 2010): 105–23, https://doi.org/10.1057/biosoc.2009.7.

190 **opioid-blocking medication Nalline:** Robinson v. California, 370 U.S. 660, 82 S.Ct. 1417 (1962). Also described in Nancy D. Campbell, *OD: Naloxone and the Politics of Overdose* (Cambridge, MA: MIT Press, 2019).

190 **"tolerance and physical dependency":** American Society of Addiction Medicine & National Council on Alcoholism and Drug Dependence, "Disease Definition of Alcoholism," *Annals of Internal Medicine*, 85, no. 6: 764. Also: "Our conceptualization of drug addiction was confused for decades by the fact that key drugs of abuse, such as opiates and alcohol, cause physical dependence as well as addiction. For this reason, the clinical definition of addiction became intertwined with definitions of dependence." Eric J. Nestler, "Historical Review: Molecular and Cellular Mechanisms of Opiate and Cocaine Addiction," *Trends in Pharmacological Sciences* 25, no. 4 (April 2004): 210–18, https://doi.org/10.1016/j.tips.2004.02.005. See also Alexander, *Globalization of Addiction*, 51n.

191 **Fleischl-Marxow loved it:** Howard Markel, *An Anatomy of Addiction: Sigmund Freud, William Halsted, and the Miracle Drug, Cocaine* (New York: Vintage, 2011), chap. 4. "Magical substance" appears in Freud's June 2, 1884, letter to Martha Bernays, as quoted in Markel, *Anatomy of Addiction*, 81.

191 **eminent German physician Friedrich Erlenmeyer:** White, *Slaying the Dragon*, 147.

191 **Freud hung a photo:** Markel, *Anatomy of Addiction*, loc. 1246, 1461 of 6798; chap. 4.

192 **"I need a lot of cocaine":** Sigmund Freud, letter to Wilhelm Fliess, June 12, 1895, in *The Complete Letters of Sigmund Freud to Wilhelm Fliess* (Psychoanalytic Electronic Publishing, n.d.), https://www.pep-web.org/document.php?id=zbk.042.0131a.

194 **Bellevue Hospital's first female case:** Rasmussen, *On Speed*, 98.

194 **they fled for Texas:** Morgan, *Literary Outlaw*, 167.

195 **"rather sleepless night":** Rasmussen, *On Speed*, 12.

196 **the white plastic empties:** Rasmussen, *On Speed*, 46, 98.

196 **stimulants were just "mentally addicting":** Rasmussen, "Maurice Seevers," 110.

196 **warfare for centuries:** Hans Neumann, "Beer as a Means of Compensation for Work in Mesopotamia during the Ur III Period," in *Drinking in Ancient Societies: History of Culture of Drinks in Ancient Near East*, ed. L. Milano (Padua: Propylaeum, 1994): 321–31; Peter Andreas, *Killer High: A History of War in Six Drugs* (New York: Oxford University Press, 2020), 17; Brecher, *Consumers Union Report*, 272.

196 **widespread use of *synthetic* drugs:** Andreas, *Killer High*, 6–7.

196 **35 million methamphetamine tablets:** Rasmussen, *On Speed*, 54–59. See also Norman Ohler, *Blitzed: Drugs in the Third Reich*, trans. Shaun Whiteside (New York: Houghton Mifflin Harcourt, 2017), 29–72.

196 **Though some soldiers hallucinated:** Rasmussen, *On Speed*, 70–87. See also Ohler, *Blitzed*, 52–63.

196 **appreciate the dangers of addiction:** Rasmussen, *On Speed*, 55.

197 **not "any pharmacologic action":** Rasmussen, *On Speed*, 100, 115, 141.

197 **age of affluence:** Jill Lepore, *These Truths: A History of the United States* (New York: W. W. Norton, 2018), 527, 592.

197 **$300 million to $2.3 billion:** Julie Donohue, "A History of Drug Advertising: The Evolving Roles of Consumers and Consumer Protection." *Milbank Quarterly* 84, no. 4 (2006): 659–99; Rasmussen, *On Speed*, 113.

198 **Sackler pioneered momentous innovations:** Barry Meier, *Pain Killer: An Empire of Deceit and the Origin of America's Opioid Epidemic* (New York: Random House, 2003), 52. See also Patrick Radden Keefe, "The Family That Built an Empire of Pain," *New Yorker*, October 30, 2017.

199 **secretly addicted to secobarbital (Seconal):** H. Frank Fraser et al., "Death Due to Withdrawal of Barbiturates," *Annals of Internal Medicine* 38, no. 6 (June 1953): 1319–25, https://doi.org/10.7326/0003-4819-38-6-1319.

199 **reported clinically significant anxiety:** David Herzberg, *Happy Pills in America: From Miltown to Prozac* (Baltimore: Johns Hopkins University Press, 2009), 51.

199 **twenty-four doses per person:** Harris Isbell et al., "Chronic Barbiturate Intoxication: An Experimental Study," *Archives of Neurology and Psychiatry* 64, no. 1 (1950): 1–28, https://doi.org/10.1001/archneurpsyc.1950.02310250007001.

199 **white and well-off consumers:** David Herzberg, *White Market Drugs: Big Pharma and the Hidden History of Addiction in America* (Chicago: University of Chicago Press, 2020), 142–67.

200 **"no matter how addiction is defined":** Harris Isbell, "Addiction to Barbiturates and the Barbiturate Abstinence Syndrome," *Annals of Internal Medicine* 33, no. 1 (1950): 108–21.

201 **middle-class white people:** Musto, *American Disease*, 213.

201 **supported in this effort by pharmaceutical companies:** Courtwright, "Century of American Narcotic Policy," 10; Herzberg, *Happy Pills*, 93–97.

201 **others, called "pharmaceuticals":** Herzberg, *White Market Drugs*, chap. 3. See also Herzberg, "Entitled to Addiction? Pharmaceuticals, Race, and America's First Drug War," *Bulletin of the History of Medicine* 91, no. 3 (Fall 2017): 586–623.

202 **mass incarceration and the opioid crisis:** Herzberg, *White Market Drugs*, 1–17.

202 **emulating his idol, Charlie "Bird" Parker:** Hugh Wyatt, *Sonny Rollins: Meditating on a Riff* (New York: Kamama Books, 2018), 97, 136; George W. Goodman, "Sonny Rollins at Sixty-Eight," *Atlantic*, July 1999, https://www.theatlantic.com/magazine/archive/1999/07/sonny-rollins-at-sixty-eight-9907/377697/.

202 **coroner estimated his age:** "Charlie Parker Biography," *PBS* (website), October 19, 2003, http://www.pbs.org/wnet/americanmasters/charlie-parker-about-charlie-parker/678/.

202 **as many as 75 percent:** Lewis MacAdams, *Birth of the Cool: Beat, Bebop, and the American Avant Garde* (New York: Free Press, 2001), loc. 607 of 4206, Kindle, citing Jazz historian Lincoln Collier.

202 **"the carnage was immense":** Jill Jonnes, *Hep-Cats, Narcs, and Pipe Dreams: A History of America's Romance with Illegal Drugs* (Baltimore: Johns Hopkins University Press, 1999), 135.

203 **early years of Narcotics Anonymous:** White, *Slaying the Dragon*, 331, 343.

203 **a first cannabis offense:** Paul P. Kennedy, "Nearly 500 Seized in Narcotics Raids across the Nation," *New York Times*, January 5, 1952, https://www.nytimes.com/1952/01/05/archives/nearly-500-seized-in-narcotics-raids-across-the-nation-arrests-here.html; Courtwright, "Century of American Narcotic Policy," 20.

203 **Racially restrictive housing policies:** Lepore, *These Truths*, 529–30; Ibram X. Kendi, *Stamped from the Beginning: The Definitive History of Racist Ideas in America* (New York: Public Affairs, 2016), 358–59; Courtwright, "Century of American Narcotic Policy," 17–20.

203 **"inner city" was marred:** Eric C. Schneider, "Introduction: Requiem for the City," in *Smack: Heroin and the American City* (Philadelphia: University of Pennsylvania Press, 2013), ix–xvi.

203 **"practically 100% among Negro people":** Anslinger and Chapman, "Narcotic Addiction," 182, quoted by Courtwright, "Century of American Narcotic Policy," 21.

204 **leading cause of death:** Isbell et al., "Chronic Barbiturate Intoxication," 1–28; Herzberg, "Entitled to Addiction?," 610–11.

204 **one in twenty American adults:** Rasmussen, *On Speed*, 3–4. See also Nicolas Rasmussen, "America's First Amphetamine Epidemic 1929–1971," *American Journal of Public Health* 98, no. 6 (June 2008): 974–85, https://dx.doi.org/10.2105%2FAJPH.2007.110593.

204 **5 percent of all Americans:** Herzberg, *White Market Drugs*, 186.

204 **the pharmaceutical/drug divide:** Herzberg, *White Market Drugs*, 171. See also Courtwright, "Century of American Narcotic Policy," 21.

204 **shot his wife, Joan Vollmer:** Morgan, *Literary Outlaw*, loc. 3959.

205 **"the most useless such establishment":** William Burroughs Jr., "Life with Father," *Esquire*, September 1, 1971, https://classic.esquire.com/article/1971/9/1/life-with-father.

Chapter Nine

211 **crime just to be addicted:** Details of the case taken from testimony at Robinson's trial: Transcript of Record, Robinson v. California, Supreme Court of the United States, October Term, 1961, no. 554. Audio of Supreme Court arguments available at "Robinson v. California," Oyez (website), accessed March 4, 2021, https://www.oyez.org/cases/1961/554. See also the Supreme Court decision itself: Robinson v. California, 370 U.S. 660 (1962), 82 S.Ct. 1417 (1962), as well as Erik Luna, "The Story of *Robinson*: From Revolutionary Constitutional Doctrine to Modest Ban on Status Crimes," in *Criminal Law Stories*, ed. Donna Coker and Robert Weisberg (New York: Foundation Press, 2013), 47–56, and Nancy D. Campbell, *OD: Naloxone and the Politics of Overdose* (Cambridge, MA: MIT Press, 2019), 64. On racial bias in traffic stops, see, for example, "Findings," Stanford Open Policing Initiative (website), accessed March 4, 2021, https://openpolicing.stanford.edu/findings/.

212 **The court took Robinson's case:** Of note, the California court's decision actually invited a further challenge to the criminalization of addiction as a status. For composition of court: "Robinson v. California," Oyez.

213 **"willfully and voluntarily":** Brief of Appellee at 8, Robinson v. California, 370 US 660 (1962); "Foreign Fire": Transcript of Oral Argument, April 17, 1962, Robinson v. California, https://www.oyez.org /cases/1961/554.

213 **"burned at the stake or hanged":** Robinson v. California, 370 U.S. 660, 82 S.Ct. 1417 (1962).

214 **New York Academy of Medicine advocated:** David F. Musto, *The American Disease: Origins of Narcotic Control*, 3rd ed. (New York: Oxford University Press, 1999), 338n44; *Drug Addiction, Crime or Disease? Interim and Final Reports of the Joint Committee of the American Bar Association and the American Medical Association* (Bloomington: Indiana University Press, 1961), Appendix A, http://www .druglibrary.org/schaffer/library/studies/dacd/Default.htm.

214 **Kolb fired off a blistering rebuke:** Lawrence Kolb, "Let's Stop This Narcotics Hysteria!," *Saturday Evening Post*, July 28, 1956, https://www.saturdayeveningpost.com/2016/09/narcotics-hysteria -criminalization-drug-addiction/.

214 **addiction as a learning process:** Alfred R. Lindesmith, *Addiction and Opiates* (Chicago: Aldine, 1968).

214 **recommending experiments in maintenance treatment:** *Drug Addiction, Crime or Disease?*; William L. White, *Slaying the Dragon: The History of Addiction Treatment and Recovery in America*, 2nd ed. (Chicago: Lighthouse Institute, 2014), 351; Rufus King, *The Drug Hang-Up: America's Fifty-Year Folly* (Springfield, IL: Bannerstone House, 1972); David T. Courtwright, Herman Joseph, and Don Des Jarlais, *Addicts Who Survived: An Oral History of Narcotic Use in America before 1965* (Knoxville: University of Tennessee Press, 2012), 297–98.

214 **vitriolic attack against the report:** David T. Courtwright, "A Century of American Narcotic Policy," in *Treating Drug Problems*, vol. 2, ed. D. R. Gerstein and H. J. Harwood (Washington, DC: National Academies Press, 1992), 25; King, *Drug Hang-Up*, chap. 18.

215 **long since died of an overdose:** "Drug Case Victory Won after Death of Addict," *Los Angeles Times*, June 26, 1962, quoted in Jordan Mylet, "The Mark of a Criminal: 'Vag Addicts,' Police Power, and Civil Rights in Postwar America," *Points in History* (blog), June 18, 2020, https://pointshistory.com /2020/06/18/the-mark-of-a-criminal-vag-addicts-police-power-and-civil-rights-in-postwar-america/.

220 **its own "Imperial Marines":** Rod A. Janzen, *The Rise and Fall of Synanon: A California Utopia* (Baltimore: Johns Hopkins University Press, 2001), 24, 134, 223.

221 **"It's Synanon! Synanon got me!":** Hillel Aron, "The Story of This Drug Rehab-Turned-Violent Cult Is *Wild, Wild Country*–Caliber Bizarre," *Los Angeles Magazine*, April 23, 2018, https://www.lamag .com/citythinkblog/synanon-cult/.

221 **eighteen vials of antivenom:** Janzen, *Rise and Fall of Synanon*, 135.

221 **so drunk on Chivas Regal:** Aron, "Drug Rehab-Turned-Violent Cult."

221 **devoted AA member in 1956:** Claire D. Clark, *Recovery Revolution: The Battle over Addiction Treatment in the United States* (New York: Columbia University Press, 2017), 10, 20; Janzen, *Rise and Fall of Synanon*, 10.

221 **called him Dad:** Aron, "Drug Rehab-Turned-Violent Cult."

221 **ultimately too soft:** Paul Morantz has written his own book on Synanon, *From Miracle to Madness* (Los Angeles: Cresta Publications, 2014). It is fascinating reading. See pages 34–35 for an extended discussion of Dederich's philosophical interests and his early years.

221 **known as "cross-talk":** Ernest Kurtz, "Whatever Happened to Twelve-Step Programs?," in *The Collected Ernie Kurtz* (New York: Authors Choice, 2008), 145–76.

221 **form of extreme group therapy:** Clark, *Recovery Revolution*, 23.

222 **"brains washed out":** Charles Dederich, quoted in Janzen, *Rise and Fall of Synanon*. Also on brainwashing: David Deitch, an early leader in the TC movement, speculates that Dederich was directly inspired by the reports of POWs from the Korean War. See David A. Deitch, "Treatment of Drug Abuse in the Therapeutic Community: Historical Influences, Current Considerations, and Future Outlook," in *Drug Use in America: Problem in Perspective*, vol. 4, *Treatment and Rehabilitation*, ed. National Commission on Marihuana and Drug Abuse (Washington, DC: Government Printing Office, 1973), 158–75.

222 **network of complexes:** Claire Clark, "'Chemistry Is the New Hope': Therapeutic Communities and Methadone Maintenance, 1965–71," *Social History of Alcohol and Drugs* 26, no. 2 (Summer 2012): 192–216, https://doi.org/10.1086/SHAD26020192.

222 **severe discipline for months:** Deitch, "Treatment of Drug Abuse," 164–65; William L. White and William R. Miller, "The Use of Confrontation in Addiction Treatment: History, Science and Time for Change," *Counselor* 8, no. 4 (March 2009): 12–30. Journalist Kevin Heldman gives a compelling firsthand description of some of the TC strategies he experienced in the early 1980s. See Kevin Heldman, "Rehab as Skinner Box, Boys Town and Hogan's Heroes: Attempts to Turn Burnouts, Gangstas, and

Misfits into Dale Carnegie through Scrubbing Floors, Wearing Diapers, and Sitting Motionless on a Bench for a Month," Journalism Works Project, accessed March 4, 2021, http://journalismworksproject .org/rehab1.html; J. D. Dickey, "The Dark Legacy of a Rehab Cult," *Fix*, May 9, 2012, https://www .thefix.com/content/aa-cults-synanon-legacy0009?page=all; Kerwin Kaye, *Enforcing Freedom* (New York: Columbia University Press, 2019), 132.

223 **Therapeutic communities filled this void:** Clark, *Recovery Revolution*, 43–45; Nancy D. Campbell, James P. Olsen, and Luke Walden, *The Narcotic Farm: The Rise and Fall of America's First Prison for Drug Addicts* (Lexington: University of Kentucky Press, 2021), 72–78, 102–3.

223 **"make your bed":** "Hazelden Betty Ford Foundation History," Hazelden Betty Ford Foundation (website), accessed March 4, 2021, https://www.hazeldenbettyford.org/about-us/history. See also Damian McElrath, *Hazelden: A Spiritual Odyssey* (n.p., Hazelden Foundation, 1987), 30.

223 **one of the first Christmases:** White, *Slaying the Dragon*, 264. See also William L. White, "Hazelden Foundation," in *Alcohol and Temperance in Modern History: A Global Encyclopedia*, vol. 1, *A–L*, ed. Jack S. Blocker, Ian R. Tyrrell, and David M. Fahey (Santa Barbara, CA: ABC-CLIO, 2003), 190.

223 **This model of a structured curriculum:** White, *Slaying the Dragon*, 263–73. See also Clark, *Recovery Revolution*, 184–87.

224 **regularly fail because of stigma:** Robin Room, "Stigma, Social Inequality and Alcohol and Drug Use," *Drug and Alcohol Review* 24, no. 2 (March 2005): 143–55, https://doi.org/10.1080/095952305 00102434.

224 **"hot seat" in group therapy:** White and Miller, "Use of Confrontation," 16–18.

225 **formally opposed "abusive" techniques:** Maia Szalavitz, "The Cult That Spawned the Tough-Love Teen Industry," *Mother Jones*, September/October 2007, https://www.motherjones.com/politics/2007 /08/cult-spawned-tough-love-teen-industry/.

225 **the worst example:** Kaye, *Enforcing Freedom*, 150–54.

225 **counterproductive, provoking more resistance:** White and Miller, "Use of Confrontation," 21–23. But for complications and contextual considerations, see Douglas L. Polcin, "Rethinking Confrontation in Alcohol and Drug Treatment: Consideration of the Clinical Context," *Substance Use & Misuse* 38, no. 2 (February 2003): 165–84, https://www.tandfonline.com/doi/abs/10.1081/ja-120017243?journalCode =isum20.

225 **offer equivalent results:** Lesley A. Smith, Simon Gates, and David Foxcroft, "Therapeutic Communities for Substance Related Disorder," *Cochrane Database of Systematic Reviews*, no. 1 (2006): CD005338, https://doi.org/10.1002/14651858.CD005338.pub2. Therapeutic community proponents often cite the statistic that 90 percent of those who complete the (months- or even yearslong) treatment and "graduate" remain drug-free, but that's misleading. Only a minority of those screened for admission are accepted at all (sometimes as many as four out of five are turned away), and even out of the few who get in, most don't finish—the average client stays only about one-third of the prescribed time. White, *Slaying the Dragon*, 324–25, 467. See also Fabián Fiestas and Javier Ponce, "Eficacia de las Comunidades Terapéuticas en el Tratamiento de Problemas por Uso de Sustancias Psicoactivas: Una Revisión Sistemática," *Revista Peruana de Medicina Experimental y Salud Pública* 29, no. 1 (March 2012): 12–20, https://doi.org/10.1590/s1726 -46342012000100003; Marion Malivert et al., "Effectiveness of Therapeutic Communities: A Systematic Review," *European Addiction Research* 18, no. 1 (2012): 1–11, https://doi.org/10.1159/000331007.

225 **reconfigure ideas about the self:** George De Leon, "The Therapeutic Community: Toward a General Theory and Model," in *Therapeutic Community: Advances in Research and Application*, NIDA Research Monograph 144, ed. F. M. Tims, George De Leon, and N. Jainchill (Washington, DC: U.S. Department of Health and Human Services, 1994), 16. Consider also Alisa Stevens, "'I Am the Person Now I Was Always Meant to Be': Identity Reconstruction and Narrative Reframing in Therapeutic Community Prisons," *Criminology & Criminal Justice* 12, no. 5 (2012): 527–47, as well as Owen Flanagan, "Identity and Addiction," as discussed in chap. 5 of this book.

228 **some form of coercion:** Carl Erik Fisher, "People Struggling with Addiction Need Help. Does Forcing Them into Treatment Work?," *Slate*, January 18, 2018, https://slate.com/technology/2018/01 /coerced-treatment-for-addiction-can-work-if-you-coerce-correctly.html.

230 **leader for compassionate, nuanced care:** David T. Courtwright, "The Prepared Mind: Marie Nyswander, Methadone Maintenance, and the Metabolic Theory of Addiction," *Addiction* 92, no. 3 (March 1997): 257–65, https://doi.org/10.1111/j.1360-0443.1997.tb03196.x.

230 **fierce optimism and respect:** See, in particular, Marie Nyswander, *The Drug Addict as a Patient* (New York: Grune & Stratton, 1956), 70–84, https://catalog.hathitrust.org/Record/001565298.

230 **"oneness of perception":** Nat Hentoff, "The Treatment of Patients–I," *New Yorker*, June 19, 1965, https://www.newyorker.com/magazine/1965/06/26/i-the-treatment-of-patients.

231 **"truly epidemic sea of misery":** Courtwright, Joseph, and Des Jarlais, *Addicts Who Survived*, 332.

231 **began with basic research:** Ivan Oransky, "Vincent Dole," *Lancet* 368, no. 9540 (September 2006): 984, https://doi.org/10.1016/S0140-6736(06)69402-6. Also Courtwright, "Prepared Mind," 257–58.

231 **extremely slow-acting opioid:** Richard K. Ries et al., *The ASAM Principles of Addiction Medicine*, 5th ed. (New York: Wolters-Kluwer, 2014), 140.

232 **newly invigorated, even "normal":** White, *Slaying the Dragon*, 353–54; Courtwright, "Prepared Mind," 259.

232 **"From two slugabeds":** "Methadone Maintenance: How Much, for Whom, for How Long?," *Medical World News*, March 17, 1972, 53–63, quoted in Eric C. Schneider, *Smack: Heroin and the American City* (Philadelphia: University of Pennsylvania Press, 2013), 167.

232 **dropped a bombshell report:** Vincent P. Dole and Marie Nyswander, "A Medical Treatment for Diacetylmorphine (Heroin) Addiction: A Clinical Trial with Methadone Hydrochloride," *JAMA* 193, no. 8 (August 1965): 646–50, https://doi.org/10.1001/jama.1965.03090080008002.

233 **"treatment offers hope of freedom":** Walter Cronkite, *CBS Evening News*, August 11, 1966, quoted in David T. Courtwright, *Dark Paradise: A History of Opiate Addiction in America* (Cambridge, MA: Harvard University Press, 2001), 164; Nat Hentoff, "The Treatment of Patients–II," *New Yorker*, July 3, 1965, https://www.newyorker.com/magazine/1965/07/03/the-treatment-of-patients.

233 **twenty-two patients expanded to 128:** Vincent P. Dole, Marie E. Nyswander, and Mary Jeanne Kreek, "Narcotic Blockade," *Archives of Internal Medicine* 118, no. 4 (October 1966): 304–9, http://doi.org/10.1001/archinte.1966.00290160004002; Marie E. Nyswander, "The Methadone Treatment of Heroin Addiction," *Hospital Practice* 2, no. 4 (April 1967): 27–33, https://doi.org/10.1080/21548331.1967.11707753.

233 **Manhattan General Hospital:** Courtwright, Joseph, and Des Jarlais, *Addicts Who Survived*, 340. Manhattan General was later absorbed into Beth Israel Hospital, which subsequently developed one of the largest methadone programs in the country (though the original Manhattan General building, like St. Vincent's, across town, was turned into luxury apartments).

233 **"best available answer":** Schneider, *Smack*, 168, 171.

233 **biological code of mental illness:** Nikolas Rose and Joelle M. Abi-Rached, "The Neuromolecular Brain," in *Neuro: The New Brain Sciences and the Management of the Mind* (Princeton: Princeton University Press, 2013), 25–52.

234 **scientific model of mental illness:** David Healy, "Twisted Thoughts and Twisted Molecules," in *The Creation of Psychopharmacology* (Cambridge, MA: Harvard University Press, 2002), 178–225. See also Rose and Abi-Richard, *Neuro*, 10, on electrical to chemical; also Peter Conrad, "The Shifting Engines of Medicalization," *Journal of Health and Social Behavior* 46, no. 1 (March 2005): 3–14, https://doi.org/10.1177%2F002214650504600102.

234 **"gratify and perpetuate their addiction":** David P. Ausubel, "The Dole-Nyswander Treatment of Heroin Addiction," *JAMA* 195, no. 11 (March 1966): 949–50, https://doi.org/10.1001/jama.1966.03100110117032.

234 **"Those are not addicts":** Courtwright, Joseph, and Des Jarlais, *Addicts Who Survived*, 335.

234 **"white, middle class America":** Schneider, *Smack*, 170.

234 **"narcotize the whole ghetto population":** William Raspberry, "Methadone Use: Another Blunder," *Washington Post*, May 11, 1971, A19, quoted in Helena Hansen and Samuel K. Roberts, "Two Tiers of Biomedicalization: Methadone, Buprenorphine, and the Racial Politics of Addiction Treatment," in *Critical Perspectives on Addiction*, ed. Julie Netherland, vol. 14, *Advances in Medical Sociology* (Emerald Group, 2012), 79–102, https://doi.org/10.1108/S1057-6290(2012)0000014008.

234 **"symptoms but not the disease":** "Drug vs. Drug; Methadone Treatment for Heroin Addiction Sparks a Controversy," *Wall Street Journal*, September 9, 1969, quoted in Schneider, *Smack*, 170.

234 **"Our objecti꞉e is to rehabilitate":** Vincent P. Dole and Marie Nyswander, "The Treatment of Heroin Addiction," *JAMA* 195, no. 11 (March 1966): 189, https://doi.org/10.1001/jama.1966.03100110140055.

235 **a "neurological susceptibility":** Vincent P. Dole and Marie E Nyswander, "Heroin Addiction—a Metabolic Disease," *Archives of Internal Medicine* 120, no. 1 (July 1967): 19–24, https://doi.org/10.1001/archinte.1967.00300010021004.

235 **"blockade" against further drug use:** Courtwright, *Dark Paradise*, 164–65.

235 **Dole himself admitted:** See extended discussion in Schneider, *Smack*, 168.

235 **pluralistic approach to addiction treatment:** One such exception was Jerome "Jerry" Jaffe, a psychiatrist and Narco grad who had established a one-stop, "multimodality" treatment program in Chicago, incorporating therapeutic communities, methadone maintenance, and other professional services. *Narcotics and Drug Abuse: Hearings Before the Special Subcommittee on Alcoholism and Narcotics of the Committee on Labor and Public Welfare United States Senate*, 91st Cong. 5939D at 181 (1969) (statement

of Jerome Jaffe, assistant professor, Department of Psychiatry, University of Chicago), http://www
.williamwhitepapers.com/pr/dlm_uploads/1969-Dr.-Jerome-Jaffe-Testimony-on-Illinois-Drug
-Abuse-Program.pdf.

236 **"ghetto malady":** "Life on Two Grams a Day," *Life* 68, no. 6 (February 20, 1970): 24–32. In general,
see Schneider, *Smack*, 142–56.

236 **Nixon deftly connected:** Ibram X. Kendi, *Stamped from the Beginning: The Definitive History of Racist
Ideas in America* (New York: Public Affairs, 2016), 405–11.

236 **"problem is really the blacks":** Harry R. Haldeman, *The Haldeman Diaries: Inside the Nixon White
House* (New York: Berkeley Books, 1995), 66; John Ehrlichman, *Witness to Power: The Nixon Years*
(New York: Simon & Schuster, 1982), 232.

237 **"second civil war":** Richard Nixon, "Drugs Our Second Civil War: Cut the Chain of Greed, Poverty,
Self-Indulgence," *Los Angeles Times*, April 12, 1990, https://www.latimes.com/archives/la-xpm-1990
-04-12-me-1267-story.html. See also Richard Davenport-Hines, *The Pursuit of Oblivion: A Global
History of Narcotics* (London: Weidenfeld & Nicolson, 2001), loc. 8197 of 13059; Myles Ambrose, interview transcript from a 2000 episode of *Frontline*, PBS, https://www.pbs.org/wgbh/pages/frontline
/shows/drugs/interviews/ambrose.html.

237 **education, research, and treatment:** Regarding his 1969 special message to Congress on the "drug
problem," see 115 Cong. Rec. S19353 (1969) (The Drug Problem—Message from the President),
https://www.govinfo.gov/content/pkg/GPO-CRECB-1969-pt14/pdf/GPO-CRECB-1969-pt14-7-2
.pdf.

Chapter Ten

238 **only one in twenty people:** Noa Krawczyk et al., "Only One in Twenty Justice-Referred Adults in Specialty Treatment for Opioid Use Receive Methadone or Buprenorphine," *Health Affairs* 36, no. 12 (December 2017): 2046–53, https://doi.org/10.1377/hlthaff.2017.0890. Access to addiction treatment in the
criminal legal system is abysmal overall, and it is a rapidly developing issue. See "Public Policy Statement
on Treatment of Opioid Use Disorder," American Society of Addiction Medicine, July 15, 2020, https://
www.asam.org/docs/default-source/public-policy-statements/2020-statement-on-treatment
-of-oud-in-correctional-settings.pdf.

239 **push-ups in the snow:** See Keri Blakinger, "New York Prisons Offer 'Tough Love' Boot Camp Programs. But Prisoners Say They're 'Torture' and 'Hell,'" *Appeal*, May 21, 2019, https://theappeal.org
/new-york-prisons-offer-tough-love-boot-camp-programs-but-prisoners-say-theyre-torture-and-hell/.

240 **third-most-pressing problem:** David J. Bellis, *Heroin and Politicians: The Failure of Public Policy to
Control Addiction in America* (Westport, CT: Greenwood Press, 1981), 19.

240 **twelfth-most-important problem:** Kristen Bialik, "State of the Union 2019: How Americans See
Major National Issues," Pew Research Center (website), February 4, 2019, https://www.pewresearch
.org/fact-tank/2019/02/04/state-of-the-union-2019-how-americans-see-major-national-issues/.

240 **enlisted personnel had tried heroin:** Lee N. Robins, *The Vietnam Drug User Returns: Final Report*,
Special Action Office Monograph, Series A, no. 2 (Washington, DC: Special Action Office for Drug
Abuse Prevention, 1974), https://files.eric.ed.gov/fulltext/ED134912.pdf. For more on domestic fears of
addicted Vietnam vets, see Eric C. Schneider, *Smack: Heroin and the American City* (Philadelphia:
University of Pennsylvania Press, 2013), 159–62; Grischa Metlay, "Federalizing Medical Campaigns
against Alcoholism and Drug Abuse," *Milbank Quarterly* 91, no. 1 (March 2013): 123–62, https://doi
.org/10.1111/milq.12004.

240 **vials of 95-percent-pure heroin:** Jill Jonnes, *Hep-Cats, Narcs, and Pipe Dreams: A History of America's
Romance with Illegal Drugs* (Baltimore: Johns Hopkins University Press, 1999), 272. See also Morgan
F. Murphy and Robert H. Steele, *The World Heroin Problem: Report of Special Study Mission* (Washing-
ton, DC: Government Printing Office, 1971), https://books.google.com/books?id=FgZiNcTOVZgC;
Schneider, *Smack*, 161–62. On the Golden Triangle and CIA: Richard Davenport-Hines, *The Pursuit
of Oblivion: A Global History of Narcotics* (London: Weidenfeld & Nicolson, 2001), loc. 8233 of 13059;
Suzanna Reiss, *We Sell Drugs: The Alchemy of US Empire* (Oakland: University of California Press,
2014).

240 **In 1971, two congressmen:** Metlay, "Federalizing Medical Campaigns," 144; Murphy and Steele,
World Heroin Problem, 18.

240 **$2 billion in property crime:** Davenport-Hines, *Pursuit of Oblivion*, loc. 8225.

240 **treatment rather than law enforcement:** "Thirty Years of America's Drug War," *Frontline*, PBS, accessed April 11, 2021, https://www.pbs.org/wgbh/pages/frontline/shows/drugs/cron/index.html#9.

240 **first drug czar:** Karst J. Besteman, "Federal Leadership in Building the National Drug Treatment System," in *Treating Drug Problems*, vol. 2, ed. D. R. Gerstein and H. J. Harwood (Washington, DC: National Academies Press, 1992), 63–88. See also Nancy D. Campbell, James P. Olsen, and Luke Walden, *The Narcotic Farm: The Rise and Fall of America's First Prison for Drug Addicts* (Lexington: University of Kentucky Press, 2021), 190, and Metlay, "Federalizing Medical Campaigns," 145.

241 **"the first therapeutic president":** Kevin Yuill, "Another Take on the Nixon Presidency: The First Therapeutic President?," *Journal of Policy History* 21, no. 2 (April 2009): 138–62, https://doi.org /10.1017/S089803060909006X; David T. Courtwright, *Dark Paradise: A History of Opiate Addiction in America* (Cambridge, MA: Harvard University Press, 2001), 171.

241 **quashing the Mexican experiment:** "The Year Mexico Legalized Drugs," *HistoryExtra*, August 6, 2019, https://www.historyextra.com/period/modern/1940-the-year-mexico-legalised-drugs/. Mexico's foreign ministry had insisted the program was successful, before it was strong-armed into stopping. See also Benjamin Smith, "The Dialectics of Dope: Leopoldo Salazar Viniegra, the Myth of Marijuana, and Mexico's State Drug Monopoly," in *Prohibitions and Psychoactive Substances in History, Culture and Theory*, ed. Susannah Wilson (London: Taylor & Francis, 2019), 111–32.

241 **no real basis in law:** Linder v. United States, 268 U.S. 5 (1925).

241 **"You ought to take me to court":** David T. Courtwright, Herman Joseph, and Don Des Jarlais, *Addicts Who Survived: An Oral History of Narcotic Use in America before 1965* (Knoxville: University of Tennessee Press, 2012), 337–38.

241 **ardent methadone advocates urged:** William L. White, *Slaying the Dragon: The History of Addiction Treatment and Recovery in America*, 2nd ed. (Chicago: Lighthouse Institute, 2014), 360.

242 **bought 280 milligrams of methadone:** Richard Severo, "Ethics of Methadone Use Questioned," *New York Times*, April 18, 1971, https://www.nytimes.com/1971/04/18/archives/ethics-of-methadone-use -questioned-ethics-of-methadone-use-is.html. See also Schneider, *Smack*, 176–77, for more problems with methadone expansion.

242 **"the stupidity of thinking":** Courtwright, Joseph, and Des Jarlais, *Addicts Who Survived*, 338.

242 **flurry of amendments and regulations:** In particular, the Narcotic Addict Treatment Act of 1974, Pub. L. No. 93-281, 88 Stat. 124, https://www.govinfo.gov/content/pkg/STATUTE-88/pdf/STATUTE -88-Pg124.pdf (originally called the "Methadone Diversion Control Act"). See also Schneider, *Smack*, 170; David T. Courtwright, "The Controlled Substances Act: How a 'Big Tent' Reform Became a Punitive Drug Law," *Drug and Alcohol Dependence* 76, no. 1 (October 2004): 9–15, https://doi.org /10.1016/j.drugalcdep.2004.04.012. On racial associations, see Julie Netherland and Helena Hansen, "White Opioids: Pharmaceutical Race and the War on Drugs That Wasn't," *BioSocieties* 12, no. 2 (June 2017): 217–38, https://dx.doi.org/10.1057%2Fbiosoc.2015.46.

242 **arm of law enforcement:** Schneider, *Smack*, 178; Helena Hansen and Samuel K. Roberts, "Two Tiers of Biomedicalization: Methadone, Buprenorphine, and the Racial Politics of Addiction Treatment," in *Critical Perspectives on Addiction*, ed. Julie Netherland, vol. 14, *Advances in Medical Sociology* (London: Emerald, 2012), 86–92.

242 **"sounding like a Republican":** David T. Courtwright, "The Prepared Mind: Marie Nyswander, Methadone Maintenance, and the Metabolic Theory of Addiction," *Addiction* 92, no. 3 (March 1997): 260.

242 **methadone treatment has significant problems:** White, *Slaying the Dragon*, 501–2.

243 **stark racial disparities:** Philippe Bourgois, "Disciplining Addictions: The Bio-Politics of Methadone and Heroin in the United States," *Culture, Medicine and Psychiatry* 24, no. 2 (2000): 165–95.

243 **Black and Puerto Rican community groups:** Nancy D. Campbell, *OD: Naloxone and the Politics of Overdose* (Cambridge, MA: MIT Press, 2019), 96–97; Thomas F. Brady, "St. Luke's Yields on Drug Facility," *New York Times*, January 18, 1970, https://www.nytimes.com/1970/01/18/archives/st-lukes -yields-on-drug-facility-plan-to-aid-young-addicts-ends-a.html; Olga Khazan, "How Racism Gave Rise to Acupuncture for Addiction Treatment," *Atlantic*, August 3, 2018, https://www.theatlantic .com/health/archive/2018/08/acupuncture-heroin-addiction/566393/.

243 **treated as inevitable and expected:** Netherland and Hansen, "White Opioids"; Campbell, *OD*, 287. On how the "war on crime" has positioned law enforcement, criminal legal institutions, and jails as the primary public program in many low-income communities, see Elizabeth Hinton, *From the War on Poverty to the War on Crime: The Making of Mass Incarceration in America* (Cambridge, MA: Harvard University Press, 2016).

243 **"poor fit for the suburban spread":** This quote comes from Alan Leshner, then head of NIDA. 145 Cong. Rec. S1091 (daily ed. January 28, 1999) (October 5, 1998 reply from NIDA Director, Dr. Alan Leshner), https://www.congress.gov/congressional-record/1999/01/28/senate-section/article/S1076-3; Hansen and Roberts, "Two Tiers of Biomedicalization," 92–97; Netherland and Hansen, "White Opioids," 13–14.

243 **roughly 90 percent:** Westat and the Avisa Group, *The SAMSHA Evaluation of the Impact of the DATA Waiver Program*, Task Order 277-00-6111 (Washington, DC: Center for Substance Abuse Treatment, 2006), 3–10, https://www.samhsa.gov/sites/default/files/programs_campaigns/medication_assisted /evaluation-impact-data-waiver-program-summary.pdf; Helena Hansen and Julie Netherland, "Is the Prescription Opioid Epidemic a White Problem?," *American Journal of Public Health* 106, no. 12 (December 2016): 2127–29, https://doi.org/10.2105/AJPH.2016.303483.

244 **still far more likely:** Pooja A. Lagisetty et al., "Buprenorphine Treatment Divide by Race/Ethnicity and Payment," *JAMA Psychiatry* 76, no. 9 (May 2019): 979–81, https://doi.org/10.1001/jamapsychiatry.2019.0876. White people received the medication at 12.7 million office-based treatment visits from 2012 to 2015, as compared with 363,000 visits for all others. For regional and socioeconomic disparities, see also Pashmineh Azar et al., "Rise and Regional Disparities in Buprenorphine Utilization in the United States," *Pharmacoepidemiology and Drug Safety* 29, no. 6 (June 2020): 708–15, https://doi.org/10.1002/pds.4984.

244 **entirely separate system:** As just one example of the two-tiered system, in January 2019, reporters at *Politico* described an addiction treatment setting where patients with private insurance go upstairs to an inpatient facility that offers medication treatment, counseling, and follow-up services, and patients who can't pay for treatment or who are there on a criminal justice mandate go downstairs to a boot-camp-like setting that shaves patients' heads, refuses to provide medication, and relies on confrontational therapy. Brianna Ehley and Rachel Roubein, "'I'm Trying Not to Die Right Now': Why Opioid-Addicted Patients Are Still Searching for Help," *Politico*, January 20, 2019, https://www.politico.com/story/2019/01/20/opioid -treatment-addiction-heroin-1088007. See also Allison McKim's excellent *Addicted to Rehab: Race, Gender, and Drugs in the Era of Mass Incarceration* (New Brunswick, NJ: Rutgers University Press, 2017). This, of course, has been a feature of the system for decades (see Mariana Valverde, *Diseases of the Will: Alcohol and the Dilemmas of Freedom* (New York: Cambridge University Press, 1998); Virginia Berridge, *Demons: Our Changing Attitudes to Alcohol, Tobacco, and Drugs* (New York: Oxford University Press, 2013).

244 **the "Junkie Priest":** John D. Harris, *The Junkie Priest, Father Daniel Egan, S.A.* (New York: Coward-McCann, 1964). See also Eric Pace, "Daniel Egan, 84, Drug Fighter Known as 'Junkie Priest,' Dies," *New York Times*, February 13, 2000, https://www.nytimes.com/2000/02/13/nyregion/daniel-egan-84 -drug-fighter-known-as-junkie-priest-dies.html.

244 **anti-medication attitudes in twelve-step:** See the extensive monograph by William L. White and Lisa Mojer-Torres, *Recovery-Oriented Methadone Maintenance* (Madison, WI: Great Lakes Addiction Technology Transfer Center, 2010), https://facesandvoicesofrecovery.org/wp-content/uploads/2019/06 /Recovery-Oriented-Methadone-Maintenance.pdf. See also Stephen Gilman, Marc Galanter, and Helen Dermatis, "Methadone Anonymous: A 12-Step Program for Methadone Maintained Heroin Addicts," *Substance Abuse* 22, no. 4 (2001): 247–56, https://doi.org/10.1080/08897070109511466.

244 **official communications from NA:** "Regarding Methadone and Other Drug Replacement Programs," World Service Board of Trustees Bulletin No. 29, Narcotics Anonymous World Services (website), 1996, https://na.org/?ID=bulletins-bull29. See also the pamphlet *Narcotics Anonymous and Persons Receiving Medication-Assisted Treatment* (Chatsworth, CA: NA World Services, 2016), https://www .na.org/admin/include/spaw2/uploads/pdf/pr/2306_NA_PRMAT_1021.pdf; William L. White, *Narcotics Anonymous and the Pharmacotherapeutic Treatment of Opioid Addiction in the United States* (Philadelphia: Department of Behavioral Health and Intellectual Disability Services, 2011), http://www .williamwhitepapers.com/pr/dlm_uploads/2011-NA-Medication-assisted-Treatment.pdf.

244 **"chewing your booze":** "On the Subject of Drugs, by One Who Took Them," *Grapevine*, March 1947, https://silkworth.net/wp-content/uploads/2020/07/Grapevine-Vol3-No10-Mar-1947.pdf; Ernest Kurtz, *Not God: A History of Alcoholics Anonymous* (Center City, MN: Hazelden Educational Materials, 1979), 116, 347, citing several early *Grapevine* articles.

245 **ideal of being "drug-free":** For a personal account, see Clancy Martin, "The Drunks Club: AA, the Cult That Cures," *Harper's*, December 9, 2010. For a professional discussion, see Izaak L. Williams and David Mee-Lee, "Inside the Black Box of Traditional Treatment Programs: Clearing the Air on the Original Literary Teachings of Alcoholics Anonymous (AA)," *Addiction Research & Theory* 27, no. 5 (September 2019): 412–19, https://doi.org/10.1080/16066359.2018.1540692.

245 **cut the rate of death:** Matthias Pierce et al., "Impact of Treatment for Opioid Dependence on Fatal Drug-Related Poisoning: A National Cohort Study in England," *Addiction* 111, no. 2 (February 2016): 298–308, https://doi.org/10.1111/add.13193; Luis Sordo et al., "Mortality Risk during and after Opioid Substitution Treatment: Systematic Review and Meta-Analysis of Cohort Studies," *BMJ* 257, no. 8103 (April 2017): j1550, https://doi.org/10.1136/bmj.j1550. See also Sarah E. Wakeman et al., "Comparative Effectiveness of Different Treatment Pathways for Opioid Use Disorder," *JAMA Network Open* 3, no. 2 (February 2020): e1920622, https://doi.org/10.1001/jamanetworkopen.2019.20622.

245 **more than forty thousand patients:** Wakeman et al., "Comparative Effectiveness." Extended-release naltrexone also has data in its favor for reducing relapse; ultimately, it is important for the practicing clinician to have options, because no treatment works for all patients. Joshua D. Lee et al., "Comparative Effectiveness of Extended-Release Naltrexone versus Buprenorphine-Naloxone for Opioid Relapse Prevention (X:BOT): A Multicentre, Open-Label, Randomised Controlled Trial," *Lancet* 391, no. 10118 (January 2018): 309–18, https://doi.org/10.1016/S0140-6736(17)32812-X.

245 **In 2012, Hazelden announced:** German Lopez, "There's a Highly Successful Treatment for Opioid Addiction. But Stigma Is Holding It Back," *Vox*, November 15, 2017, https://www.vox.com/science-and-health/2017/7/20/15937896/medication-assisted-treatment-methadone-buprenorphine-naltrexone.

245 **does not allow its clients:** See its original stance at "Methadone vs Suboxone in Opioid Treatment: Hazelden Betty Ford Foundation's View on Use," Hazelden Betty Ford Foundation (website), October 28, 2016, https://web.archive.org/web/20161105110130/https://www.hazeldenbettyford.org/articles/methadone-vs-suboxone-opioid-treatment. "While methadone is very effective and useful for certain populations, most people in methadone maintenance programs commonly don't have an abstinence orientation, which can result in continued use of benzodiazepines, cocaine, alcohol, marijuana, and other drugs. This is not in keeping with our abstinence-based, Twelve Step model." This is still their current position, albeit with slightly different wording: "Suboxone v. Methadone v. Naltrexone in Opioid Addiction Treatment," Hazelden Betty Ford Foundation (website), December 12, 2019, https://www.hazeldenbettyford.org/articles/methadone-vs-suboxone-opioid-treatment.

245 **National Commission on Marihuana and Drug Abuse:** United States Commission on Marihuana and Drug Abuse, *Marihuana: A Signal of Misunderstanding: First Report* (Washington, DC: Government Printing Office, 1972). The volume is still relevant today, especially sec. V, 127–68.

245 **Nixon, predictably, ignored the report:** David F. Musto, *The American Disease: Origins of Narcotic Control*, 3rd ed. (New York: Oxford University Press, 1999), 256n29.

245 **In 1975, the Ford administration:** Domestic Council Drug Abuse Task Force, *White Paper on Drug Use: September 1975* (Washington, DC: Government Printing Office, 1975), https://www.ojp.gov/pdffiles1/Photocopy/38406NCJRS.pdf.

246 **increasingly restrictive and punitive measures:** Herzberg describes the CSA as a potentially radical possibility for rethinking drug reform, but one that was overcome by the later punitive developments. David Herzberg, *White Market Drugs: Big Pharma and the Hidden History of Addiction in America* (Chicago: University of Chicago Press, 2020), chaps. 5–6. See also Leo Beletsky, "Controlled Substances Act at 50: A Blueprint for Reform," Northeastern University School of Law Research Paper No. 370-2020 (February 25, 2020), https://dx.doi.org/10.2139/ssrn.3544384; Courtwright, "The Controlled Substances Act," 9–15; Joseph F. Spillane, "Debating the Controlled Substances Act," *Drug and Alcohol Dependence* 76, no. 1 (October 2004): 17–29, https://doi.org/10.1016/j.drugalcdep.2004.04.011.

246 **powerful new law enforcement tools:** Dan Baum, *Smoke and Mirrors: The War on Drugs and the Politics of Failure* (New York: Little, Brown, 1996), 68, referring to BNDD.

246 **"hunted to the end of the earth":** Baum, *Smoke and Mirrors*, 72.

246 **to $217 million in 1974:** *Congressional Resource Guide to the Federal Effort on Narcotics Abuse and Control 1969–1976, Part 1: A Report of the Select Committee on Narcotics Abuse and Control*, SCNAC-95-2-2 (Washington, DC: Government Printing Office, 1978), 250, https://www.ojp.gov/pdffiles1/Digitization/48337NCJRS.pdf.

246 **created the Drug Enforcement Administration:** Jonnes, *Hep-Cats*, 296–97.

247 **in 1973, Nelson Rockefeller:** Gene Spagnoli, "Rocky Asks Life for Pushers," *New York Daily News*, January 3, 1973, sec. C; Jessica Neptune, "Harshest in the Nation: The Rockefeller Drug Laws and the Widening Embrace of Punitive Politics," *Social History of Alcohol and Drugs* 26, no. 2 (Summer 2012): 1–22, https://doi.org/10.1086/SHAD26020170.

247 **"tougher penalties and stronger weapons":** Richard Nixon, "Radio Address about the State of the Union Message on Law Enforcement and Drug Abuse Prevention," March 10, 1973, https://www.presidency.ucsb.edu/documents/radio-address-about-the-state-the-union-message-law-enforcement-and-drug-abuse-prevention.

247 **political scientist James Q. Wilson suggested:** James Q. Wilson, "If Every Criminal Knew He Would Be Punished If Caught," *New York Times*, January 28, 1973, https://www.nytimes.com/1973/01/28/archives/if-every-criminal-knew-he-would-be-punished-if-caught-but-he-doesnt.html.

247 **more enforcement-oriented tools:** Hinton, *From the War on Poverty*. See also Kerwin Kaye, *Enforcing Freedom* (New York: Columbia University Press, 2019), 52.

247 **Hughes, the senator:** Bart Barnes, "Harold Hughes Dies at 74," *Washington Post*, October 25, 1996, https://www.washingtonpost.com/archive/local/1996/10/25/harold-hughes-dies-at-74/5c2e1ca8-ce34 -4d3f-93f4-d684ba9f1e5b/.

247 **Hughes led a congressional charge:** Nancy Olson, *With a Lot of Help from Our Friends: The Politics of Alcoholism* (Lincoln, NE: Writers Club Press, 2003), 110–17.

248 **"in the guise of helping them":** Harold Hughes, North American Congress on Alcohol and Drug Problems, San Francisco, California, December 13, 1974, quoted in Olson, *With a Lot of Help*, 457–58. See also Harold A. Mulford, *Alcoholism in Wonderland: A Memoir* (self-pub, 2001), http://www .williamwhitepapers.com/pr/Mulford%20Memoir%202001.pdf; "Public Figures Take Part in Program at Conference," NIAAA Information and Feature Service, October 1, 1974, 5, https://books .google.com/books?id=DFUsrIfed8sC.

248 **quintupled from 1973 to 1977:** White, *Slaying the Dragon*, 376–83, 391. Other developments included federal legislation and increased population of people seeking treatment. On legislation: Constance Weisner and Robin Room, "Financing and Ideology in Alcohol Treatment," *Social Problems* 32, no. 2 (December 1984): 167–84, https://doi.org/10.2307/800786. On increased population: Robin Room, "Treatment-Seeking Populations and Larger Realities," in *Alcoholism Treatment in Transition*, ed. Griffith Edwards and Marcus Grant (London: Croom Helm, 1980), 205–24. The budget of the NIAAA grew from a paltry $6.5 million in 1970 to $214 million in 1975. William Grimes, "Morris Chafetz, 87, Dies; Altered View of Alcoholism," *New York Times*, October 21, 2011, https://www .nytimes.com/2011/10/21/us/morris-chafetz-87-dies-altered-view-of-alcoholism.html. By 1977, specialty alcoholism treatment facilities delivered an estimated $700 million worth of services, and general health facilities spent an additional $2 billion. Leonard Saxe et al., *Health Technology Case Study 22: The Effectiveness and Costs of Alcoholism Treatment* (Washington, DC: Government Printing Office, 1983), 59, https://www.princeton.edu/~ota/disk3/1983/8307/8307.pdf.

248 **well over a million people:** *Special Report to the U.S. Congress on Alcohol and Health from the Secretary of Health and Human Services* (Rockville, MD: National Institute on Alcohol Abuse and Alcoholism, 1981).

248 **Desperate for staff:** Ernie Kurtz calls it a "mad race for money." See Kurtz, "Whatever Happened to Twelve-Step Programs?," in *The Collected Ernie Kurtz* (New York: Authors Choice, 2008), 151. Note also White, *Slaying the Dragon*, 396, on everyone being diagnosed with the same condition. William L. White, "Lost Vision: Addiction Counseling as Community Organization," *Alcoholism Treatment Quarterly* 19, no. 4 (2001): 1–32, https://psycnet.apa.org/doi/10.1300/J020v19n04_01.

249 **"if you *don't* go to AA":** John Schwarzlose, quoted in Nan Robertson, *Getting Better: Inside Alcoholics Anonymous* (New York: William Morrow, 1988), 210.

249 **addiction was changing drastically:** William R. Miller, "Alcoholism: Toward a Better Disease Model," *Psychology of Addictive Behaviors* 7, no. 2 (1993): 129–36, https://doi.org/10.1037/0893-164X.7.2.129.

249 **without lowering their use:** Katie Witkiewitz et al., "What Is Recovery?," *Alcohol Research: Current Reviews* 40, no. 3 (September 2020): 1–12, https://doi.org/10.35946/arcr.v40.3.01.

250 **"abstinence violation effect":** Susan Curry, G. Alan Marlatt, and Judith R. Gordon, "Abstinence Violation Effect: Validation of an Attributional Construct with Smoking Cessation," *Journal of Consulting and Clinical Psychology* 55, no. 2 (1987): 145–49, https://psycnet.apa.org/doi/10.1037/0022-006X.55.2 .145; G. Alan Marlatt and Dennis M. Donovan, eds., *Relapse Prevention: Maintenance Strategies in the Treatment of Addictive Behaviors* (New York: Guilford Press, 2005).

250 **Pike rallied his CEO friends:** Burt A. Folkart, "Thomas P. Pike; Industrialist Led Fight against Alcoholism," *Los Angeles Times*, August 3, 1993, https://www.latimes.com/archives/la-xpm-1993 -08-03-mn-19647-story.html; Olson, *With a Lot of Help*, 51, 92; Sally Brown and David R. Brown, *A Biography of Mrs. Marty Mann: The First Lady of Alcoholics Anonymous* (Center City, MN: Hazelden, 2011), 282; "Pike, Thomas P.: Records, 1955–58," February 16, 1972, Dwight D. Eisenhower Library, Abilene, Kansas, https://web.archive.org/web/20170125043425/https://www.eisenhower.archives.gov /research/finding_aids/pdf/Pike_Thomas_Records.pdf.

251 **"obsession of every abnormal drinker":** *Alcoholics Anonymous*, 4th ed. (New York: Alcoholics Anonymous World Services, 2001), 30.

251 **"fought like a tiger":** Olson, *With a Lot of Help*, 257. See also David J. Armor, J. Michael Polich, and Harriet B. Braiker, *Alcoholism and Treatment* (Santa Monica CA: RAND Corporation, 1976), https:// www.rand.org/pubs/reports/R1739.html; Ron Roizen, "Comment on the 'Rand Report,'" *Journal of Studies on Alcohol* 38, no. 1 (January 1977): 170–78, https://doi.org/10.15288/jsa.1977.38.152.

251 **the director refused:** Morris E. Chafetz, *The Tyranny of Experts: Blowing the Whistle on the Cult of Expertise* (Lanham, MD: Madison Books, 1996), 113.

251 **"unprincipled, and playing Russian roulette":** NCA press release, July 1, 1976, reproduced in David J. Armor, I. Michael Polich, and Harriet B. Stambul, *Alcoholism and Treatment* (New York: John Wiley & Sons, 1978), 232–33.

251 **"a lot of people will die":** Dr. Nicholas A. Pace, president, New York City chapter of the National Council on Alcoholism, quoted in Jane Brody, "Study on Alcoholics Called 'Misleading,'" *New York Times*, June 11, 1976, https://www.nytimes.com/1976/06/11/archives/study-on-alcoholics-called-misleading -alcoholic-study-held.html.

251 **Enoch Gordis, a future director:** Quoted in Robertson, *Getting Better*, 192.

251 **AA Big Book itself recognized:** *Alcoholics Anonymous*, 31. "We do not like to pronounce any individual as alcoholic," and it acknowledges that not all substance problems necessarily fit into their framework and that there are many other roads to recovery.

251 **Mark and Linda Sobell:** Mark B. Sobell and Linda C. Sobell, "Individualized Behavior Therapy for Alcoholics," *Behavior Therapy* 4, no. 1 (January 1973): 49–72, https://doi.org/10.1016/S0005 -7894(73)80074-7; Sobell and Sobell, "Second Year Treatment Outcome of Alcoholics Treated by Individualized Behavior Therapy: Results," *Behaviour Research and Therapy* 14, no. 3 (January 1, 1976): 195–215, https://doi.org/10.1016/0005-7967(76)90013-9; Sobell and Sobell, *Behavioral Treatment of Alcohol Problems: Individualized Therapy and Controlled Drinking* (New York: Springer, 1978). There was an independent three-year follow-up of their study, which was consistent with what the Sobells reported: Glenn R. Caddy, Harold J. Addington Jr., and David Perkins, "Individualized Behavior Therapy for Alcoholics: A Third Year Independent Double-Blind Follow-Up," *Behaviour Research and Therapy* 16, no. 5 (1978): 345–62, https://doi.org/10.1016/0005-7967(78)90004-9.

252 **job performance showed improvement, too:** Sobell and Sobell, "Individualized Behavior Therapy for Alcoholics," table 7.

252 **disillusioned former patient:** Roizen, "Comment on the 'Rand Report,'" 171.

252 **"Beyond any reasonable doubt, it's fraud":** Philip M. Boffey, "Alcoholism Study under New Attack," *New York Times*, June 28, 1982, https://www.nytimes.com/1982/06/28/us/alcholism-study-under-new -attack.html.

252 **CBS show *60 Minutes*:** Robert E. Haskell, "Realpolitik in the Addictions Field: Treatment-Professional, Popular-Culture Ideology, and Scientific Research," *Journal of Mind and Behavior* 14, no. 3 (Summer 1993): 257–76, https://www.jstor.org/stable/43853765.

253 **completely exonerated the Sobells:** At this point in their career, the Sobells were at the prestigious Addiction Research Foundation, in Toronto, which conducted a monthslong investigation into the allegations of fraud. The resulting 143-page report came to the "clear and unequivocal" conclusion that the Sobells had acted with scientific and personal integrity. Bernard M. Dickens et al., *Report of the Committee of Enquiry into Allegations Concerning Drs. Linda & Mark Sobell* (Toronto: Alcoholism and Drug Addiction Research Foundation, 1982). Other investigations are described in G. Alan Marlatt, "The Controlled-Drinking Controversy: A Commentary," *American Psychologist* 38, no. 10 (October 1983): 1097–110, https://doi.org/10.1037//0003-066x.38.10.1097; Mark B. Sobell and Linda C. Sobell, "Moratorium on Maltzman," *Journal of Studies on Alcohol* 50, no. 5 (1989): 473–80; Ron Roizen, "The Great Controlled-Drinking Controversy," in *Recent Developments in Alcoholism*, vol. 5, ed. Marc Galanter (New York: Plenum, 1987), 245–79.

253 **without total abstinence:** Witkiewitz et al., "What Is Recovery?," 4. For further discussion of this issue of "controlled drinking," see Nick Heather and Ian Robertson's classic book *Controlled Drinking* (London: Methuen, 1981), as well as Marlatt, "Controlled-Drinking Controversy."

253 **binary "loss of control":** For example, people diagnosed as alcoholics were given unlimited access to alcohol but moderated their intake according to rewards and inconveniences; in other words, expectations and not the amount of alcohol in the drink drove the amount people with alcoholism consumed. By 1981, there was enough evidence on "controlled drinking" for Heather and Robertson to publish their classic book on the subject, with hundreds of supportive references, and there were similar findings for drug addiction, such as the researcher Norman Zinberg's classic finding that "chippers" regularly used heroin in a controlled way. Heather and Robertson, *Controlled Drinking*, particularly chap. 3; Herbert Fingarette, *Heavy Drinking: The Myth of Alcoholism as a Disease* (Berkeley: University of California Press, 1988), 35–38; Norman E. Zinberg, Wayne M. Harding, and Miriam Winkeller, "A Study of Social Regulatory Mechanisms in Controlled Illicit Drug Users," *Journal of Drug Issues* 7, no. 2 (April 1977): 117–33, https://doi.org/10.1177%2F002204267700700203.

253 **evidence-based treatments for addiction:** William R. Miller, "Motivation for Treatment: A Review with Special Emphasis on Alcoholism," *Psychological Bulletin* 98, no. 1 (1985): 85–107, https://content .apa.org/doi/10.1037/0033-2909.98.1.84; William R. Miller and Stephen Rollnick, *Motivational*

Interviewing: Preparing People to Change Addictive Behavior (New York: Guilford Press, 1991); Miller interview: William R. Miller, "Warm Turkey: Other Routes to Abstinence," interview by Andrew C. Page, *Journal of Substance Abuse Treatment* 8, no. 4 (January 1991): 227–32, https://doi.org/10.1016 /0740-5472(91)90043-A; White, *Slaying the Dragon*, 465; Marlatt and Donovan, *Relapse Prevention*.

253 **Marsha Keith Schuchard:** Baum, *Smoke and Mirrors*, 88–89, based on his interview with Keith Schuchard; Emily Dufton, Grass *Roots: The Rise and Fall and Rise of Marijuana in America* (New York: Basic Books, 2017), 90. See also Musto, *American Disease*, 264.

254 **most people in the late seventies:** For example, in 1978, the perception among high school seniors that cannabis was harmful reached a low point of 35 percent. Musto, *American Disease*, 264.

254 **"welfare queens" and "strapping young bucks":** See, for example, "'Welfare Queen'" Becomes Issue in Reagan Campaign," *New York Times*, February 15, 1976, https://www.nytimes.com/1976/02/15 /archives/welfare-queen-becomes-issue-in-reagan-campaign-hitting-a-nerve-now.html.

254 **"drug problem" as a moral issue:** Musto, *American Disease*, 265–67; Baum, *Smoke and Mirrors*, 140–41.

255 **solution was individual responsibility:** David Farber, *Crack: Rock Cocaine, Street Capitalism, and the Decade of Greed* (New York: Cambridge University Press, 2019), 129–62, https://doi.org/10.1017 /9781108349055.

255 **"self-help, voluntary initiatives":** Keith Humphreys, *Circles of Recovery: Self-Help Organizations for Addictions* (New York: Cambridge University Press, 2004), 149–76.

255 **Mothers Against Drunk Driving:** Craig Reinarman, "The Social Construction of an Alcohol Problem," *Theory and Society* 17, no. 1 (January 1, 1988): 91–120, https://doi.org/10/b55kvt. MADD was thus attractive to, and cozy with, industry interests—both Anheuser-Busch and Miller Brewing made significant contributions.

255 **widened the pharmaceutical/drug divide:** Herzberg, *White Market Drugs*, chap. 7.

255 **the role of law enforcement:** This was true below the federal level as well, of course. See Donna Murch, "Crack in Los Angeles: Crisis, Militarization, and Black Response to the Late Twentieth-Century War on Drugs," *Journal of American History* 102, no. 1 (June 2015): 162–73, https://doi.org /10.1093/jahist/jav260.

255 **"taking down the surrender flag":** Ronald Reagan, "Remarks on Signing Executive Order 12368, Concerning Federal Drug Abuse Policy Functions," June 24, 1982, American Presidency Project, University of California, Santa Barbara, https://www.presidency.ucsb.edu/documents/remarks-signing -executive-order-12368-concerning-federal-drug-abuse-policy-functions. See also Baum, *Smoke and Mirrors*, 166.

255 **budgets of federal agencies grew:** "Staffing and Budget," Drug Enforcement Administration (website), accessed February 24, 2021, https://www.dea.gov/staffing-and-budget. Between 1979 and 1984, the DEA budget grew from $200 million to well over $300 million. Also important, the Reagan drug war enabled new connections between the military and domestic law enforcement. Hinton, *From the War on Poverty*, 311.

255 **expansion in asset forfeiture laws:** Eric L. Jensen and Jurg Gerber, "The Civil Forfeiture of Assets and the War on Drugs: Expanding Criminal Sanctions While Reducing Due Process Protections," *Crime & Delinquency* 42, no. 3 (1996): 421–34, https://doi.org/10.1177%2F0011128796042003005.

255 **"almost instantaneous addiction":** Arnold Washton, quoted in "Kids and Cocaine," *Newsweek*, March 17, 1986, discussed in Craig Reinarman and Harry G. Levine, "Crack in the Rearview Mirror: Deconstructing Drug War Mythology," *Social Justice* 31, nos. 1/2 (2004): 182–99, https://www.jstor .org/stable/29768248. See also Ibram X. Kendi, *Stamped from the Beginning: The Definitive History of Racist Ideas in America* (New York: Public Affairs, 2016), 434; Michelle Alexander, *The New Jim Crow* (New York: New Press, 2012), 5; Jacob Sullum, "Smackdown!," *Reason*, June 1, 2003, https://reason .com/2003/06/01/smackdown-2/.

256 **"national crusade against drugs":** Ronald Reagan, "Remarks Announcing the Campaign against Drug Abuse and a Question-and-Answer Session with Reporters," White House Rose Garden, August 4, 1986, Ronald Reagan Presidential Library and Museum, https://www.reaganlibrary.gov /archives/speech/remarks-announcing-campaign-against-drug-abuse-and-question-and-answer-session.

256 **radical sentencing disparities:** Kendi, *Stamped from the Beginning*, 435. On sentencing. Musto, *American Disease*, 273. See also Neptune, "Harshest in the Nation."

256 **largest system of incarceration on earth:** Roy Walmsley, *World Prison Population List*, 12th ed. (London: Institute for Criminal Policy Research, 2018), https://www.prisonstudies.org/sites/default/files /resources/downloads/wppl_12.pdf.

256 **more than twice as likely:** *Crime in the United States: 2019* (Washington, DC: Federal Bureau of Investigation), Table 43, https://ucr.fbi.gov/crime-in-the-u.s/2019/crime-in-the-u.s.-2019/topic-pages/tables

/table-43. The degree to which drug arrests contribute to mass incarceration is a contested topic in criminology—i.e., whether drug laws are a main driver of mass incarceration, versus just one small component of a much larger and more complex system. Consider John Pfaff, *Locked In: The True Causes of Mass Incarceration—and How to Achieve Real Reform* (New York: Basic Books, 2017), arguing against the conclusions of Michelle Alexander's *New Jim Crow*. (Also consider the important distinction between people exposed to the system and the total proportion of incarcerated people at a given time: Jonathan Rothwell, "Drug Offenders in American Prisons: The Critical Distinction between Stock and Flow," *Brookings* (blog), November 25, 2015, https://www.brookings.edu/blog/social-mobility-memos/2015/11/25/drug-offenders-in-american-prisons-the-critical-distinction-between-stock-and-flow/.) Suffice to say that the war on drugs, and particularly the moral panic around drugs, was one important component of mass incarceration—at the very least, a powerful driver of attitudes about punishment.

256 **DARE (Drug Abuse Resistance Education):** DARE was founded by Daryl Gates, chief of the Los Angeles Police Department. For a taste of his approach, consider how Gates, testifying before the Senate Judiciary Committee in 1990, said that "the casual drug user ought to be taken out and shot." Gates, quoted in Davenport-Hines, *Pursuit of Oblivion*, locs. 1073–74 of 13059.

257 **White House officials lined up to urinate:** Cornelius Friesendorf, *US Foreign Policy and the War on Drugs: Displacing the Cocaine and Heroin Industry* (New York: Routledge, 2007), 81; Eleanor Clift, "Drug Testing for Reagan, Top Aides to Begin Monday," *Los Angeles Times*, August 8, 1986, https://www.latimes.com/archives/la-xpm-1986-08-08-mn-1846-story.html.

257 **"Where the fuck is the White House?":** Craig Reinarman and Harry G. Levine, eds., *Crack in America: Demon Drugs and Social Justice* (Berkeley: University of California Press, 1997), 22. The special agent in charge of the DEA's Washington office later admitted, "We had to manipulate him to get him down there. It wasn't easy. Corinne Purtill, "US Agents Lured a Teen near the White House to Sell Drugs So George H. W. Bush Could Make a Point," *Quartz*, December 2, 2018, https://qz.com/1481809/george-h-w-bush-had-a-teen-set-up-to-lure-sell-drugs-near-white-house/.

258 **number was 54 percent:** "War: 1 Percent. Drugs: 54 Percent," *New York Times*, September 28, 1989, https://www.nytimes.com/1989/09/28/opinion/war-1-percent-drugs-54-percent.html.

259 **fifteen thousand specialized treatment programs:** Substance Abuse and Mental Health Services Administration, *National Survey of Substance Abuse Treatment Services (N-SSATS): 2019. Data on Substance Abuse Treatment Facilities* (Rockville, MD: Substance Abuse and Mental Health Services Administration, 2020); Substance Abuse and Mental Health Services Administration, *Key Substance Use and Mental Health Indicators in the United States: Results from the 2019 National Survey on Drug Use and Health* (Washington, DC: Department of Health and Human Services, 2020), 54; ResearchandMarkets.com, "United States Addiction Rehab Industry Report 2020: SAMHSA Survey Findings, Major Trends & Issues, Operating Ratios, Competitor Profiles, and More," GlobeNewswire News Room, January 29, 2020, http://www.globenewswire.com/news-release/2020/01/29/1976908/0/en/United-States-Addiction-Rehab-Industry-Report-2020-SAMHSA-Survey-Findings-Major-Trends-Issues-Operating-Ratios-Competitor-Profiles-and-More.html. For a compelling description of what it's like for families to find treatment today, see David Sheff, *Clean* (New York: Houghton Mifflin Harcourt, 2013), 129–34, reporting in part on the experience of Gary Mendell (of the nonprofit Shatterproof).

259 **"Body brokers":** Peter Haden, "'Body Brokers' Get Kickbacks to Lure People with Addictions to Bad Rehab," *NPR*, August 15, 2017, https://www.npr.org/sections/health-shots/2017/08/15/542630442/body-brokers-get-kickbacks-to-lure-people-with-addictions-to-bad-rehab.

259 **just there to urinate:** David Segal, "In Pursuit of Liquid Gold," *New York Times*, December 27, 2017, www.nytimes.com/interactive/2017/12/27/business/urine-test-cost.html.

259 **disconnected from evidence-based practices:** CASA Columbia, *Addiction Medicine: Closing the Gap between Science and Practice* (New York: Columbia University Press, 2012), https://drugfree.org/reports/addiction-medicine-closing-the-gap-between-science-and-practice/. To be specific, many are doubly non-evidence-based: there are evidence-based interventions they aren't using, and the practices they do use often lack an evidence base.

260 **resume substance use:** John F. Kelly and William L. White, *Addiction Recovery Management: Theory, Research and Practice (Current Clinical Psychiatry)* (New York: Humana Press, 2011), introduction, chap. 16.

260 **criminal legal referrals:** White, *Slaying the Dragon*, 434; Kaye, *Enforcing Freedom*, 3–16; Weisner and Room, "Financing and Ideology in Alcohol Treatment," 176.

260 **treatment related to drunk driving:** Weisner and Room, "Financing and Ideology in Alcohol Treatment," 176–77.

260 **massive arrest-to-treatment pipeline:** Substance Abuse and Mental Health Services Administration, Center for Behavioral Health Statistics and Quality, *Treatment Episode Data Set (TEDS): 2017. Admissions to and Discharges from Publicly-Funded Substance Use Treatment* (Rockville, MD: Substance Abuse and Mental Health Services Administration, 2019), 57–58, https://www.samhsa.gov/data/sites/default/files/cbhsq-reports/TEDS-2017.pdf. See also Kaye, *Enforcing* Freedom, 3–16, for a discussion of this arrest-to-treatment pipeline.

260 **coercive approach spread outward:** White, *Slaying the Dragon*, 392–93.

260 **"alcoholics are liars":** R. S. Greenberger, "Sobering Methods: Firms Are Confronting Alcoholic Executives with Threat of Firing," *Wall Street Journal*, 1983, quoted in William L. White and William R. Miller, "The Use of Confrontation in Addiction Treatment: History, Science and Time for Change," *Counselor* 8, no. 4 (March 2009): 3.

261 **terminating treatment when people relapse:** For example, in 2014, there were more than 100,000 cases of forced termination, more than 7 percent of all treatment cases during that year. For further discussion: Izaak L. Williams and David Mee-Lee, "Inside the Black Box of Traditional Treatment Programs: Clearing the Air on the Original Literary Teachings of Alcoholics Anonymous," *Addiction Research & Theory* 27, no. 5 (2019): 412–19, https://doi.org/10.1080/16066359.2018.1540692, citing SAMHSA data. Again see Sheff, *Clean*, 129–34, for a personal description of forced termination.

261 **AA never insisted:** William L. White and Ernest Kurtz, "A Message of Tolerance and Celebration: The Portrayal of Multiple Pathways of Recovery in the Writings of Alcoholics Anonymous Co-Founder Bill Wilson," *Selected Papers of William L. White*, 2010, http://smtp.williamwhitepapers.com/pr/dlm_uploads/2010-Bill-Wilson-on-Multiple-Pathways-of-Recovery.pdf. White and Kurtz have documented numerous statements from Bill Wilson to this effect, e.g., "AA has no monopoly on reviving alcoholics." "The roads to recovery are many . . . Any story or theory of recovery from one who has trod the highway is bound to contain much truth." "Upon therapy for the alcoholic himself, we surely have no monopoly." "In no circumstances should members feel that Alcoholics Anonymous is the know-all and do-all of alcoholism."

261 **often the *only* treatment goal:** Katie Witkiewitz and Jalie A. Tucker, "Abstinence Not Required: Expanding the Definition of Recovery from Alcohol Use Disorder," *Alcoholism: Clinical & Experimental Research* 44, no. 1 (January 2020): 36–40, https://doi.org/10.1111/acer.14235.

262 **declined by more than 70 percent:** Tami L. Mark and Rosanna M. Coffey, "The Decline in Receipt of Substance Abuse Treatment by the Privately Insured, 1992–2001," *Health Affairs* 23, no. 6 (November 2004): 157–62, https://doi.org/10.1377/hlthaff.23.6.157; White, *Slaying the Dragon*, 401.

262 **"a nice bulldozer":** Maia Szalavitz, "The Rehab Industry Needs to Clean Up Its Act. Here's How," *Huff-Post*, February 12, 2016, https://www.huffpost.com/entry/the-rehab-industry-needs-clean-up_b_9210542.

263 **"How many people have to die?":** Randy Shilts, *And the Band Played On: Politics, People, and the AIDS Epidemic*, 20th Anniversary Edition (New York: St. Martin's Press, 2007), 265–86.

263 **Cancer patients demanded:** Siddhartha Mukherjee, *Emperor of All Maladies: A Biography of Cancer* (New York: Scribner, 2010), 321–23.

263 **A "consumer movement":** Paul S. Appelbaum, *Almost a Revolution: Mental Health Law and the Limits of Change* (New York: Oxford University Press, 1994).

263 **patients' bills of rights:** Paul Starr, *The Social Transformation of American Medicine: The Rise of a Sovereign Profession and the Making of a Vast Industry* (New York: Basic Books, 1982), 389.

263 **first generation of harm reduction activists:** Maia Szalavitz has recently written an excellent history of the harm reduction movement in the United States, based on hundreds of interviews, detailed research, and her own first-person account of drug use. Maia Szalavitz, *Undoing Drugs: The Untold Story of Harm Reduction and the Future of Addiction* (New York: Hachette Go, forthcoming). See also Campbell, *OD*, 142, 202; Pat O'Hare, "Merseyside, the First Harm Reduction Conferences, and the Early History of Harm Reduction," *International Journal of Drug Policy* 18 (2007): 141–44.

264 **"frenzied and desperate minutes before injecting":** Joyce Purnick, "Koch Bars Easing of Syringe Sales in AIDS Fight," *New York Times*, October 4, 1985, https://www.nytimes.com/1985/10/04/nyregion/koch-bars-easing-of-syringe-sales-in-aids-fight.html.

264 **legal and public relations battles:** Szalavitz, *Undoing Drugs*, chap. 5; Reinarman and Levine, *Crack in America;* Nancy D. Campbell and Susan J. Shaw, "Incitements to Discourse: Illicit Drugs, Harm Reduction, and the Production of Ethnographic Subjects," *Cultural Anthropology* 23, no. 4 (November 2008): 688–717; Warwick Anderson, "The New York Needle Trial: The Politics of Public Health in the Age of AIDS," *American Journal of Public Health* 81, no. 11 (November 1991): 1506–18.

264 **"wash your mouth out with soap":** Campbell, *OD*, 140.

264 **Federal law banned funding:** Of note, the ban was briefly lifted, then reinstated in 2011. Sarah Barr, "Needle-Exchange Programs Face New Federal Funding Ban," *Kaiser Health News* (blog), December

21, 2011, https://khn.org/news/needle-exchange-federal-funding/. On studies: "Syringe Services Programs (SSPs) FAQs," CDC (website), updated May 23, 2019, https://www.cdc.gov/ssp/syringe-services -programs-faq.html.

265 **range of evidence-based practices:** The evidence for naloxone, drug checking, and syringe service programs is extremely strong and supported by the CDC: "CDC Health Alert Advisory: Increase in Fatal Drug Overdoses across the United States Driven by Synthetic Opioids before and during the COVID-19 Pandemic," CDC Health Alert Network, December 17, 2020, https://emergency.cdc.gov/han/2020/pdf /CDC-HAN-00438.pdf; "Reverse Overdose to Prevent Death," CDC (website), updated October 2, 2020, https://www.cdc.gov/drugoverdose/prevention/reverse-od.html; "Syringe Services Programs (SSPs) Fact Sheet," CDC (website), May 23, 2019, https://www.cdc.gov/ssp/syringe-services-programs -factsheet.html. Safe consumption facilities are more controversial and often face community opposition, but they also have strong evidence in their favor: *Overdose Prevention in New York City: Supervised Injection as a Strategy to Reduce Opioid Overdose and Public Injection* (New York: New York City Health, 2018), https://www1.nyc.gov/assets/doh/downloads/pdf/public/supervised-injection-report.pdf.

265 **"harm reduction therapy":** Szalavitz, *Undoing Drugs*, chap. 13. Andrew Tatarsky and G. Alan Marlatt, "State of the Art in Harm Reduction Psychotherapy: An Emerging Treatment for Substance Misuse," *Journal of Clinical Psychology* 66, no. 2 (2010): 117–22, https://doi.org/10.1002/jclp.20672.

265 **a "stepped care" model:** Mark Sobell and Linda C. Sobell, "It Is Time for Low-Risk Drinking Goals to Come Out of the Closet," *Addiction* 106, no. 10 (October 2011): 1715–74, https://doi.org/10.1111 /j.1360-0443.2011.03509.x. For example, medications are still useful for people who are unwilling or unable to engage in psychosocial support. Kathleen M. Carroll and Roger D. Weiss, "The Role of Behavioral Interventions in Buprenorphine Maintenance Treatment: A Review," *American Journal of Psychiatry* 174, no. 8 (August 2017): 738–47, https://doi.org/10.1176/appi.ajp.2016.16070792. Stephen A. Martin et al., "The Next Stage of Buprenorphine Care for Opioid Use Disorder," *Annals of Internal Medicine* 169, no. 9 (October 23, 2018): 628–35, https://doi.org/10.7326/M18-1652. This in fact is the official guidance for New York State–certified addiction treatment programs: Marc Manseau, *Standards for Person-Centered Medication Treatment at OASAS Certified Programs* (Albany: New York State Office of Alcoholism and Substance Abuse Services, 2019), https://oasas.ny.gov/system/files/documents /2019/10/medical-standards-for-certified-programs.pdf.

265 **stated as a philosophy:** This is my own necessarily imperfect distillation of statements about harm reduction made by leading stakeholders. See "Principles of Harm Reduction," National Harm Reduction Coalition (website), accessed March 5, 2021, https://harmreduction.org/about-us/principles-of -harm-reduction/; "About HRI," Harm Reduction International (website), accessed March 5, 2021, https://www.hri.global/about. For further critical discussion of harm reduction as a philosophy and movement, see Helen Keane, "Critiques of Harm Reduction, Morality and the Promise of Human Rights," *International Journal of Drug Policy* 14, no. 3 (2003): 227–32, https://doi.org/10.1016/S0955 -3959(02)00151-2; Bernadette Pauly, "Harm Reduction through a Social Justice Lens," *International Journal of Drug Policy* 19, no. 1 (2008): 4–10, https://doi.org/10.1016/j.drugpo.2007.11.005; Tara Marie Watson et al., "Critical Studies of Harm Reduction: Overdose Response in Uncertain Political Times," *International Journal of Drug Policy* 76 (2020): 102615, https://doi.org/10.1016/j.drugpo.2019.102615.

266 **Democratic Party's commitment:** For example, the notorious 1994 crime bill. Dan Baum, "Epilogue: Night and Day: 1993–1994," in *Smoke and Mirrors*, 329–37. On the continued opposition to harm reduction measures in treatment and research in the 1990s, see Campbell, *OD*, 174–81.

266 **"can't arrest our way out":** Gil Kerlikowske, interview with Michael Martin, "Drug Control Policy Director Talks Prevention," *NPR*, July 16, 2010, https://www.npr.org/templates/story/story.php?storyId =128567349; Amanda Gardner, "White House Drug Policy Shifts Strategy," *MedicineNet*, April 17, 2012, https://www.medicinenet.com/script/main/art.asp?articlekey=157198; Zachary A. Siegel, "We've Been Fighting the Drug War for 50 Years. So Why Aren't We Winning?," *Appeal*, June 4, 2018, https:// theappeal.org/weve-been-fighting-the-drug-war-for-50-years-so-why-arent-we-winning/.

266 **was finally lifted in 2016:** Audie Cornish, "Congress Ends Ban on Federal Funding for Needle Exchange Programs," *NPR*, January 8, 2016, https://www.npr.org/2016/01/08/462412631/congress-ends-ban-on -federal-funding-for-needle-exchange-programs. On investments in naloxone: Campbell, *OD*, 181

Chapter Eleven

269 **plague of soldiers:** "Federalizing Medical Campaigns against Alcoholism and Drug Abuse," *Milbank Quarterly* 91, no. 1 (March 2013): 140–47; Matthew Pembleton, *Containing Addiction: The Federal Bureau of Narcotics and the Origins of America's Global Drug War* (Amherst: University of Massachusetts

Press, 2017), 289–90; John E. Helzer, "Significance of the Robins et al. Vietnam Veterans Study," *American Journal on Addictions* 19, no. 3 (May–June 2010): 218–21, https://doi.org/10.1111/j.1521 -0391.2010.00044.x.

269 **testing positive each month:** Lee N. Robins et al., "Vietnam Veterans Three Years after Vietnam: How Our Study Changed Our View of Heroin," *American Journal on Addictions* 19, no. 3 (May–June 2010): 203–11, https://doi.org/10.1111/j.1521-0391.2010.00046.x; Eric C. Schneider, *Smack: Heroin and the American City* (Philadelphia: University of Pennsylvania Press, 2013), 162–63.

269 **Jaffe also wanted to understand:** Jerry Jaffe, interview by Nancy Campbell, 1998, Oral History of Substance Abuse Research Project, Bentley Historical Library, University of Michigan, Ann Arbor. Other useful descriptions of the studies: Robins et al., "Vietnam Veterans"; Wayne Hall and Megan Weier, "Lee Robins' Studies of Heroin Use among US Vietnam Veterans," *Addiction* 112, no. 1 (2017): 176–80, https://doi.org/10.1111/add.13584; Jerome H. Jaffe, "A Follow-Up of Vietnam Drug Users: Origins and Context of Lee Robins' Classic Study," *American Journal on Addictions* 19, no. 3 (May 2010): 212–14, https://doi.org/10.1111/j.1521-0391.2010.00043.x.

270 **only 1 percent were addicted:** Robins et al., "Vietnam Veterans," 206. The key 1970s papers: Lee N. Robins, "A Follow-up Study of Vietnam Veterans' Drug Use," *Journal of Drug Issues* 4, no. 1 (January 1974): 61–63, https://doi.org/10.1177/002204267400400107; Lee N. Robins, Darlene H. Davis, and Donald W. Goodwin, "Drug Use by U.S. Army Enlisted Men in Vietnam: A Follow-Up on Their Return Home," *American Journal of Epidemiology* 99, no. 4 (April 1, 1974): 235–49, https://doi.org /10.1093/oxfordjournals.aje.a121608; Lee N. Robins, Darlene H. Davis, and David N. Nurco, "How Permanent Was Vietnam Drug Addiction?," *American Journal of Public Health* 64, no. S12 (December 1974): 38–43, https://doi.org/10.2105/AJPH.64.12_Suppl.38; Lee N. Robins, "Narcotic Use in Southeast Asia and Afterward: An Interview Study of 898 Vietnam Returnees," *Archives of General Psychiatry* 32, no. 8 (August 1975): 955–61, https://doi.org/10.1001/archpsyc.1975.01760260019001.

270 **no more than 12 percent:** Robins, Davis, and Goodwin, "Drug Use," 242–43.

270 **recovery without any treatment:** Robins et al., "Vietnam Veterans," 207.

270 **incredulity and outright denial:** Jaffe, "A Follow-up of Vietnam Drug Users," 213.

271 **reliable and rigorously classified entities:** For example, through such means as the "Feighner Criteria" and the Research Diagnostic Criteria, which formed the basis of the *DSM*, today's huge compendium of diagnostic criteria. Kenneth S. Kendler, Rodrigo A. Muñoz, and George Murphy, "The Development of the Feighner Criteria: A Historical Perspective," *American Journal of Psychiatry* 167, no. 2 (2010): 134–42.

271 **equated physical dependence with addiction:** To meet Robins's criteria for addiction, subjects had to meet three of the following four criteria: (1) frequency of use, (2) presence of withdrawal symptoms, (3) length of withdrawal symptoms, and (4) self-report of "believes he was addicted." The self-report of addiction, of course, could also simply reflect the popular understanding of addiction as tolerance and dependence and not the subjective sense of loss of control. Robins, "Narcotic Use in Southeast Asia and Afterward," 955.

271 **discrete and relatively uniform condition:** On the central tenets and endurance of the folk psychology of addiction, see E. Mansell Pattison, Mark B. Sobell, and Linda C. Sobell, *Emerging Concepts of Alcohol Dependence* (New York: Springer, 1977), 10. Robin Room, "Social Science Research and Alcohol Policy Making," in *Alcohol: The Development of Sociological Perspectives on Use and Abuse*, ed. Paul Roman (New Brunswick, NJ: Rutgers Center of Alcohol Studies, 1991), 311–35.

272 **"great majority of alcohol addicts":** E. M. Jellinek, "Phases in the Drinking History of Alcoholics: Analysis of a Survey Conducted by the Official Organ of Alcoholics Anonymous," *Quarterly Journal of Studies on Alcohol* 7, no. 1 (1946): 1–88, https://doi.org/10.15288/QJSA.1946.7.1; and E. M. Jellinek, "Phases of Alcohol Addiction," *Quarterly Journal of Studies on Alcohol* 13, no. 4 (1952): 673–84, https:// doi.org/10.15288/qjsa.1952.13.673. See also Trysh Travis, *Language of the Heart* (Chapel Hill: University of North Carolina, 2009), 38–39; Robin Room, "Governing Images of Alcohol and Drug Problems: The Structure, Sources, and Sequels of Conceptualizations of an Intractable Problem" (PhD diss., University of California, Berkeley, 1978), 55–57; Ron Roizen, "The Great Controlled-Drinking Controversy," in *Recent Developments in Alcoholism*, vol. 5, ed. Marc Galanter (New York: Plenum, 1987), 257–59.

272 **upward slope of "rehabilitation":** M. M. Glatt, "Group Therapy in Alcoholism," *British Journal of Addiction* 54, no. 2 (1958): 133–48.

272 **recapitulated the classic temperance tale:** Several others have made this observation. See, for example, John Crowley, ed., *Drunkard's Progress: Narratives of Addiction, Despair, and Recovery* (Baltimore: Johns Hopkins University Press, 1999), 1, 20.

272 **"the most widely diffused artifact":** Room, "Governing Images of Alcohol and Drug Problems," 55–56. See, for example, "Stages of Alcoholism," Hazelden Betty Ford Foundation (website), March 13, 2019, https://www.hazeldenbettyford.org/articles/stages-of-alcoholism.

273 **hundreds of Boston-area men:** George Vaillant, *The Natural History of Alcoholism* (Cambridge, MA: Harvard University Press, 1983).

274 **rate of comorbidity:** Bridget F. Grant et al., "Prevalence and Co-Occurrence of Substance Use Disorders and Independent Mood and Anxiety Disorders: Results from the National Epidemiologic Survey on Alcohol and Related Conditions," *Archives of General Psychiatry* 61, no. 8 (August 1, 2004): 807–16, https://doi.org/10.1001/archpsyc.61.8.807; Harry Man Xiong Lai et al., "Prevalence of Comorbid Substance Use, Anxiety and Mood Disorders in Epidemiological Surveys, 1990–2014: A Systematic Review and Meta-Analysis," *Drug and Alcohol Dependence* 154 (September 1, 2015): 1–13, https://doi.org/10.1016/j.drugalcdep.2015.05.031. Some outlier studies have comorbidity rates approaching or even at 100 percent: Rosemary E. F. Kingston, Christina Marel, and Katherine L. Mills, "A Systematic Review of the Prevalence of Comorbid Mental Health Disorders in People Presenting for Substance Use Treatment in Australia," *Drug and Alcohol Review* 36, no. 4 (2017): 527–39, https://doi.org/10.1111/dar.12448.

274 **comorbidity across all psychiatric disorders:** Ronald C. Kessler et al., "Prevalence, Severity, and Comorbidity of 12-Month DSM-IV Disorders in the National Comorbidity Survey Replication," *Archives of General Psychiatry* 62, no. 6 (June 1, 2005): 617–27, https://doi.org/10.1001/archpsyc.62.6.617. For cross-cultural findings also showing high rates of comorbidity, see Oleguer Plana-Ripoll et al., "Exploring Comorbidity within Mental Disorders among a Danish National Population," *JAMA Psychiatry* 76, no. 3 (March 1, 2019): 259, https://doi.org/10.1001/jamapsychiatry.2018.3658; Annika Steffen et al., "Mental and Somatic Comorbidity of Depression: A Comprehensive Cross-Sectional Analysis of 202 Diagnosis Groups Using German Nationwide Ambulatory Claims Data," *BMC Psychiatry* 20, no. 1 (March 30, 2020): 142, https://doi.org/10.1186/s12888-020-02546-8.

274 **improve without any interventions:** Jalie A. Tucker, Susan D. Chandler, and Katie Witkiewitz, "Epidemiology of Recovery from Alcohol Use Disorder," *Alcohol Research* 40, no. 3 (2020): 2, https://doi.org/10.35946/arcr.v40.3.02.

274 **stop using them by age thirty:** Gene M. Heyman, "Addiction and Choice: Theory and New Data," *Frontiers in Psychiatry* 4 (2013), https://doi.org/10.3389/fpsyt.2013.00031.

274 **age thirty-seven, approximately 75 percent:** Gene M. Heyman, *Addiction: A Disorder of Choice* (Cambridge, MA: Harvard University Press, 2009), 67–83. Over the course of someone's lifetime, the estimated chance that a severe substance problem will go into remission is stratospheric: 83.7 percent for nicotine, 90.6 percent for alcohol, 97.2 percent for cannabis, and 99.2 percent for cocaine. Catalina Lopez-Quintero et al., "Probability and Predictors of Remission from Life-Time Nicotine, Alcohol, Cannabis or Cocaine Dependence: Results from the National Epidemiologic Survey on Alcohol and Related Conditions," *Addiction* 106, no. 3 (2011): 657–69, https://doi.org/10.1111/j.1360-0443.2010.03194.x. See also Wilson M. Compton et al., "Prevalence, Correlates, Disability, and Comorbidity of DSM-IV Drug Abuse and Dependence in the United States: Results from the National Epidemiologic Survey on Alcohol and Related Conditions," *Archives of General Psychiatry* 64, no. 5 (2007): 566–76, https://doi.org/10.1001/archpsyc.64.5.566.

274 **when far narrower criteria are used:** Jerome C. Wakefield and Mark F. Schmitz, "The Harmful Dysfunction Model of Alcohol Use Disorder: Revised Criteria to Improve the Validity of Diagnosis and Prevalence Estimates," *Addiction* 110, no. 6 (June 2015): 931–42, https://doi.org/10.1111/add.12859. Jerome C. Wakefield and Mark F. Schmitz, "Corrigendum: How Many People Have Alcohol Use Disorders? Using the Harmful Dysfunction Analysis to Reconcile Prevalence Estimates in Two Community Surveys," *Frontiers in Psychiatry* 5, no. 144 (2014), https://doi.org/10.3389/fpsyt.2014.00144.

275 **massive funding into drug research:** Scott Vrecko, "Birth of a Brain Disease: Science, the State and Addiction Neuropolitics," *History of the Human Sciences* 23, no. 4 (August 2010): 52–67, https://doi.org/10.1177/0952695110371598. Generally, on the discovery of the opioid receptor, see David Healy, *The Creation of Psychopharmacology* (Cambridge, MA: Harvard University Press, 2002), 211.

276 **researchers at Narco had hypothesized:** Nancy D. Campbell, *Discovering Addiction: The Science and Politics of Substance Abuse Research* (Ann Arbor: University of Michigan Press, 2007), 211.

276 **electric organ of an electric eel:** David Healy, "Twisted Thoughts and Twisted Molecules," in *The Creation of Psychopharmacology* (Cambridge, MA: Harvard University Press, 2002), 210.

276 **the first verified receptor:** Candace B. Pert and Solomon H. Snyder, "Opiate Receptor: Demonstration in Nervous Tissue," *Science* 179, no. 4077 (March 1973): 1011–14, https://doi.org/10.1126/science.179.4077.1011.

276 **John Hughes and Hans Kosterlitz:** Snyder, Hughes, and Kosterlitz, but not Pert, were given the 1978 Lasker Award, one of the most prestigious prizes in all of medicine. Pert objected, claiming she originated the work and even fought for it over objections and threatened cancellation by Snyder, and it became an international controversy, with echoes of other men taking credit for women's scientific work, like Katherine Johnson and Rosalind Franklin. "Lasker Award Stirs Controversy," *Science* 203, no. 4378 (January 1979): 341, https://doi.org/10.1126/science.216074.

276 **an era of "receptor fever":** Campbell, *Discovering Addition*, 210. Also Nancy D. Campbell, "Multiple Commitments: Heterogeneous Histories of Neuroscientific Addiction Research," in *The Routledge Handbook of Philosophy and Science of Addiction*, ed. Hanna Pickard and Serge H. Ahmed (New York: Routledge, 2019), 240–50.

276 **damaged the receptor system:** A. Goldstein, "Opioid Peptides (Endorphins) in Pituitary and Brain," *Science* 193, no. 4258 (September 1976): 7, https://doi.org/10.1126/science.959823.

276 *New York Times* **proclaimed:** Harold M. Schinieck Jr., "Opiate-Like Substances in Brain May Hold Clue to Pain and Mood," *New York Times*, October 2, 1977, https://www.nytimes.com/1977/10/02/archives/opiatelike-substances-in-brain-may-hold-clue-to-pain-and-mood.html.

277 **natural "runner's high":** Julie Deardorff, "Chasing Facts on Runners' High," *Chicago Tribune*, October 10, 2003, https://www.chicagotribune.com/news/ct-xpm-2003-10-12-0310120504-story.html.

277 **Billy's addiction might stem from:** William S. Burroughs Jr., *Cursed from Birth*, ed. David Ohle (Brooklyn: Soft Skull Press, 2006), 190.

277 **failed to find consistent changes:** Eric J. Nestler, "Historical Review: Molecular and Cellular Mechanisms of Opiate and Cocaine Addiction," *Trends in Pharmacological Sciences* 25, no. 4 (April 2004): 210–18, https://doi.org/10.1016/j.tips.2004.02.005. "Early [receptor] research failed to find consistent changes in opioid receptors, monoamine transporters and other targets that could account for drug tolerance and dependence."

277 **"we must plead failure":** Solomon H. Snyder, "You've Come a Long Way, Baby!," in *The Opiate Receptors*, ed. Gavril W. Pasternak (New York: Springer, 2010), 4. See also Nancy D. Campbell, *OD: Naloxone and the Politics of Overdose* (Cambridge, MA: MIT Press, 2019), 43-44.

277 **genetic factors increased the risk:** Donald Goodwin, *Is Alcoholism Hereditary? One in Six Families in America Is Affected by Alcoholism. Here Is the Answer to Their Most Pressing Question* (New York: Random House, 1988).

277 **excited articles in the popular press:** See, for example, Margot Slade and Wayne Biddle, "Ideas and Trends; Inheriting Alcoholism," *New York Times*, July 25, 1982, https://www.nytimes.com/1982/07/25/weekinreview/ideas-and-trends-inheriting-alcoholism.html; Lucinda Franks, "A New Attack on Alcoholism," *New York Times*, October 20, 1985, https://www.nytimes.com/1985/10/20/magazine/a-new-attack-on-alcoholism.html; Sandra Blakeslee, "Scientists Find Key Biological Causes of Alcoholism," *New York Times*, https://www.nytimes.com/1984/08/14/science/scientists-find-key-biological-causes-of-alcoholism.html.

277 **"scientists should have perfected":** Andrew Purvis, "Medicine: DNA and the Desire to Drink," *Time*, April 30, 1990, http://content.time.com/time/subscriber/article/0,33009,969965,00.html.

277 **coverage as a blatant overpromise:** Stanton Peele, "Second Thoughts about a Gene for Alcoholism," *Atlantic*, August 1990, https://www.peele.net/lib/atlcgene.html. See also Gabor Maté, "It's Not in the Genes," in *In the Realm of Hungry Ghosts* (Berkeley: North Atlantic Books, 2010), 211–31, for extended useful discussion of genetic narratives.

278 **treatment industry and popular authors:** For example, in the 1989 book *Getting Better*, by Nan Robertson, the vast majority of her chapter on medical research, titled "The Disease," focuses on how addiction genetics legitimizes the disease concept. Nan Robertson, *Getting Better: Inside Alcoholics Anonymous* (New York: William Morrow, 1988), 183–209.

278 **only one of many factors:** William R. Miller and David J. Atencio, "Free Will as a Proportion of Variance," in *Are We Free? Psychology and Free Will*, ed. John Baer, James C. Kaufman, and Roy F. Baumeister (New York: Oxford University Press, 2008), 275–95.

278 **heritability of addiction:** A. Agrawal et al., "The Genetics of Addiction—a Translational Perspective," *Translational Psychiatry* 2, no. 7 (July 2012): e140, https://doi.org/10.1038/tp.2012.54; Mary-Anne Enoch, "Genetic Influences on the Development of Alcoholism," *Current Psychiatry Reports* 15, no. 11 (November 2013): 412, https://doi.org/10.1007/s11920-013-0412-1; Dana B. Hancock et al., "Human Genetics of Addiction: New Insights and Future Directions," *Current Psychiatry Reports* 20, no. 2 (March 2018): 8, https://doi.org/10.1007/s11920-018-0873-3; Richard C. Crist, Benjamin C. Reiner, and Wade H. Berrettini, "A Review of Opioid Addiction Genetics," in "Genetics," special issue, *Current Opinion in Psychology* 27 (June 2019): 31–35, https://doi.org/10.1016/j.copsyc.2018.07.014.

278 **"the importance of the environment":** Robert Plomin, quoted by Charles C. Mann, "Behavioral Genetics in Transition: A Mass of Evidence—Animal and Human—Shows That Genes Influence Behavior. But the Attempt to Pin Down Which Genes Influence Behaviors Has Proved Frustratingly Difficult," *Science* 264, no. 5166 (June 17, 1994): 1686–90, https://doi.org/10.1126/science.8209246.

279 **everything beyond the brain:** Keith Humphreys et al., "Brains, Environments, and Policy Responses to Addiction," *Science* 356, no. 6344 (June 2017): 1237–38, https://doi.org/10.1126/science.aan0655.

279 **five different types of *Trunksucht*:** Friedrich-Wilhelm Kielhorn, "The History of Alcoholism: Brühl-Cramer's Concepts and Observations," *Addiction* 91, no. 1 (January 1996): 123–24.

279 **various "oinomanias," or wine manias:** William B. Carpenter, *On the Use and Abuse of Alcoholic Liquors, in Health and Disease* (Philadelphia, 1855), 45, https://books.google.com/books?id= V-sPAAAAYAAJ; Thomas F. Babor and Richard J. Lauerman, "Classification and Forms of Inebriety: Historical Antecedents of Alcoholic Typologies," in *Recent Developments in Alcoholism*, vol. 4, ed. Marc Galanter (New York: Plenum, 1986), 113–44. Babor has found thirty-nine different classification systems published from 1850 to 1941.

280 **actually complicating the disease notion:** E. M. Jellinek, *The Disease Concept of Alcoholism* (New York: Hillhouse Press, 1960), 36; Penny Booth Page, "E. M. Jellinek and the Evolution of Alcohol Studies: A Critical Essay," *Addiction* 92, no. 12 (December 1997): 1619–37, https://doi.org/10.1111 /j.1360-0443.1997.tb02882.x; John F. Kelly, "E. M. Jellinek's Disease Concept of Alcoholism," *Addiction* 114, no. 3 (September 2018): 555–59, https://doi.org/10.1111/add.14400.

280 **based on inherited traits:** Thomas F. Babor and Raul Caetano, "Subtypes of Substance Dependence and Abuse: Implications for Diagnostic Classification and Empirical Research," *Addiction* 101, no. S1 (2006): 104–10, https://doi.org/10.1111/j.1360-0443.2006.01595.x.

280 **different, powerful influences on addiction:** Victor M. Hesselbrock and Michie N. Hesselbrock, "Are There Empirically Supported and Clinically Useful Subtypes of Alcohol Dependence?," *Addiction* 101, no. S1 (2006): 97–103, https://doi.org/10.1111/j.1360-0443.2006.01596.x; Lia Nower et al., "Subtypes of Disordered Gamblers: Results from the National Epidemiologic Survey on Alcohol and Related Conditions," *Addiction* 108, no. 4 (January 3, 2013): 789–98, https://doi.org/10.1111/add.12012.

281 **almost entirely determined by trauma:** Timothy D. Brewerton and Kathleen Brady, "The Role of Stress, Trauma, and PTSD in the Etiology and Treatment of Eating Disorders, Addictions, and Substance Use Disorders," in *Eating Disorders, Addictions and Substance Use Disorders*, ed. Timothy D. Brewerton and Amy Baker Dennis (New York: Springer, 2014), 379–404.

281 **no one dominant cause of addiction:** Lorenzo Leggio et al., "Typologies of Alcohol Dependence: From Jellinek to Genetics and Beyond," *Neuropsychology Review* 19, no. 1 (2009): 115–29, https://doi .org/10.1007/s11065-008-9080-z; Mark Griffiths, "A 'Components' Model of Addiction within a Biopsychosocial Framework," *Journal of Substance Use* 10, no. 4 (2005): 191–97, https://doi.org/10.1080 /14659890500114359; Mark D. Griffiths and Michael Larkin. "Conceptualizing Addiction: The Case for a 'Complex Systems' Account," *Addiction Research & Theory* 12, no. 2 (2004): 99–102, https://doi .org/10.1080/1606635042000193211; James MacKillop and Lara A. Ray, "The Etiology of Addiction," in *Integrating Psychological and Pharmacological Treatments for Addictive Disorders*, 1st ed., ed. James MacKillop et al., (New York: Routledge, 2017), 32–53, https://doi.org/10.4324/9781315683331-2; Matt Field, Nick Heather, and Reinout W. Wiers, "Indeed, Not Really a Brain Disorder: Implications for Reductionist Accounts of Addiction," *Behavioral and Brain Sciences* 42 (2019): e9, https://doi.org /10.1017/S0140525X18001024.

281 **categorical, fixed entities:** Nick Haslam, "Psychiatric Categories as Natural Kinds: Essentialist Thinking about Mental Disorder," *Social Research* 67, no. 4 (Winter 2000); Peter Zachar and Kenneth S. Kendler, "Psychiatric Disorders: A Conceptual Taxonomy," *American Journal of Psychiatry* 164, no. 4 (April 2007): 557–65, https://doi.org/10.1176/ajp.2007.164.4.557; Kathryn Tabb, "Psychiatric Progress and the Assumption of Diagnostic Discrimination," *Philosophy of Science* 82, no. 5 (December 2015): 1047–58, https://doi.org/10.1086/683439.

281 **not ground truths about reality:** Howard J. Shaffer et al., "Toward a Syndrome Model of Addiction: Multiple Expressions, Common Etiology," *Harvard Review of Psychiatry* 12, no. 6 (2004): 367–74, https://doi.org/10.1080/10673220490905705; Paige M. Shaffer and Howard J. Shaffer, "Reconsidering Addiction as Syndrome" in Pickard and Ahmed, eds., *Handbook of Philosophy and Science of Addiction*, 106.

283 **no essential boundary:** This, in the end, was the researcher George Vaillant's conclusion in 1995, after revisiting his own decades of natural history studies on alcoholism. He acknowledged that alcoholism wasn't strictly a disease in the sense of being neatly separable from the rest of the population or caused by one clear set of biological factors, but he argued that the disease metaphor was still a useful

organizing concept, if you didn't take it too seriously. "Just as light can consist of both waves and particles, just so alcoholism can exist both as one end of a continuum of drinking problems and as a specific disorder." George Vaillant, *The Natural History of Alcoholism Revisited* (Cambridge, MA: Harvard University Press, 1995), 376.

283 **most clearly on display:** Richard Rohr, *Breathing Underwater: Spirituality and the Twelve Steps* (Cincinnati: St. Anthony Messenger Press, 2011), xviii. "Alcoholics just have their powerlessness visible for all to see."

283 **also in obesity and gambling:** This, particularly the role of the dorsal and ventral striatum, is discussed at length by Marc Lewis, *The Biology of Desire: Why Addiction Is Not a Disease* (New York: Public Affairs, 2015), 126. See also Barry J. Everitt and Trevor W. Robbins, "From the Ventral to the Dorsal Striatum: Devolving Views of Their Roles in Drug Addiction," *Neuroscience & Biobehavioral Reviews* 37, no. 9 (November 2013): 1946–54, https://doi.org/10.1016/j.neubiorev.2013.02.010; Oren Contreras-Rodríguez et al., "Ventral and Dorsal Striatum Networks in Obesity: Link to Food Craving and Weight Gain," *Biological Psychiatry* 81, no. 9 (May 2017): 789–96, https://doi.org/10.1016/j.biopsych.2015.11.020; Kent C. Berridge, "The Debate over Dopamine's Role in Reward: The Case for Incentive Salience," *Psychopharmacology* 191, no. 3 (April 2007): 391–431, https://doi.org/10.1007/s00213-006-0578-x; Kent C. Berridge and Morten L. Kringelbach, "Pleasure Systems in the Brain," *Neuron* 86, no. 3 (May 2015).

Conclusion

286 **integrating substance use disorder treatment:** "A Growing Impetus for Integration," in *Facing Addiction in America: The Surgeon General's Report on Alcohol, Drugs, and Health* (Washington, DC: Office of the Surgeon General, 2016), chap. 6, http://www.ncbi.nlm.nih.gov/books/NBK424857/.

287 **only about one in ten:** Michael A. Hoge et al., "Mental Health and Addiction Workforce Development: Federal Leadership Is Needed to Address the Growing Crisis," *Health Affairs* 32, no. 11 (November 2013): 2005–12, https://doi.org/10.1377/hlthaff.2013.0541. See also "Addiction Treatment: Improving Quality and Capacity," Shatterproof (website), accessed March 5, 2021, https://www.shatterproof.org/advocacy/federal-addiction-treatment-improving; *ASAM Advocacy Roadmap: February 2020* (Washington, DC: American Society of Addiction Medicine, 2020), https://www.asam.org/docs/default-source/advocacy/asam_report_feb2020_final.pdf.

288 **fewer than 10 percent:** "Practitioner and Program Data," SAMHSA (website), accessed March 5, 2021, https://www.samhsa.gov/medication-assisted-treatment/practitioner-resources/DATA-program-data; "Professionally Active Physicians," Kaiser Family Foundation (website), updated September 2020, https://www.kff.org/other/state-indicator/total-active-physicians/. Eligible providers also include nurse practitioners and physician assistants, so as of February 2021, the number is approximately 6 percent of eligible providers. See also Justin Berk, "To Help Providers Fight the Opioid Epidemic, 'X the X Waiver,'" *Health Affairs* (blog), March 5, 2019, https://www.healthaffairs.org/do/10.1377/hblog20190301.79453/full/.

288 **Biden administration has committed:** Regina LaBelle, "Announcing President Biden's New Team and Priorities at ONDCP," American Academy of Addiction Psychiatry (website), February 4, 2021, https://www.aaap.org/announcing-president-bidens-new-team-and-priorities-at-ondcp/.

288 **25 percent of waivered physicians:** Cindy Parks Thomas et al., "Prescribing Patterns of Buprenorphine Waivered Physicians," *Drug and Alcohol Dependence* 181 (December 1, 2017): 213–18, https://doi.org/10.1016/j.drugalcdep.2017.10.002; Stacey C. Sigmon, "The Untapped Potential of Office-Based Buprenorphine Treatment," *JAMA Psychiatry* 72, no. 4 (April 1, 2015): 395, https://doi.org/10.1001/jamapsychiatry.2014.2421.

288 **surveys about the barriers:** Eliza Hutchinson et al., "Barriers to Primary Care Physicians Prescribing Buprenorphine," *Annals of Family Medicine* 12, no. 2 (March 2014): 128–33, https://doi.org/10.1370/afm.1595. See also Wendy Kissin et al., "Experiences of a National Sample of Qualified Addiction Specialists Who Have and Have Not Prescribed Buprenorphine for Opioid Dependence," *Journal of Addictive Diseases* 25, no. 4 (November 2006): 91–103, https://doi.org/10.1300/J069v25n04_09; Cindy Parks Thomas et al., "Use of Buprenorphine for Addiction Treatment: Perspectives of Addiction Specialists and General Psychiatrists," *Psychiatric Services* 59, no. 8 (August, 2008): 909–16, https://doi.org/10.1176/ps.2008.59.8.909.

290 **wide variety of recovery experiences:** William L. White and Ernest Kurtz, "The Varieties of Recovery Experience," *International Journal of Self-Help and Self Care* 3, no. 1–2 (2006): 21–61; William L. White, "Addiction Recovery: Its Definition and Conceptual Boundaries," *Journal of Studies on Alcohol* 33, no. 3 (October 2007): 229–41, https://doi.org/10.1016/j.jsat.2007.04.015.

291 **little less than half:** John F. Kelly et al., "Prevalence and Pathways of Recovery from Drug and Alcohol Problems in the United States Population: Implications for Practice, Research, and Policy," *Drug and Alcohol Dependence* 181 (December 2017): 162–69, https://doi.org/10.1016/j.drugalcdep.2017.09.028. Regarding "multiple pathways of recovery," people also switch back and forth between those different sources of support, suggesting more of a dynamic interplay than the linear term "pathways" suggests.

291 **70 percent improve without interventions:** Jalie A. Tucker, Susan D. Chandler, and Katie Witkiewitz, "Epidemiology of Recovery from Alcohol Use Disorder," *Alcohol Research* 40, no. 3 (2020): 4–7.

292 **such as opioid use disorder:** Aaron L. Sarvet and Deborah Hasin, "The Natural History of Substance Use Disorders," *Current Opinion in Psychiatry* 29, no. 4 (July 2016): 250–57, https://doi.org/10.1097/YCO.0000000000000257; Lauren A. Hoffman, Corrie Vilsaint, and John F. Kelly, "Recovery from Opioid Problems in the US Population: Prevalence, Pathways, and Psychological Well-Being," *Journal of Addiction Medicine* 14, no. 3 (June 2020): 207–16, https://doi.org/10.1097/ADM.0000000000000561. It's worth noting that people with OUD seeking care should be offered psychosocial treatment, but a decision to decline psychosocial treatment or an absence of psychosocial treatment should not preclude medication treatment: "The ASAM National Practice Guideline for the Treatment of Opioid Use Disorder: 2020 Focused Update," *Journal of Addiction Medicine* 14, no. 2S (March 2020): 1–91, https://doi.org/10.1097/ADM.0000000000000633.

292 **broad definition of recovery:** For a discussion that traces the Sobells through to contemporary definitions of recovery, see Katie Witkiewitz et al., "What Is Recovery?," *Alcohol Research: Current Reviews* 40, no. 3 (September 2020).

292 **undergoing a paradigm shift:** Mark Sobell and Linda C. Sobell, "The Aftermath of Heresy: A Response to Pendery et al.'s (1982) Critique of 'Individualized Behavior Therapy for Alcoholics,'" *Behaviour Research and Therapy* 22, no. 4 (1984): 413–40, https://doi.org/10.1016/0005-7967(84)90084-6.

292 **an inclusive definition of recovery:** William L. White, "Recovery: Old Wine, Flavor of the Month or New Organizing Paradigm?," *Substance Use & Misuse* 43, no. 12–13 (October 2008): 1987–2000, https://doi.org/10.1080/10826080802297518; Jason Schwartz, "Revisiting Recovery-Oriented Harm Reduction (Part 3)," *Recovery Review* (blog), May 17, 2019, https://recoveryreview.blog/category/recovery-oriented-harm-reduction/.

292 **measures of well-being increase exponentially:** John F. Kelly, M. Claire Greene, and Brandon G. Bergman, "Beyond Abstinence: Changes in Indices of Quality of Life with Time in Recovery in a Nationally Representative Sample of U.S. Adults," *Alcoholism, Clinical and Experimental Research* 42, no. 4 (April 2018): 770–80, https://doi.org/10.1111/acer.13604. See also Witkiewitz et al., "What Is Recovery?," 1, 7.

293 **evidence of physical brain changes:** See especially the extended discussion in Carl L. Hart, *Drug Use for Grown-Ups: Chasing Liberty in the Land of Fear* (New York: Penguin Press, 2021), chap. 4. For more on how brain-based explanations can be stigmatizing: Bill White, "Hijacked Brains & the Question of Social Stigma," *Selected Papers of William L. White* (blog), September 13, 2013, http://www.williamwhitepapers.com/blog/2013/09/hijacked-brains-the-question-of-social-stigma.html. Media and marketing examples of equating brain changes with permanence abound; see, for example, Alex Orlando, "Can We Reverse the Brain Damage That Drug Use Causes?," *Discover*, December 15, 2019, https://www.discovermagazine.com/mind/can-we-reverse-the-brain-damage-that-drug-use-causes; "Effects of Drugs and Alcohol on the Brain: Causes of Brain Damage," American Addiction Centers (website), updated September 3, 2019, https://americanaddictioncenters.org/alcoholism-treatment/brain-damage.

293 **The brain does change:** A separate but closely related issue is to what extent substances directly cause brain injury. If anything, the most brain-toxic drug is alcohol, but otherwise, the vast majority of addiction-related brain injury is related to the consequences of addiction rather than the drugs themselves: injuries from fights or falls, hypoxic injury from overdoses, and infections from nonsterile injections. Even the notion that methamphetamine causes lasting neuronal cell damage, widely publicized by the press and treatment center advertising, has not held up under scrutiny. Carl L. Hart et al., "Is Cognitive Functioning Impaired in Methamphetamine Users? A Critical Review," *Neuropsychopharmacology* 37, no. 3 (February 2012): 586–608, https://doi.org/10.1038/npp.2011.276. There is also some evidence for the damaging effects of cocaine on blood vessels, as well as other less commonly used drugs such as nitrous oxide. Michael B. Erwin et al., "Cocaine and Accelerated Atherosclerosis: Insights from Intravascular Ultrasound," *International Journal of Cardiology* 93, no. 2 (2004): 301–3, https://doi.org/10.1016/S0167-5273(03)00170-0.

293 **brain undergoes significant changes:** Marc Lewis, "Brain Change in Addiction as Learning, Not Disease," *New England Journal of Medicine* 379, no. 16 (October 18, 2018): 1551–60, https://doi.org/10.1056/NEJMra1602872; Marc Lewis, "Addiction and the Brain: Development, Not Disease," *Neuroethics* 10, no. 1 (May 18, 2017): 1–12, https://doi.org/10.1007/s12152-016-9293-4.

293 **volumes increased even further:** Colm G. Connolly et al., "Dissociated Grey Matter Changes with Prolonged Addiction and Extended Abstinence in Cocaine Users," *PloS ONE* 8, no. 3 (2013): e59645, https://doi.org/10.1371/journal.pone.0059645. Other studies on biological correlates of recovery: Scott J. Moeller and Martin P. Paulus, "Toward Biomarkers of the Addicted Human Brain: Using Neuroimaging to Predict Relapse and Sustained Abstinence in Substance Use Disorder," *Progress in Neuro-Psychopharmacology and Biological Psychiatry* 80, part B (January 2018): 143–54, https://www.ncbi.nlm.nih.gov/pmc/articles/PMC5603350/; Ryan P. Bell, Hugh Garavan, and John J. Foxe, "Neural Correlates of Craving and Impulsivity in Abstinent Former Cocaine Users: Towards Biomarkers of Relapse Risk," *Neuropharmacology* 85 (October 2014): 461–70, https://dx.doi.org/10.1016%2Fj.neuropharm.2014.05.011.

295 **much of an evidence base:** "IFS, an Evidence-Based Practice," Foundation for Self Leadership, accessed February 25, 2021, https://foundationifs.org/news-articles/79-ifs-an-evidence-based-practice.

297 **deep brain stimulation:** Tony R. Wang et al., "Deep Brain Stimulation for the Treatment of Drug Addiction," *Neurosurgical Focus* 45, no. 2 (August 2018): E11, https://doi.org/10.3171/2018.5.FOCUS18163; "First Trial in US to Use Deep Brain Stimulation to Fight Opioid Addiction," *Medical Xpress*, November 5, 2019, https://medicalxpress.com/news/2019-11-trial-deep-brain-opioid-addiction.html.

297 **replace her depression:** Lone Frank, *The Pleasure Shock* (New York: Penguin, 2018), 107–8.

299 **pain and purpose:** Steven C. Hayes, *A Liberated Mind* (New York: Avery, 2019), 23.

299 **"recovery capital":** William L. White and William Cloud, "Recovery Capital: A Primer for Addictions Professionals," *Counselor* 9, no. 5 (2008): 29; Emily A. Hennessy, "Recovery Capital: A Systematic Review of the Literature," *Addiction Research & Theory* 25, no. 5 (October 2017): 349–60, https://doi.org/10.1080/16066359.2017.1297990; William Cloud and Robert Granfield, "Conceptualizing Recovery Capital: Expansion of a Theoretical Construct," *Substance Use & Misuse* 43, no. 12–13 (2008): 1971–86, https://doi.org/10.1080/10826080802289762; David Best and Alexandre B. Laudet, *The Potential of Recovery Capital* (Peterborough, UK: Citizen Power Peterborough, 2019), https://facesandvoicesofrecovery.org/wp-content/uploads/2019/06/The-Potential-of-Recovery-Capital.pdf.

299 **have more psychological struggles:** Kelly, Greene, and Bergman, "Beyond Abstinence."

Image Credits

p. 27: Wellcome Collection, London.

p. 45: The Metropolitan Museum of Art, New York, Harris Brisbane Dick Fund.

p. 51: Independence National Historical Park.

p. 59: Jonathan Jones, University of North Carolina Bullitt Lecture, December 4, 2018, http://archives.hsl.unc.edu/bullitt-lectures/20181204-Jones.pdf.

p. 80: Emory University, Manuscript, Archives and Rare Book Library.

p. 84: Library of Congress Print and Photographs Online Catalog.

p. 115: New York Public Library.

p. 127: University of South Florida Visitor Collections.

p. 131: *The New York Times* Digital Collections.

p. 172: Image courtesy of Stepping Stones Archive at Stepping Stones—Historic Home of Bill & Lois Wilson, Katonah, NY.

p. 172: Image courtesy of Stepping Stones Archive at Stepping Stones—Historic Home of Bill & Lois Wilson, Katonah, NY, LBW 206, Box 13, Folder 5, Item 27.

p. 181: U.S. National Library of Medicine Digital Collections.

p. 186: Roadshow Attractions, pulled from Wikimedia Commons.

p. 199: Courtesy of Nicolas Rasmussen, as cited in "Making the First Anti-Depressant: Amphetamine in American Medicine, 1929–1950," *History of Medicine and Allied Sciences* 61 (2006): 288–323.

p. 226: Getty, Bettmann Archive.

IMAGE CREDITS

p. 236: Courtesy of The Rockefeller University, New York. Photograph by Inglent Grütner.

p. 257: White House Photographic Collection, 1/20/1981–1/20/1989.

p. 273: Aistė Šlikienė.

p. 273: Library of Congress Print and Photographs Online Catalog.

Index

INDEX